UNDERSTANDING AND MANAGING Oncologic Emergencies

Traditional and Emerging

Edited by

Megan Hoffman,
DNP, APRN, AOCNS®, AGCNS-BC, EBP-C

Jennie Matays,
DNP, APRN-CNS, CCNS, CCRN, EBP-CH, FCNS

Oncology Nursing Society
Pittsburgh, Pennsylvania

ONS Publications Department
Publisher and Director of Publications: Lynn Nace, BA
Acquisitions Editor: Dave Burns, BA, FLTA
Staff Editor II: Andrew Petyak, BA, PMP
Design and Production Administrator: Dany Sjoen

Library of Congress Cataloging-in-Publication Data
Names: Hoffman, Megan editor | Matays, Jennie editor
Title: Understanding and managing oncologic emergencies: traditional and emerging/ edited by Megan Hoffman, DNP, APRN, AOCNS, AGCNS-BC, EBP-C, and Jennie Matays, DNP, APRN-CNS, CCNS, CCRN, EBP-CH, FCNS.
Description: First edition. | Pittsburgh, Pennsylvania: Oncology Nursing Society, [2026] | Includes bibliographical references and index. |
Identifiers: LCCN 2025051463 | ISBN 9781635930757 paperback | ISBN 9781635930764 ebook
Subjects: LCSH: Cancer--Nursing
Due to a government shutdown in September 2025, this information was not finalized at the time of publication.

Publisher's Note

This book is published by the Oncology Nursing Society (ONS). ONS neither represents nor guarantees that the practices described herein will, if followed, ensure safe and effective patient care. The recommendations contained in this book reflect ONS's judgment regarding the state of general knowledge and practice in the field as of the date of publication. The recommendations may not be appropriate for use in all circumstances. Those who use this book should make their own determinations regarding specific safe and appropriate patient care practices, taking into account the personnel, equipment, and practices available at the hospital or other facility at which they are located. The editors and publisher cannot be held responsible for any liability incurred as a consequence from the use or application of any of the contents of this book. Figures and tables are used as examples only. They are not meant to be all-inclusive, nor do they represent endorsement of any particular institution by ONS. Mention of specific products and opinions related to those products do not indicate or imply endorsement by ONS. Websites mentioned are provided for information only; the hosts are responsible for their own content and availability. Unless otherwise indicated, dollar amounts reflect U.S. dollars.

ONS publications are originally published in English. Publishers wishing to translate ONS publications must contact ONS about licensing arrangements. ONS publications cannot be translated without obtaining written permission from ONS. (Individual tables and figures that are reprinted or adapted require additional permission from the original source.) Because translations from English may not always be accurate or precise, ONS disclaims any responsibility for inaccuracies in words or meaning that may occur as a result of the translation. Readers relying on precise information should check the original English version.

Printed in the United States of America

ONS
Oncology Nursing Society

Innovation • Excellence • Advocacy • Inclusivity

Contributors

Editors

Megan Hoffman, DNP, APRN, AOCNS®, AGCNS-BC, EBP-C
Nurse Leader
Memorial Sloan Kettering Cancer Center
New York, New York

Jennie Matays, DNP, APRN-CNS, CCNS, CCRN, EBP-CH, FCNS
Magnet Program Director
Kaiser Permanente Roseville
Roseville, California

Authors

Hamza Abid, MS, APRN-CNS, AOCNS®, OCN®
Manager, Inpatient Oncology
Sutter Health–Mills-Peninsula Medical Center
Burlingame, California
Chapter 10. Tumor Lysis Syndrome

Linda Bloom, MPA, RN, OCN®
Clinical Nurse IV Perioperative Services
Memorial Sloan Kettering Cancer Center
New York, New York
Chapter 7. Increased Intracranial Pressure

Joaquin Buitrago, PhD, RN, OCN®
Nurse Professional Development Specialist
University of Texas MD Anderson Cancer Center
Texas Woman's University
Houston, Texas
Chapter 7. Increased Intracranial Pressure

Liffy I. Cherian, MSN, APRN, AGCNS-BC, OCN®
Lead Advanced Practice Provider
Oncology Acute Care, Infusion Services and Clinical Trial Unit
University of Texas Southwestern University Hospital
Dallas, Texas
Chapter 8. Hypercalcemia of Malignancy

Diane G. Cope, PhD, APRN, BC, AOCNP®
Oncology Nurse Practitioner
Florida Cancer Specialists and Research Institute
Fort Myers, Florida
Chapter 9. Syndrome of Inappropriate Antidiuretic Hormone Secretion; Chapter 11. Bleeding; Chapter 12. Venous Thromboembolism; Chapter 13. Disseminated Intravascular Coagulation

Mary Elizabeth Davis, DNP, RN, CHPN®, AOCNS®
Clinical Nurse Specialist
Memorial Sloan Kettering Cancer Center
New York, New York
Chapter 14. Febrile Neutropenia

Katie Dombrowski, DNP, AGNP-C
Senior Medical Science Liaison
AbbVie
Tampa, Florida
Chapter 15. Sepsis and Septic Shock

Lisa Feldsien, BSN, RN, OCN®
Staff Nurse – Radiation Oncology
Baptist Health Paducah
Paducah, Kentucky
Chapter 6. Spinal Cord Compression

Kristin Marie Ferguson, DNP, MBA, RN, OCN®, CGNC
Senior Director, Strategic Operations: BMT and Cellular Therapy
MedStar Georgetown University Hospital
Washington, DC
Chapter 16. Hypersensitivity Reactions

Sara Gomes, MSc, RN
Adjunct Professor
University of Coimbra
Nursing School of University of Coimbra
Coimbra, Portugal
Chapter 2. Superior Vena Cava Syndrome

Whitney Houser, MSN, RN, OCN®
Nursing Professional Development Lead
Huntsman Cancer Institute
University of Utah
Salt Lake City, Utah
Chapter 17. Immune-Related Adverse Events

Vivian Huang, MS, RN, CNS, AGCNS-BC, OCN®, TCTCN™
Clinical Nurse Specialist
Hematology, Blood and Marrow Transplant, and Cellular Therapy
University of California, San Francisco
San Francisco, California
Chapter 17. Immune-Related Adverse Events

Melissa A. Kerr, MSN-Ed, RN, OCN®
Registered Nurse–Senior
Texas Oncology–Keller
Fort Worth, Texas
Chapter 1. Cardiac Tamponade

Patryk Madrid, DNP, FNP-C
Nurse Practitioner
Johns Hopkins University
Baltimore, Maryland
Chapter 3. Pleural Effusion

Michelle K. Maiers, MSN, RN, AGPCNP-BC, OCN®
Clinical Nurse Educator
Inova Health System
Fairfax, Virginia
Chapter 14. Febrile Neutropenia

Luciana Lopes Manfredini, PhD, BSN
Project Consultant and Professor
Einstein Hospital Israelita
São Paulo, Brazil
Chapter 15. Sepsis and Septic Shock

Christina Matousek, DNP, RN, OCN®
Patient Education Specialist
Smilow Cancer Hospital
New Haven, Connecticut
Chapter 16. Hypersensitivity Reactions

Colleen McCracken, MSN, RN, CMSRN, CHPN, OCN®, NPD-BC
System Educator, Registered Nurse
Froedtert ThedaCare Health
Milwaukee, Wisconsin
Chapter 10. Tumor Lysis Syndrome

Allison Mitchell, BSN, RN, OCN®
Oncology RN Navigator
Avera Cancer Institute
Sioux Falls, South Dakota
Chapter 4. Bowel Obstruction; Chapter 5. Urinary Obstruction

Lindsay Muratore, DNP, FNP-BC, OCN®
Family Nurse Practitioner
University of Maryland Neurology Care Center
Baltimore, Maryland
Chapter 1. Cardiac Tamponade

Jennifer C. Myers, DNP, MSN, RN, ANP-BC
Manager of Advanced Practice Providers/Adult Nurse Practitioner
Washington University School of Medicine – Department of Radiation Oncology
St. Louis, Missouri
Chapter 6. Spinal Cord Compression

Brenda S. Nettles, DNP, MS, ACNP-BC, AOCNP®, CNE
Assistant Professor and Nurse Practitioner
Johns Hopkins School of Nursing
Baltimore, Maryland
Chapter 4. Bowel Obstruction; Chapter 5. Urinary Obstruction

Chinomso Nwozichi, PhD, RN, CMSRN, OCN®, FAAN
Assistant Professor of Nursing
Kennesaw State University, Wellstar School of Nursing
Kennesaw, Georgia
Chapter 9. Syndrome of Inappropriate Antidiuretic Hormone Secretion

Megan O'Neil, DNP, APRN, FNP-C, OCN®
Oncology Nurse Practitioner
NantHealth
Philadelphia, Pennsylvania
Assistant Professor
Rocky Mountain University of Health Professions
Provo, Utah
Chapter 16. Hypersensitivity Reactions

Cindy Stern, MSN, RN, CCRP
Advanced Practice Nurse
Independent Consultant
Philadelphia, Pennsylvania
Chapter 8. Hypercalcemia of Malignancy

Abigail Tesar, BSN, RN, OCN®, TCTCN™
Assistant Nurse Manager
St. Luke's Health System
Boise, Idaho
Chapter 11. Bleeding; Chapter 12. Venous Thromboembolism; Chapter 13. Disseminated Intravascular Coagulation

Kelli Thoele, PhD, RN
Clinical Research Scientist
Eli Lilly and Company
Indianapolis, Indiana
Chapter 3. Pleural Effusion

Disclosure

Editors and authors of books and guidelines provided by the Oncology Nursing Society are expected to disclose to the readers any significant financial interest or other relationships with the manufacturer(s) of any commercial products.

A vested interest may be considered to exist if a contributor is affiliated with or has a financial interest in commercial organizations that may have a direct or indirect interest in the subject matter. A "financial interest" may include, but is not limited to, being a shareholder in the organization; being an employee of the commercial organization; serving on an organization's speakers bureau; or receiving research funding from the organization. An "affiliation" may be holding a position on an advisory board or some other role of benefit to the commercial organization. Vested interest statements appear in the front matter for each publication.

Contributors are expected to disclose any unlabeled or investigational use of products discussed in their content. This information is acknowledged solely for the information of the readers.

The contributors provided the following disclosure and vested interest information:

Liffy I. Cherian, MSN, APRN, AGCNS-BC, OCN®: Association of Cancer Care Centers, consultant or advisory role

Mary Elizabeth Davis, DNP, RN, CHPN®, AOCNS®: Hospice and Palliative Nurses Association, consultant or advisory role, other remuneration

Kristin Marie Ferguson, DNP, MBA, RN, OCN®, CGNC: American Nurses Association, consultant or advisory role; Northside Hospital Cancer Institute Oncology Nursing Symposium, honoraria

Colleen McCracken, MSN, RN, CMSRN, CHPN, OCN®, NPD-BC: Scripps Cancer Center, honoraria

Brenda S. Nettles, DNP, MS, ACNP-BC, AOCNP®, CNE: *Clinical Journal of Oncology Nursing*, employment or leadership position

Kelli Thoele, PhD, RN: Eli Lilly and Company, employment or leadership position, stock ownership, other remuneration

Contents

Preface

The management of oncologic emergencies represents one of the most challenging and time-sensitive aspects of cancer care. As cancer incidence continues to rise globally and patients live longer with advanced disease due to novel therapeutics, clinicians across specialties increasingly encounter acute, life-threatening complications of malignancy and its treatment. Rapid recognition and timely intervention can mean the difference between a manageable complication and a life-threatening deterioration. Yet, despite the frequency of these crises, evidence-based guidance tailored to real-world clinical settings remains fragmented. This book was developed to address that gap, offering a comprehensive, practical, and up-to-date resource for nurses involved in the acute management of patients with cancer.

This edition, featuring a new subtitle, provides a structured, systems-based approach to the recognition, diagnosis, and management of the full spectrum of oncologic emergencies. Core chapters address classic and frequently encountered conditions, and each section integrates current evidence, diagnostic algorithms, and interprofessional management strategies—organized into key areas to guide both emergent stabilization and the coordination of comprehensive, patient-centered cancer care.

Significant updates distinguish this edition from its predecessors. New chapters on bowel and urinary obstructions, febrile neutropenia, and immune-related adverse events reflect the evolving landscape of oncology practice. The authors highlight clinical pearls, decision-making frameworks, and the role of nursing assessment and intervention in optimizing outcomes. Wherever possible, recommendations align with current guidelines while acknowledging the realities of diverse healthcare environments.

We hope that this book serves not only as a reference but also as a teaching tool, bridging the knowledge between oncology nursing, emergency and critical care nursing, and general clinical practice to support nurses in delivering timely, evidence-based care during oncologic emergencies. By empowering nurses to act swiftly and confidently, we aim to improve both survival and quality of life for patients confronting the most urgent complications of cancer and its treatment.

Megan Hoffman, DNP, APRN, AOCNS®, AGCNS-BC, EBP-C
Jennie Matays, DNP, APRN-CNS, CCNS, CCRN, EBP-CH, FCNS

Acknowledgment

We are deeply grateful to the mentors who have guided our paths, the colleagues who have shared their wisdom and support, and the patients and families whose strength and stories remind us why we do this work.

SECTION I

STRUCTURAL EMERGENCIES

Melissa A. Kerr, MSN-Ed, RN, OCN®,
and Lindsay Muratore, DNP, FNP-BC, OCN®

CHAPTER 1

Cardiac Tamponade

FAST FACTS

- **Description:** Cardiac tamponade occurs when excessive fluid accumulates in the pericardial sac and exerts extrinsic pressure on the heart, causing compression of the cardiac chambers, decreased cardiac output, circulatory collapse, and eventual death. Malignancy and procedure-related cardiac trauma are notable causes.
- **Incidence:** The exact incidence is unknown, but autopsy studies reveal that malignant pericardial effusion occurs in 21% of those affected by cardiac tamponade. Metastatic involvement of the pericardium is highest in patients with lung cancer, followed by breast cancer, lymphoma, leukemia, and melanoma.
- **Clinical Manifestations:** Symptom presentation depends on the rate and volume of pericardial fluid accumulation. Dyspnea is the cardinal symptom and may progress to orthopnea. Tachycardia, chest discomfort, and jugular venous distension are often present.
- **Risk Factors and Etiology:** Multiple risk factors contribute to the development of pericardial effusion, with malignancy representing the most prevalent cause. In patients with cancer, the etiology of pericardial effusion is often associated with drug-induced or treatment-related injury to the pericardium.
- **Pathophysiology and Patient Evaluation:** Hemodynamic consequences are determined by the magnitude of the intrapericardial pressure increase and the ability of the heart to accommodate and compensate for the changes. A detailed physical examination should be completed, noting any signs and symptoms of reduced cardiac output (e.g., tachypnea, diaphoresis, cool extremities, peripheral cyanosis).
- **Advanced Practice Considerations:** Echocardiogram is the imaging modality of choice. A chest x-ray may give an initial indication of enlarged heart size. Fluid evaluation is critical to help determine the best treatment course.
- **Treatment Modalities:** Supportive therapies with immediate pericardiocentesis can relieve symptoms and improve cardiac hemodynamics. Further treatment to prevent fluid reaccumulation and control the precipitating malignancy may include percutaneous or surgical procedures, depending on patient performance status and life expectancy.
- **Nursing Management:** The nursing role involves prompt recognition of clinical changes; astute monitoring of respiratory, cardiac, and neurologic systems; administration of medications and treatments with ongoing assessment for therapeutic response and potential complications; management of drainage catheters and other devices; pain management; care coordination; patient and caregiver education; emotional support; and discharge planning.
- **Outcomes:** Early intervention may help prolong a patient's life, although cardiac tamponade is typically associated with late-stage disease and limited survival. The average survival rate after diagnosis of pericardial effusion is four to six months.

Introduction

Cardiac tamponade occurs when an abnormal accumulation of fluid in the pericardial cavity, or a pericardial effusion, causes pressure within the pericardial cavity to rise to the point that the cardiac chambers become compressed and impair the chamber's ability to fill. This intrapericardial pressure is typically negative, allowing for low-pressure venous blood flow into the right side of the heart. The atria are lower-pressure chambers compared to the ventricles (Shelton, 2022). The progressive decline in stroke volume and cardiac output leads to inadequate perfusion of vital organs, cardiogenic shock, and circulatory collapse. Without prompt intervention, the hemodynamic consequences of cardiac tamponade are fatal (Shelton, 2022; Shirakabe et al., 2023).

Incidence

Cardiac tamponade from all causes is reported to occur in five cases per 10,000 in the United States (Chahine et al., 2021). About one-third of patients with cancer and pericardial effusion will develop cardiac tamponade (Chahine et al., 2021). The incidence of cardiac metastases leading to effusion and tamponade is likely to increase because patients with cancer are surviving longer (Nova-Camacho et al., 2023). According to Al-Ogaili et al. (2018), the two most common causes of cardiac tamponade are chronic kidney injury and malignancy, accounting for 18.4% and 17% of cases, respectively. Metastatic cancer and acute kidney injury were independent predictors of mortality.

Epidemiologic studies exploring the incidence of cardiac tamponade are lacking. The highest incidence rates of malignant pericardial effusion at autopsy were found in patients with lung cancer (33%), breast cancer (25%), and hematologic malignancies, including leukemia, Hodgkin lymphoma, and non-Hodgkin lymphoma (15%) (National Cancer Institute [NCI], 2025). Primary cardiac tumors, such as mesotheliomas or sarcomas, are very rare and account for only 0.02% of all cancer cases (Hatta et al., 2025).

Pericardial Physiology

The pericardium is a membranous sac that envelops the heart and roots of the great vessels (the aorta, superior and inferior vena cava, pulmonary artery, and pulmonary vein) and has properties that help maintain healthy cardiac function. It has two layers: the outer parietal pericardium, a thick fibrous layer composed primarily of collagen, and the inner visceral pericardium, a thin serous layer formed of a single layer of mesothelial cells and adherent to the surface of the heart (Shelton, 2022; Shirakabe et al., 2023). Between the two layers of pericardium is the pericardial space that contains 15–50 ml of an ultrafiltrate of plasma produced by the visceral pericardium (Shelton, 2022; Shirakabe et al., 2023). This fluid lubricates the pericardial membranes and prevents friction as the heart beats (Chiabrando et al., 2020). Because of its high content of collagen fibers, the pericardium is relatively inelastic but can stretch gradually over time up to a critical limit. Accumulation of pericardial fluid beyond the limit of membrane stretch results in cardiac tamponade (Chiabrando et al., 2020; Stashko & Meer, 2023).

The pattern of pericardial lymphatic drainage and the interactions with pleural lymphatics provide pathways for the spread of pulmonary diseases, such as tuberculosis and lung cancer, into the pericardium (Stashko & Meer, 2023).

The pericardium performs several crucial and complex functions to ensure the healthy performance of the heart. These functions can be categorized as mechanical, membranous, or ligamentous (Rehman et al., 2023). The pericardium also provides immune protection by acting as a barrier against the spread of infection and malignancy from nearby structures (Spangler & Gentlesk, 2019). Despite these beneficial properties, total absence of the pericardium, either due to surgical removal (i.e., pericardiectomy) or congenital absence, has minimal effects on normal cardiac function (Rehman et al., 2023).

Pericardial Effusion

A pericardial effusion is an abnormal collection of fluid in the pericardial space. Any pathologic process or procedure involving the pericardium can result in a pericardial effusion or cardiac tamponade (Stashko & Meer, 2023). A pericardial effusion creates an echo-free space between the visceral and parietal pericardium, and the width of this space is used to define the size of the effusion (Wang et al., 2025). Classifications of pericardial effusions include the following (Hoit, 2024b; Ripley, 2023; Stashko & Meer, 2023; Wang et al., 2025):

- Onset: acute (within minutes to hours), subacute (within 1–3 months), or chronic (lasting > 3 months)
- Distribution: circumferential or loculated (localized to a region of the pericardium)
- Hemodynamic impact: none, cardiac tamponade, or effusive-constrictive pericarditis
- Composition: exudate, transudate, blood, or air or gas from bacterial infections (rare)
- Size: based on echocardiographic findings related to the pericardial sac during diastole
  - Physiologic (< 5 mm): 25–50 ml
  - Small (< 10 mm): < 100 ml
  - Moderate (10–20 mm): 100–500 ml
  - Large (> 20 mm): > 500 ml

Effusions that develop from malignant involvement of the pericardium have a high risk of progressing to tamponade (Wang et al., 2025). The inflammatory response to the presence of tumor cells may stimulate the pericardium to produce excessive fluid, and lymphatic drainage from the heart may be obstructed by mediastinal lymph nodes filled with tumor cells (Hoit, 2024b; Ripley, 2023). Slow growing effusions, which are typically associated with malignancy, can become quite large before patients become symptomatic and develop tamponade (Stashko & Meer, 2023). For example, a rapid accumulation of only 150 ml may severely affect cardiac output, but 1,000 ml of slowly developing fluid might not have an impact on diastolic filling of the heart.

The presence of a pericardial effusion may represent the initial manifestation of an unsuspected cancer elsewhere in the body.

The pericardium can stretch to accommodate up to 2 L of fluid, gradually accumulating over time, before the limit of pericardial membrane stretch is exceeded and cardiac tamponade ensues. Therefore, cardiac tamponade may be considered a last drop phenomenon that is precipitated by only a slight increase in the volume of pericardial fluid (Cremer et al., 2024).

Clinical Manifestations

Symptoms of pericardial effusion and cardiac tamponade can be nonspecific, making it a difficult diagnosis, especially in patients with preexisting comorbidities. See Table 1-1 for clinical manifestations of pericardial effusion and cardiac tamponade. Patients may present with a vague combination of symptoms, such as dyspnea or cough, chest heaviness, and palpitations. Beck's triad of symptoms is most commonly seen in patients presenting with cardiac tamponade and includes hypotension, increased jugular venous pressure, and distant muffled heart sounds (Shelton, 2022; Stashko & Meer, 2023) (see Figure 1-1). These findings reflect the rapid accumulation of pericardial fluid and are seen mostly with acute tamponade rather than slowly evolving tamponade (Nair, 2021; Stashko & Meer, 2023).

Subacute cardiac tamponade is a syndrome that evolves as pericardial fluid accumulates over time and is typical of tamponade associated with malignancy (Borlaug & DeCamp, 2024b; Hoit, 2024a). Initially, patients are asymptomatic or have only vague and nonspecific symptoms. As the pericardial effusion increases in volume and exceeds the limit of pericardium stretch, symptoms appear that can resemble those of right-sided heart failure, including dyspnea on exertion progressing to orthopnea, hepatic engorgement, and peripheral edema (Stashko & Meer, 2023). Dyspnea and tachypnea reflect pulmonary congestion as well as decreased oxygen delivery to peripheral tissues. Poor organ perfusion is manifested by cool, clammy extremities, weakened peripheral pulses, cyanosis, and declining renal function with decreased urine output (Hoit, 2024a). Hypoperfusion of the brain may result in confusion, restlessness, anxiety, agitation, syncope, and a sense of impending death (Nair, 2021). Given that the signs and symptoms of cardiac tamponade are neither sensitive nor specific, it is challenging to make a diagnosis by clinical signs alone, making a transthoracic echocardiography warranted (Shelton, 2022).

Risk Factors and Etiology

Malignancy

Tumors of the heart and pericardium are rare, whether benign or malignant, but all have the potential to cause life-threatening complications related to hemodynamic compromise (Shelton, 2022; Shirakabe et al., 2023). Lung cancer is the most

TABLE 1-1
Clinical Manifestations of Pericardial Effusion and Cardiac Tamponade

Type of Tamponade	Clinical Manifestations		Contributing Factors
	Symptoms	Signs	
Acute: develops within minutes to hours	Severe dyspnea Air hunger Chest pain or heaviness Confusion Apprehension	Classic Beck triad • Hypotension (< 100 mm Hg) • Elevated jugular venous pressure • Muffled heart sounds Tachycardia (> 90 bpm) Jugular venous distension Decreased stroke volume Decreased cardiac output Hypoperfusion • Cool, clammy extremities • Peripheral cyanosis • Weak peripheral pulses • Decreased urine output or anuria Cardiogenic shock: life threatening, can occur rapidly • Jugular venous distension • Muffled heart sounds	Perforation of the pericardium following procedures: • Central line placement • Pacemaker implantation • Interventional cardiac procedures (e.g., cardiac catheterization, pericardiocentesis) • Sternal bone marrow biopsies • Thoracic surgery Rupture of the heart following myocardial infarction Dissecting aortic aneurysm Chest trauma: blunt impact or penetrating wound Malignancy: Invasive tumor bleeds into the pericardial space. Malignancy: The presence of tumor cells inflames the pericardium, causing a pericardial effusion to develop; lymphatic drainage from the heart is obstructed by mediastinal lymph nodes involved with the tumor. Cardiac tamponade physiology: Elevated intracardiac pressures impair venous return to the heart, causing the sympathetic
Subacute: evolves gradually over days to weeks	Mild • Asymptomatic initially or vague • Dyspnea (most common early symptom)	Mild: initially no hemodynamic changes or not apparent	
	Moderate • Exertional dyspnea • Chest discomfort • Cough • Fatigue • Weakness • Anorexia • Anxiety • Restlessness	Moderate • Tachycardia (> 90 bpm) • Hypotension (< 100 mm Hg) • Elevated jugular venous pressure • Jugular venous distension • Muffled heart sounds • Point of maximal impulse shifted to the left or downward	

(Continued on next page)

TABLE 1-1
Clinical Manifestations of Pericardial Effusion and Cardiac Tamponade *(Continued)*

Type of Tamponade	Clinical Manifestations: Symptoms	Clinical Manifestations: Signs	Contributing Factors
Subacute: evolves gradually over days to weeks *(Cont.)*		• Narrowing pulse pressure • Central venous pressure moderately elevated (8–12 mm Hg) • Low-voltage QRS complex • Mild peripheral edema • Mild abdominal distension • Decreased urine output	nervous system to stimulate tachycardia and vasoconstriction in an effort to increase cardiac output. Manifestations of increasing cardiac tamponade can resemble those of right-sided heart failure and reflect systemic venous and visceral congestion (e.g., dyspnea, orthopnea, cough, fatigue, weakness, peripheral edema, jugular venous distension, hepatic engorgement, anorexia). A large pericardial effusion can compress structures adjacent to the heart and lead to atypical symptoms depending on the involved structure: • Esophagus—dysphagia • Diaphragm—nausea • Phrenic nerve—hiccups • Recurrent laryngeal nerve—hoarseness
	Late • Dyspnea at rest • Orthopnea • Worsening cough • Possible disappearance of chest pain • Mental status changes • Hoarseness • Hiccups • Nausea • Dysphagia • Anxiety • Apprehension • Sense of impending doom	Late • Hypotension • Tachycardia • Increased jugular venous distension • Narrowed pulse pressure • Pulsus paradoxus • Muffled or absent heart sounds Point of maximal impulse shifted or has disappeared Central venous pressure very high (12–22 mm Hg) Electrical alternans Severe peripheral edema Severe abdominal distension Hepatojugular reflex Hypoperfusion • Cold, clammy extremities • Peripheral cyanosis • Weak pulse • Absent peripheral pulses • Poor capillary refill • Anuria • Cardiogenic shock	

Clinical manifestations occur on a continuum as accumulating pericardial fluid causes increasing intrapericardial pressure and increasingly severe hemodynamic compromise.

Note. Based on information from Borlaug & DeCamp, 2024b; Hoit, 2024a; Nair, 2021; Shelton, 2022; Stashko & Meer, 2023.

FIGURE 1-1. Beck's Triad

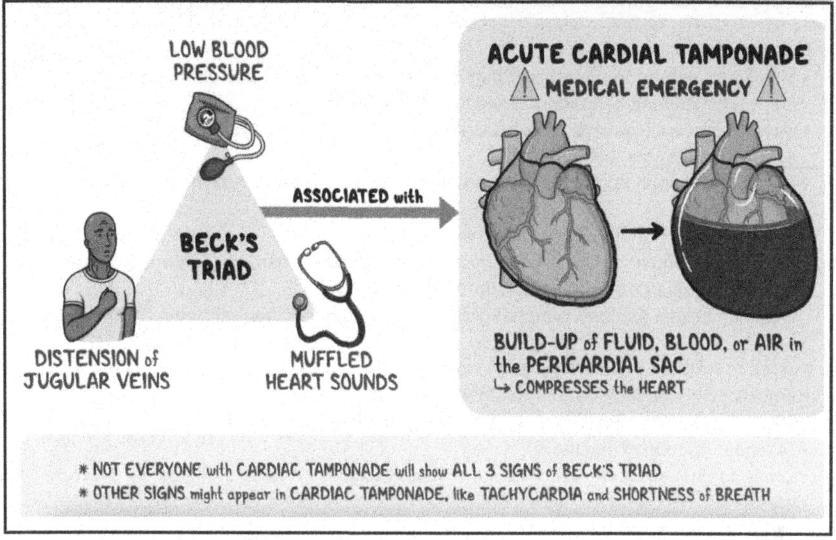

Note. From *Pericardial Tamponade: What is It, Causes, Pericardial Effusion, Signs, Diagnosis, Treatment, and More*, by A.H. Castillo; Illustrated by Abbey Richard, 2025 (https://www.osmosis.org/answers/pericardial-tamponade). Copyright 2025 by Osmosis. Reprinted with permission from Elsevier.

common cancer that spreads to the pericardium and accounts for approximately 40% of malignant pericardial effusions (Cremer et al., 2024). This is followed by breast cancer, esophageal cancer, pancreatic cancer, melanoma, and hematologic malignancies, specifically B-cell lymphoma (Chahine et al., 2021; Mori et al., 2024). Figure 1-2 provides a list of risk factors for cardiac tamponade or pericardial effusion.

Malignant involvement of the pericardium can occur through direct local extension of tumors in the chest or from the spread of tumor cells through lymphatic channels or the circulatory system (Ripley, 2023). Lymphatic drainage from the pericardium can also become obstructed when mediastinal lymph nodes are enlarged with tumor cells or damaged by the effects of prior chest radiation therapy (RT) (Mori et al., 2024).

Mesothelioma is the most common primary malignancy of the pericardium, accounting for 50% of primary pericardial tumors (Mori et al., 2024; Shelton, 2022). These tumors commonly involve the right side of the heart and lead to hemodynamic compromise (Shelton, 2022). Primary cardiac lymphomas are rare, but their incidence appears to be increasing as the population of individuals who are immunocompromised increases, including recipients of live organ transplants who receive long-term treatment with antirejection drugs, as well as individuals with HIV infection (Agudo-Quílez et al., 2024). Primary pericardial tumors can metastasize but are more often fatal because of their local malignant effects, including pericarditis with resultant cardiac tamponade, arrhythmia caused by myocardial invasion, or obstruction of the vena cava (Tyebally et al., 2020).

FIGURE 1-2. Etiologies Associated With Risk for Pericardial Effusion or Cardiac Tamponade Malignancy

Malignancy
- Metastatic spread to the pericardium (mainly through lymphatic channels): lung cancer, breast cancer, lymphoma, leukemia, melanoma
- Direct tumor extension to the pericardium: lung cancer, breast cancer, lymphoma, esophageal cancer, thymic cancer
- Mediastinal lymph nodes involved with the tumor: obstruction of lymphatic drainage from the heart
- Primary tumors of the pericardium (very rare)
  - Malignant origin: mesothelioma (most common), angiosarcomas, fibrosarcomas, rhabdomyosarcoma, malignant fibrous histiocytoma
  - Benign origin: lipomas, lymphangiomas, hemangiomas, neurofibromas, teratomas

Systemic Antineoplastic Agents
- Anthracycline agents: daunorubicin, doxorubicin
- Alkylating agents: busulfan, cyclophosphamide, ifosfamide
- Taxanes: docetaxel, paclitaxel
- Other agents: all-trans-retinoic acid, arsenic trioxide, cytosine arabinoside, 5-fluorouracil
- Targeted biotherapy agents
  - Tyrosine kinase inhibitor drugs
    * Vascular endothelial growth factor inhibitors: bevacizumab, sorafenib, sunitinib
    * Bcr-Abl inhibitors: imatinib, dasatinib, erlotinib, nilotinib, bosutinib
  - Bortezomib
  - Interleukin-2
  - Interferon alpha
  - Granulocyte macrophage–colony-stimulating factor
  - Anti–tumor necrosis factor agents

Drugs
- Anticoagulants and antithrombotics
- Thrombolytics
- Hydralazine, procainamide, methyldopa, isoniazid, phenytoin (may lead to a drug-induced lupus-like syndrome and pericardial inflammation)
- Minoxidil
- Methysergide
- Penicillins
- Phenylbutazone
- Cromolyn sodium
- Dantrolene

Chest Radiation Therapy
- Total radiation dose to mediastinum > 30–35 Gy delivered to > 30% of the pericardium

Infection
- Patients who are immunocompromised due to malignant disease or its treatment can develop opportunistic infections that affect the pericardium:
  - Viral: cytomegalovirus, HIV (most common are viral etiologies)
  - Bacterial: *Mycobacterium tuberculosis* (especially in low-income countries)
  - Fungal: *Candida*, *Aspergillus*, *Histoplasma*

(Continued on next page)

FIGURE 1-2. Etiologies Associated With Risk for Pericardial Effusion or Cardiac Tamponade Malignancy *(Continued)*

Autoimmune and Autoinflammatory Disorders
- Autoimmune connective tissue disorders
  - Systemic lupus erythematosus
  - Sjögren syndrome
  - Rheumatoid arthritis
  - Scleroderma
- Autoinflammatory disorders
  - Systemic vasculitis
  - Behçet syndrome
  - Sarcoidosis
  - Inflammatory bowel diseases

Invasive Cardiac Procedures (Iatrogenic)
- Cardiac perforation during placement of central lines, pacemaker insertion, cardiac catheterization, sternal bone marrow biopsies, percutaneous pericardiocentesis

Chest Trauma
- Blunt impact or penetrating injury

Cardiac Disease
- Dissecting aortic aneurysm (type A)
- Myocardial infarction with ventricular rupture
- Chronic heart failure
- Pulmonary hypertension

Other Conditions
- Severe hypothyroidism (myxedema)
- Uremia from end-stage renal failure
- Severe hypoalbuminemia related to advanced cirrhosis or nephrotic syndrome
- Obstruction of the thoracic duct outflow leading to the accumulation of chyle in the pericardium
  - More frequent in males than females (1.3:1)
  - Pneumonia

Note. Based on information from Hoit, 2024a; Imazio & De Ferrari, 2019; Lorenzo-Esteller et al., 2024; Mori et al., 2024.

Cardiotoxic Systemic Antineoplastic Drugs

The most common agents associated with risk for cardiotoxicity and pericardial effusion are anthracyclines, alkylating agents, and multitargeted tyrosine kinase inhibitors (Mori et al., 2024; Shelton, 2022). Anthracycline drugs (e.g., doxorubicin, daunorubicin) are commonly associated with cardiotoxicity. The median time to onset is usually 30–70 days, with some cases occurring 6 months after immunotherapy initiation (Lorenzo-Esteller et al., 2024).

Risk factors for cardiotoxicity include total lifetime cumulative drug dose greater than 450 mg/m^2, concomitant use of other agents known to have cardiotoxic effects (e.g., cyclophosphamide, 5-fluorouracil, trastuzumab, paclitaxel), history of prior or concurrent chest irradiation, increased length of time since completion of chemotherapy, and preexisting heart disease (Koutsoukis et al., 2018; Shelton, 2022). Mediastinal irradiation potentiates doxorubicin cardiotoxicity, even when the therapies are not delivered concomitantly (Koutsoukis et al., 2018). Alkylating agents (e.g., busulfan, cyclophosphamide, ifosfamide) can cause dose-related injury to cardiac endothelial tissue, possibly resulting in acute pericarditis with effusions and potentially cardiac tamponade (Koutsoukis et al., 2018).

Immune checkpoint inhibitors have been increasingly associated with the development of pericardial effusions, including frequently administered monoclonal antibodies, specifically HER2-targeted therapies (e.g., astrastuzumab, pertuzumab), as well as tyrosine kinase inhibitors that target vascular endothelial growth factors and receptors (e.g., bevacizumab, sunitinib) (Adashek et al., 2025). Cardiac immune-related adverse events were severe in more than 80% of cases in an analysis from the World Health Organization (Salem et al., 2018). The anti–programmed cell death 1 antibody nivolumab specifically has been associated with higher rates of pericardial effusion (Mori et al., 2024). The cardiac immune-related adverse events after immune checkpoint inhibitor administration could be caused by an increase in the size of micrometastasis from T-cell infiltration, also known as pseudoprogression (Adashek et al., 2025).

Commonly used non-antineoplastic drugs associated with the potential for pericardial effusion and cardiac tamponade include anticoagulants, thrombolytics, hydralazine, procainamide, methyldopa, isoniazid, minoxidil, phenytoin, methysergide, penicillins, phenylbutazone, cromolyn sodium, and dantrolene (NCI, 2025; Strimel et al., 2025; Wang et al., 2025).

Thoracic Radiation Therapy

RT delivered to the mediastinum can contribute to the development of pericardial disease (Hoit, 2024a; Wang et al., 2025). About 20%–55% of all patients with cancer undergo RT as part of their treatment regimen, with about half for curative intent. Complications occur in about 6%–30% of patients, and there does not seem to be a safe heart dose (von Kemp & Cosyns, 2023). In general, individuals at the most significant risk for radiation-induced pericarditis are 15- to 20-year survivors of Hodgkin lymphoma or early-stage breast cancer (particularly on the left side) who were treated with chest irradiation at a younger age (Curigliano et al., 2016; Wang et al., 2025).

Risk factors for cardiac damage following thoracic irradiation are usually related to the total radiation dose the heart receives, the volume of the heart exposed to radiation, radiation technique, younger age at exposure, longer time since exposure, and use of concurrent or anthracycline-based chemotherapy, endocrine therapy, or trastuzumab (Adashek et al., 2025; Mori et al., 2024; Shelton, 2022).

Although the concomitant use of RT with systemic or surgical agents has synergistic effects and can improve patient outcomes in terms of tumor control and survival, it can potentiate cardiovascular side effects (von Kemp & Cosyns, 2023). The risk of pericarditis worsens from 5% to 50% when the dose is increased from 40 Gy to 50 Gy, with the risk being highest when more than 30% of the heart is exposed (Lorenzo-Esteller et al., 2024). RT can damage the pericardial cells by prolonged inflammation, which can lead to fibrotic changes that stiffen the pericardium and lead to restricted cardiac movement (Ning et al., 2017; von Kemp & Cosyns, 2023).

Pericarditis usually appears 6–12 months following RT but can also occur many years later and manifest as chest pain and a friction rub or chronic toxicity (von Kemp & Cosyns, 2023). Pericardial disease is the most common RT complication, and long-term follow-up for cancer survivors should include an appropriate cardiac workup if symptoms are present (Ning et al., 2017; von Kemp & Cosyns, 2023).

Infection

Any pathogen can infect the pericardium and lead to the development of pericardial effusions or cardiac tamponade, including viruses, bacteria, and parasites (Hoit, 2024b). Patients with cancer who are immunocompromised because of the disease process or antineoplastic therapies are at increased risk for developing opportunistic infections that can lead to pericardial effusions and cardiac tamponade. Viral etiologies in these patients are most common (e.g., cytomegalovirus), followed by bacterial (e.g., *Mycobacterium* tuberculosis) and fungal sources (e.g., *Candida, Aspergillus*) (Keyvanfar et al., 2024). The mainstays of treatment are usually nonsteroidal anti-inflammatory drugs, colchicine, and corticosteroids. In severe cases, a pericardiocentesis is needed (Lorenzo-Esteller et al., 2024). Colchicine is recommended for three months to prevent recurrence for all patients who have their first episode of acute pericarditis (Cremer et al., 2024; Lorenzo-Esteller et al., 2024).

Interventional Cardiac Procedures and Trauma

Invasive cardiac procedures and thoracic surgery can cause bleeding into the pericardial space that results in acute cardiac tamponade. Incidence of these occurrences depends on the patients' comorbidities, sex, age, and operator skills (Adamczyk et al., 2019). Procedures associated with risk for cardiac perforation include placement of central lines, pacemaker insertion, cardiac catheterization, sternal bone marrow biopsies, and pericardiocentesis (Spangler & Gentlesk, 2019). The right atrium is the most common site of perforation from the catheter placement (Spangler & Gentlesk, 2019).

Prognosis

The development of pericardial effusion in patients usually indicates an advanced stage of the disease, and survival among these patients rarely exceeds 12 months, with mortality reaching around 80% by this time period (Chahine et al., 2021). Patients with a nonmalignant cause of pericardial effusion have a mortality rate less than 15% (Stashko & Meer, 2023). The prognosis for survival mostly depends on the type of tumor causing the effusion and its chemosensitivity.

Compensatory Mechanisms

The compensatory cardiac response to decreased venous return to the heart and increased vascular resistance is an increase in sympathetic tone that stimulates tachycardia, vasoconstriction, and increased cardiac contractility to maintain cardiac output and blood pressure (Stashko & Meer, 2023). Oncology nurses must be aware that the presence of tachycardia indicates that compensatory mechanisms may become overwhelmed, and hemodynamic collapse and cardiogenic shock may be imminent without intervention (Kaplan, 2018).

Pathophysiology and Patient Evaluation

Changes Associated With Cardiac Tamponade

Fluid accumulating in the pericardium leads to alterations in the normal intrapericardial pressure-volume dynamics that influence filling of the cardiac chambers and cardiac output. The hemodynamic consequences of a pericardial effusion are primarily determined by the magnitude of the intrapericardial pressure increase (rather than the amount of accumulated fluid) and the ability of the heart to accommodate and compensate for the changes. As pericardial fluid effusion increases in volume, it causes the intrapericardial pressure to rise until the filling of the chambers of the heart during diastole becomes impaired. The cardiac chambers with the lowest intracardiac pressures are affected first, usually in the sequence of right atrium, right ventricle, and left atrium (Hoit, 2024a; Shelton, 2022). Eventually, the increasing intrapericardial pressure equalizes with the pressures within the cardiac chambers, abolishing the pressure gradients needed for cardiac filling. At this point, the cardiac chambers become compressed, and the hemodynamic consequences of cardiac tamponade become clinically evident (Rehman et al., 2023).

Patient Assessment

History

Oncology nurses should ask about the type and stage of cancer, date of diagnosis, and cardiotoxic treatments received, such as chest radiation that included the mediastinum or chemotherapy and biotherapy agents (Adashek et al., 2025). Patients without a known history of cancer should be assessed for cancer risk factors, with particular attention paid to those associated with lung and breast cancers (e.g., smoking, asbestos exposure, family history of breast cancer), as these cancers pose the greatest risk for tamponade (Stashko & Meer, 2023). Nurses should also question patients about the chronology of symptom onset and about preexisting medical conditions that may cause pericardial effusion or mimic its effects, such as recent myocardial infarction, autoimmune disorders, or renal failure (Adasehk et al., 2025; Stashko & Meer, 2023).

Physical Examination

The common manifestations associated with tamponade (e.g., dyspnea, tachycardia, elevated jugular venous pressure) may not present in all patients and can also occur with other pathologic conditions (Hoit, 2024a).

FIGURE 1-3. Jugular Venous Distension

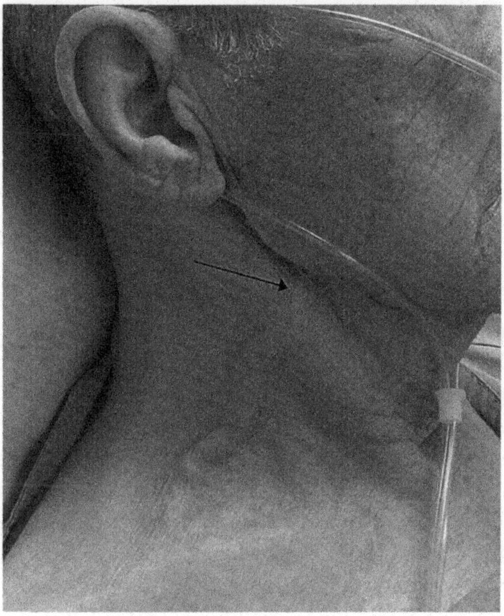

Note. Image courtesy of James Heilman (https://commons.wikimedia.org/wiki/File:Elevated_JVP.JPG). Licensed under CC BY-SA 3.0 (https://creativecommons.org/licenses/by-sa/3.0/deed.en).

On physical examination, patients with tamponade appear uncomfortable, with signs reflecting varying degrees of reduced cardiac output and shock, including tachypnea, diaphoresis, cool extremities, and a later sign of peripheral cyanosis (Stashko & Meer, 2023). The physical examination includes assessment of blood pressure and pulse, noting fluctuations with inspiration, heart rate and rhythm, heart sounds, respiratory rate, the presence of jugular venous distension, peripheral edema, the presence or absence of engorgement of abdominal organs, and mental status (Shelton, 2022; Stashko & Meer, 2023). Jugular venous distension may not be apparent (see Figure 1-3) unless patients are dehydrated or hypovolemic. Distension of superficial veins of the forehead and scalp may be noted as well (Hoit, 2024a; Wang et al., 2025).

A pulsus paradoxus is considered the most helpful clinical test for cardiac tamponade, with a sensitivity of 98% and specificity of 83% (Hoit, 2024a). It is an exaggerated decrease in systolic blood pressure of more than 10 mm Hg during inspiration compared to the normal physiologic reduction of less than 10 mm Hg during inspiration (Van Dam et al., 2024). Pulsus paradoxus is traditionally assessed using a manual cuff sphygmomanometer. The steps involved in this specific measurement include the following (Hoit, 2024a; Van Dam et al., 2024):

- Have the patient lie supine with the head of the examination table elevated 30°–45°.
- Instruct the patient to breathe normally (rather than deeply).
- Apply a manual blood pressure cuff to the patient's arm.
- Inflate the cuff to at least 20 mm Hg above the highest systolic pressure previously auscultated.
- Deflate the cuff slowly until the first Korotkoff sound (indicating the systolic pressure) is heard on expiration (intermittently), and note this value. This sound corresponds to the higher systolic blood pressure (e.g., 120 mm Hg).
- Continue to slowly deflate the cuff (about 5 mm Hg/second) until Korotkoff sounds are audible during both inspiration and expiration (with every heartbeat), and record this point. This is the lower systolic pressure (e.g., 105 mm Hg).

- Calculate the difference in systolic pressures between the intermittent and persistent Korotkoff sounds (e.g., 120 mm Hg – 105 mm Hg = 15 mm Hg).
- In this example, pulsus paradoxus is present; the measured difference between the pressure readings is 15 mm Hg, which exceeds the normal physiologic decrease of < 10 mm Hg during inspiration.

Advanced Practice Considerations

Laboratory Studies

Although not diagnostic for cardiac tamponade, blood test results may aid in determining the etiology of a pericardial effusion. A complete blood count with differential may reveal an infectious process causing pericarditis. Elevated cardiac biomarkers, including creatine kinase and isoenzyme levels, may be seen in patients with myocardial infarction or cardiac trauma. Renal function test results may indicate an effusion associated with uremia. Coagulation studies to evaluate prothrombin time and activated partial thromboplastin time are helpful to assess bleeding as a cause of the effusion or evaluate risk for bleeding during therapeutic fluid drainage interventions. Test results for inflammatory markers, including erythrocyte sedimentation rate, C-reactive protein, antinuclear antibody assay, and rheumatoid factor, can help diagnose autoimmune conditions. Thyroid-stimulating hormone levels are useful to assess for hypothyroidism as a cause of pericardial effusion. Testing for HIV infection and tuberculosis may assist in determining the etiology in appropriate patients (Agudo-Quílez et al., 2024; Nair, 2021; Stashko & Meer, 2023).

Electrocardiography

An electrocardiogram can provide helpful information, but most changes are nonspecific (Lorenzo-Esteller et al., 2024). Findings that should raise suspicion for cardiac tamponade are sinus tachycardia, low-voltage QRS complexes, nonspecific ST and T wave changes, and atrial dysrhythmia (Lorenzo-Esteller et al., 2024). An electrocardiogram can rule out myocardial infarction or myopericarditis because presentation is similar to cardiac tamponade (Stashko & Meer, 2023).

Imaging Studies

Echocardiography

Echocardiography is the imaging method of choice for the diagnosis of cardiac tamponade because it is widely available, noninvasive, and can provide information about the size and location of the effusion and the level of impairment to cardiac functioning (Mudra et al., 2024). A two-dimensional echocardiogram is recommended because it visualizes movement of the structures of the heart in real time, can detect as little as 15 ml of effusion, and identifies abnormalities of cardiac anatomy or movement (Ripley, 2023). It also serves as a valuable guide to optimal site selection for percutaneous drainage of the effusion by revealing the size of the effusion (Ripley, 2023). The classic echocardiographic sign of cardiac tamponade is collapse of the right atrium and right ventricle during diastole or left-sided chamber collapse (Hoit, 2024a). Echocardiography is used on a repeated basis to monitor the cardiac status of patients with pericardial effusions who do not require immediate intervention and will be followed over time (Borlaug & DeCamp, 2024a).

FIGURE 1-4. Chest X-Ray Demonstrating Cardiac Tamponade From Malignancy

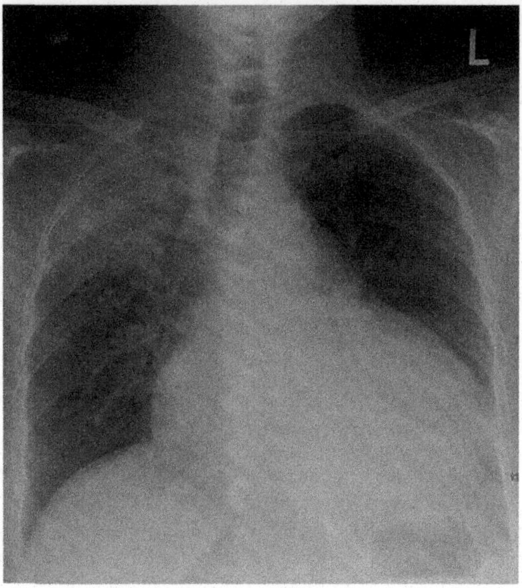

Bulbous heart and primary lung cancer appear in the right upper lobe.

Note. Image courtesy of James Heilman (https://commons.wikimedia.org/wiki/File:Tamponade.PNG). Licensed under CC BY-SA 3.0 (https://creativecommons.org/licenses/by-sa/3.0/deed.en).

Chest Radiography

Chest radiography is not a definitive diagnostic test for cardiac tamponade. However, it may reveal an enlarged, rounded cardiac silhouette, often referred to as a water bottle heart, indicating a pericardial effusion (see Figure 1-4). At least 200 ml of pericardial fluid is required for detection, and a normal chest x-ray does not rule out the condition (Hoit, 2024a). It has been observed that an enlarged cardiac silhouette appears in about 70% of patients with pericardial effusion and tamponade (Hoit, 2024a). Chest x-rays can also reveal concomitant pleural effusions; however, limitations make them insufficiently sensitive or specific for confirming cardiac tamponade.

Pericardial Fluid Analysis

Understanding the underlying cause of pericardial effusion is crucial for guiding treatment and assessing prognosis. Benign effusion can occur in patients with cancer due to infections, autoimmune disease, or post-RT injury. Pericardial fluid is obtained during a percutaneous tap of the pericardium, known as pericardiocentesis. It is then sent to a laboratory for cytologic analysis to determine whether it is malignant.

Routine laboratory tests performed on pericardial fluid should include cytology, Gram stain, bacterial and fungal culture, acid-fast bacilli, glucose, total protein count, and complete blood cell count with differential (Farinde et al., 2025; Hoit, 2024b). See Table 1-2 for analysis of pericardial fluid.

TABLE 1-2
Characteristics of Pericardial Effusions

Effusion Type	Associated Etiology
Sanguineous: bloody	Nonspecific; does not necessarily indicate active bleeding Most often associated with malignancy, renal failure with uremia, and dialysis in the United States, and with tuberculosis in low-income countries Cardiac injury due to chest trauma, heart surgery, procedure-related cardiac perforation, anticoagulation, and acute rheumatic fever
Purulent: cloudy, white-yellow, yellow, or straw colored	Suggestive of increased capillary leakage and leukocytosis, indicating infections (natural or postoperative)
Turbid: gold paint color	Cholesterol-rich effusion; associated with tuberculosis infection, rheumatoid arthritis, and severe hypothyroidism (myxedema)
Chylous: milky	Associated with the involvement of the lymphatic system Chylopericardium (effusion of chylous fluid from the digestion of fats in the intestinal tract) from trauma or surgical injury to the thoracic duct or obstruction by a malignant tumor

Note. Based on information from Farinde et al., 2025; Hoit, 2024b.

Treatment Modalities

Treatment Goals

Treatment goals for malignant pericardial effusion and cardiac tamponade are tailored to a patient's condition and individual factors, including extent of hemodynamic instability, overall medical condition, presenting symptoms, type and extent of the underlying malignancy, life expectancy, and end-of-life wishes (NCI, 2025). The immediate goal is to drain pericardial fluid to restore hemodynamic stability and alleviate symptoms. For patients who are terminally ill, the goal is to return them to their home as soon as possible after a simple fluid drainage is completed to alleviate symptoms and improve quality of life (NCI, 2025). For those with a longer life expectancy or with only mild symptoms, management goals should focus on controlling the underlying malignancy and implementing procedures to prevent reaccumulation of the effusion after initial fluid drainage, aiming to prolong symptom relief (NCI, 2025).

Pericardial Drainage Methods

Pericardiocentesis

Pericardiocentesis (percutaneous needle aspiration) is the preferred initial approach for percutaneous drainage of a pericardial effusion. This procedure is the simplest and least invasive method to treat pericardial effusion, can be performed by physicians or radiologists, and serves both a therapeutic and diagnostic purpose (Willner et al., 2025). Pericardiocentesis should be performed with either an echocardiography or fluoroscopy for localized guidance in a cardiac catheterization laboratory or procedure room with local anesthesia in order to monitor hemodynamics and minimize complications; however, in emergent, life-threatening situations, it can be performed blind (Imazio & De Ferrari, 2019). Complications can occur, even with echocardiography-guided pericardiocentesis, such as puncture of a cardiac chamber, perforation of a coronary vessel, air embolism, pneumothorax, arrhythmias (usually vasovagal bradycardia), puncture of the peritoneal cavity or abdominal viscera, and death (Imazio & De Ferrari, 2019).

Removal of 50–100 ml of pericardial fluid can be enough to relieve dyspnea, increase blood pressure, and decrease pulsus parodoxus (Ripley, 2023). After pericardiocentesis is completed, patients should be placed in a telemetry-monitored bed with continuous monitoring and frequent vital sign assessments for 24–48 hours (Hoit, 2024c). Echocardiography should be repeated prior to discharge to confirm adequate fluid removal and to detect fluid reaccumulation (Hoit, 2024c).

Prolonged Fluid Drainage

Malignant pericardial effusions have a high recurrence rate. Placement of an indwelling drainage catheter into the pericardial space, in conjunction with pericardiocentesis, is routinely recommended to provide prolonged drainage over several days, as well as a route for sclerotherapy (Hoit, 2024c; Ripley, 2023). The procedure is termed a *percutaneous tube pericardiostomy.* The catheter is left in place and aspirated intermittently (every 4–6 hours) until the output of pericardial fluid decreases to less than 25–50 ml/day (Hoit, 2024c). If, after five days, the catheter has an output of 50 ml or greater in 24 hours, patients should be evaluated for a pericardial window (Hoit, 2024c). Catheter-related complications and infections can be reduced with intermittent drainage rather than continuous drainage (Borlaug & DeCamp, 2024b).

Surgical Procedures

Subxiphoid Pericardiostomy

Subxiphoid pericardiostomy, or pericardial window, is a minimally invasive surgical procedure to create a window in the pericardium to allow fluid to drain continuously from the pericardial space into the pleural cavity (Mueller, 2024). Pericardiocentesis is often performed immediately before the pericardial window surgery to drain the fluid and reduce the tamponade so that induction of general anesthesia does not precipitate cardiovascular collapse. This is important because mechanical ventilation can impair cardiac filling and output (Borlaug & DeCamp, 2024b; Hoit, 2024a). The subxiphoid pericardiostomy typically involves taking a biopsy specimen from the pericardium for histologic examination and fluid collection for analysis. After the procedure, a chest tube is inserted into the pericardial window and connected to a water seal or suction drainage. It remains in place until fluid output drops below 50 ml/day (Mueller, 2024). The presence of the chest tube causes irritation and can help form adhesions between the pericardial layers to help prevent fluid reaccumulation. Postoperative complications may include infection, bleeding, arrhythmia, cardiac arrest, myocardial infarction, and death (Mueller, 2024).

Pericardiectomy

Pericardiectomy is the surgical excision of all or part of the pericardium to allow continuous drainage of pericardial fluid into the pleural space. It is considered the definitive treatment for pericardial effusions, as it prevents the reaccumulation of fluid (Ripley, 2023). However, pericardiectomy has serious drawbacks for patients who are debilitated with limited life expectancy, including higher morbidity rates and longer recovery periods. It has not been found to be superior to the creation of a subxiphoid pericardial window. Therefore, pericardiectomy is restricted to patients with constrictive fibrous pericarditis, which may develop as a complication of RT, and is an irreversible condition for which surgery is the only treatment option (Shelton, 2022). Pericardiectomy may also be considered for patients who have recurrent symptomatic malignant pericardial effusion after failing subxiphoid pericardiostomy and pericardiocentesis (Ripley, 2023). Table 1-3 describes each type of surgical intervention.

Additional Medical Management

Medical management of cardiac tamponade is used only as an initial measure in patients who are stable until pericardial fluid can be drained to provide more long-lasting therapeutic effects (Hoit, 2024a). Interventions such as IV fluid volume repletion, inotropic drug support, or both may be used temporarily in select patients to relieve symptoms and improve clinical condition (Hoit, 2024a). Patients with malignant pericardial effusion who are hemodynamically stable and asymptomatic can often be managed safely with observation and careful monitoring of symptoms, serial echocardiograms, and avoidance of volume depletion while receiving treatment for the underlying malignancy (Hoit, 2024a). Oxygen therapy can help reduce the work of the heart and decrease patient anxiety and respiratory distress. Placing patients on bed rest in the semi-Fowler position helps to increase venous return to the heart. Diuretics are strongly contraindicated in patients with cardiac tamponade, as they reduce circulating volume and lower central venous pressure below the intrapericardial pressure, leading to impaired ventricular filling. Endotracheal intubation with positive pressure ventilation should be avoided or used with extreme caution, as increased thoracic pressure can further compromise cardiac filling, potentially causing rapid hemodynamic deterioration (Hoit, 2024a). To minimize stress and cardiac workload, pain- and anxiety-relieving medications should be administered as needed (Kaplan, 2018).

Chemotherapy

Most patients with malignant pericardial effusion and cardiac tamponade have metastatic disease, and the use of antineoplastic therapies plus pericardial window may help to prevent recurrent malignant pericardial effusion by providing long-lasting control of the underlying malignancy (Borlaug & DeCamp, 2024b). Chemotherapy

TABLE 1-3
Intervention Options for Malignancy-Related Cardiac Tamponade

Option	Comments
Percutaneous Minimally Invasive Fluid Drainage Procedures	
Pericardiocentesis	This intervention is used for emergency management in hemodynamically unstable patients and is the preferred initial approach to pericardial drainage. The procedure is both therapeutic (provides immediate symptom relief) and diagnostic (provides fluid for laboratory analysis). Echocardiographic guidance is mandatory at the bedside or in the cardiac catheterization laboratory. A needle is inserted into the pericardial sac via a subxiphoid approach toward the left shoulder. The patient receives local anesthesia. The procedure provides short-term symptom management (effusion often recurs and requires more definitive approaches). Vital signs must be monitored during the procedure. This procedure is used for life-threatening cardiac tamponade when an open procedure can not be performed promptly.
Pericardial catheter with prolonged drainage with or without pericardial sclerosis	During pericardiocentesis, a drainage catheter is inserted into the pericardial sac. The catheter remains in place for several days for prolonged pericardial drainage. Catheter patency should be maintained, accounting for drainage quantity, color, and consistency. The catheter should be flushed every 4–8 hours as needed. The patient receives local anesthesia. The procedure provides short-term symptom management. The drainage bag should be kept below the level of the heart.
Balloon pericardiotomy	A balloon is inserted into the pericardial sac under fluoroscopic guidance and inflated to create a hole in the pericardium that allows continuous fluid drainage into the pleural space. The patient receives local anesthesia. The procedure provides short-term symptom management.
Surgical Drainage Procedures	
Pericardial window (subxiphoid pericardiostomy)	A window in the pericardium is created to allow for continuous fluid drainage into the pleural space. The main indication is to manage large, recurrent malignant pericardial effusions or cardiac tamponade in patients with limited survival. A subxiphoid approach to the pericardium can be done under local anesthesia. Biopsies and fluid can be obtained for analysis. A laparoscopic video-assisted thoracoscopic surgery approach using general anesthesia may be recommended for patients with a better survival prognosis. The procedure provides long-term management in select patients.

(Continued on next page)

TABLE 1-3
Intervention Options for Malignancy-Related Cardiac Tamponade *(Continued)*

Option	Comments
Surgical Drainage Procedures *(Cont.)*	
Pericardiectomy	Surgical excision of all or part of the pericardium is performed to allow continuous fluid drainage into the pleural space and is a definitive treatment to prevent fluid reaccumulation. The procedure is performed under general anesthesia using a laparoscopic video-assisted thoracoscopic surgery or thoracotomy approach. The intervention is indicated to treat radiation-induced constrictive pericarditis and may be considered for patients with recurrent malignant pericardial effusion following pericardial window. The procedure provides long-term management in select patients.

Note. Based on information from Hoit, 2024a; Ripley, 2023; Shelton, 2022.

can be delivered directly into the pericardial sac, systemically, or through both means. Local chemotherapy is instilled into the pericardial sac, where high drug concentrations can be achieved because the space is limited; cardiac motion can promote diffusion of the drug across the cardiac surface; and reabsorption through the lymphatic vessels is slow, which produces few systemic side effects and relieves malignant obstruction in local lymphatic vessels (Shelton, 2022). Treating patients with a combination of local and systemic chemotherapy enhances survival following malignant pericardial effusion caused by solid tumors. For highly chemosensitive cancers, treatment should be administered with a combination of steroids and systemic chemotherapy.

Radiation Therapy

External beam RT is not often used to manage cardiac tamponade but as a palliative treatment for radiosensitive tumors that are adjacent to the heart, such as lymphomas, leukemias, and esophageal, lung, and breast cancers (Borlaug & DeCamp, 2024b). If malignant pericardial effusion is found in a radiosensitive tumor, a dose of 100–200 cGy is given daily for three to four weeks to help control the effusion (Shelton, 2022).

Nursing Management

Nurses have a key role in monitoring the cardiac, respiratory, and mental status of patients with cardiac tamponade or pericardial effusion and managing their complex care needs (see Figure 1-5). No special nursing measures exist to prevent cardiac tamponade; however, astute observation and a high level of suspicion can help nurses identify patients at risk or those who have a pericardial effusion or tamponade so that appropriate treatment can be instituted before life-threatening circulatory collapse. Assessment of vital signs and cardiac and respiratory status is crucial to recognition and early intervention in patients with cardiac tamponade or pericardial effusion because

FIGURE 1-5. Nursing Management of Patients With Cardiac Tamponade

Assessments

- Hemodynamic
  - Monitor blood pressure, heart rate, and rhythm.
  - Auscultate heart sounds.
  - Monitor pulse pressures (measure pulsus paradoxus).
  - Monitor echocardiogram readings. Assess for low-voltage QRS complexes, ST-T changes, and electrical alternans.
  - Assess for jugular venous distension and tissue perfusion. Assess skin for color, temperature, turgor, capillary refill, peripheral pulses, and edema.
  - Monitor urine output for oliguria.
- Pulmonary
  - Assess for dyspnea, tachypnea, and air hunger.
  - Auscultate breath sounds.
  - Check oximetry levels.
- Central nervous system: Note changes in mental status and level of consciousness related to cerebral hypoxia.
- Laboratory test results: Note electrolyte abnormalities that can adversely affect cardiac function (e.g., hyponatremia, hypokalemia, hypomagnesemia, hypocalcemia).
- Report changes in the patient's status promptly.

General Measures

- Management of dyspnea
  - Maintain the patient on bed rest with the head of the bed elevated (e.g., semi-fowler position).
  - Administer oxygen, preferably by face mask.
  - Position the patient sitting up and leaning forward, which may alleviate dyspnea by reducing abdominal pressure on the thoracic cavity.
  - Teach diaphragmatic breathing or pursed-lip breathing.
  - Administer opioids as ordered (may be concurrent with opioids for pain control); start at a low dose and titrate up as needed.
- Management of pain and anxiety
  - Provide psychosocial support to reduce anxiety and distress.
  - Teach meditation and relaxation techniques.
  - Provide comfort measures.
  - Administer analgesics and anxiolytics as ordered; note and report adverse effects.
  - Use analgesics with caution in patients with severe hypotension.
- Conservation of energy
  - Deliver nursing care on an interval basis to minimize patient fatigue.
  - Assist with activities of daily living.
  - Encourage rest periods.
  - Provide measures to reduce anxiety and associated increased oxygen demands; teach relaxation techniques, and provide comfort measures.

Medical Care Prior to Pericardial Drainage, if Indicated

- Fluid volume expansion with IV normal saline is restricted to patients who are hypervolemic. Carefully monitor for increased hemodynamic compromise during fluid infusion; have emergency resuscitation equipment available.
- Administer inotropic or vasopressor drug as ordered to increase venous return to the heart and cardiac output; assess for clinical deterioration.
- Avoid diuretics because they decrease circulating volume and lower central venous pressure.

(Continued on next page)

FIGURE 1-5. Nursing Management of Patients With Cardiac Tamponade *(Continued)*

Care Related to Pericardiocentesis

- Preparation for procedure
  - Assess the patient's bleeding and coagulation laboratory parameters; they may need correction if the procedure is not urgent.
  - Explain the planned procedure, including purpose, equipment, expected outcomes, and side effects; respond to the patient's questions.
  - Endotracheal intubation with positive-pressure ventilation is not instituted until the heart has been decompressed by fluid removal to avoid the risk of circulatory collapse.
  - Have emergency resuscitation equipment and medications nearby.
- After the procedure
  - Assess vital signs, improvement in hemodynamic status, and relief of symptoms of cardiac tamponade (e.g., decreased dyspnea).
  - Monitor for complications (e.g., cardiac puncture, pneumothorax).
  - Assess characteristics of drainage fluid if the catheter remains in place for prolonged drainage (e.g., amount, color, turbidity); send specimens for laboratory analysis.
  - For catheter care, observe patency, amount of drainage, and signs of infection at the exit site.
  - Observe signs and symptoms of fluid reaccumulation and hemodynamic compromise (e.g., dyspnea, tachycardia, hypotension, jugular venous distension, muffled heart sounds).
  - Report changes in the patient's status promptly.

Patient and Caregiver Education

- Instruct the patient on the recognition of signs and symptoms of fluid reaccumulation and the importance of prompt reporting.
- Provide instructions regarding medication management, follow-up schedule for doctor visits and repeat echocardiograms, and the importance of adequate fluid intake to prevent hypotension.
- Teach strategies to help reduce the patient's energy expenditure.
- Provide emotional support and an opportunity to ask questions.
- Help identify and support coping strategies.

Discharge Planning

- Increase activity levels, as tolerated, as signs and symptoms of tamponade resolve.
- Schedule follow-up echocardiogram and chest x-ray at one month to check for fluid reaccumulation.
- Provide referrals as needed:
  - A homecare nurse can evaluate for symptoms indicating effusion recurrence, provide education and evaluation on catheter care, arrange for home oxygen if needed, and offer assistance with activities of daily living.
  - Rehabilitation services introduce strategies to enhance patients' functional abilities and determine what modifications may be needed in the home to support limitations with activities of daily living.
  - Psychologic counseling aims to help patients manage dyspnea by teaching relaxation or distraction techniques and supporting them emotionally as they process awareness of the current prognosis of impending mortality.

Note. Based on information from Hoit, 2024a; Nair, 2021; Shelton, 2022.

their condition can deteriorate rapidly. Nursing assessment includes frequent monitoring, noting any changes in blood pressure, pulse, respiratory rate, heart rhythm, heart sounds, and pulse pressures, with additional evaluation for pulsus parodoxus, reporting any difference greater than 10 mm Hg (Kaplan, 2018). Cardiogenic shock is associated with poor peripheral and organ perfusion and tissue hypoxia. The effectiveness of cardiac output is monitored, noting skin color, temperature, turgor, capillary refill, and peripheral pulses, as well as mental status and level of consciousness, which can reflect cerebral hypoxia. Nurses should closely monitor electrolyte abnormalities (e.g., potassium, sodium, magnesium, calcium) that can adversely affect cardiac function and report changes promptly. Assessing patients' respiratory status is crucial for evaluating cardiac function, requiring nurses to auscultate breath sounds, monitor oximetry levels, and identify tamponade-related signs, such as dyspnea, tachypnea, Kussmaul sign, and hypoxemia. Patients should remain on bed rest in the semi-Fowler position to reduce abdominal pressure on the thorax, with nurses assisting in daily activities and encouraging rest to conserve energy. Nurses should assess patients for chest pain, administer prescribed analgesia, monitor for respiratory side effects, and closely observe consciousness levels (Shelton, 2022). Strategies to help reduce patients' anxiety and cardiac workload include administering antianxiety drugs, as prescribed, and providing emotional support and teaching about relaxation and distraction techniques, such as meditation, guided imagery, and deep breathing.

Cardiac tamponade is a medical emergency, and nurses should expect that patients will be sent for urgent pericardiocentesis to drain the effusion and relieve symptoms. Providing instructions and preparing patients and caregivers for all invasive procedures or transfers to the operating room are essential facets of the nursing role. After the drainage procedure, assessment of vital signs, airway, circulation, urinary output, and level of consciousness should be ongoing, along with wound care, comfort measures, reassurance, and emotional support.

Patient and caregiver education, emotional support, and reassurance are necessary to decrease anxiety and psychosocial distress and improve decision-making related to patient-specific treatment goals. By giving patients and caregivers the opportunity to ask questions, express concerns, and receive emotional support, nurses can help reduce anxiety and distress. Providing educational information and offering referrals to psychosocial specialists or clergy, as needed, can also facilitate patients' ability to cope with difficult decisions. Discharge instructions should include education on recognizing signs of malignant pericardial effusion recurrence (e.g., difficulty breathing) and treatment complications, emphasizing the need for prompt reporting, catheter care instructions, and the importance of scheduling follow-up visits with medical oncologists and other specialists.

Summary

Cardiac tamponade is a life-threatening oncologic emergency that requires rapid identification and intervention to avoid cardiovascular collapse and death. In patients with cancer, diagnosing cardiac tamponade can be challenging, as early symptoms are vague and nonspecific, vary among patients, and may be attributed to the disease, treatment side effects, or other nonmalignant conditions. Treatment goals are tailored to the extent of the disease and life expectancy, with the primary objective being symptom palliation, particularly alleviating distressing symptoms such as dyspnea by draining pericardial fluid to improve cardiac output. Nurses who are aware of cancers linked to an increased risk for malignant pericardial effusion and the signs of hemodynamic compromise associated with cardiac tamponade can facilitate early identification, allowing for timely intervention and improved patient outcomes.

The authors would like to acknowledge Marcelle Kaplan, MS, RN, CNS, for her contribution to this chapter that remains unchanged from the previous edition of this book.

References

Adamczyk, M., Wasilewski, J., Niedziela, J., Rozentryt, P., & Gąsior, M. (2019). Pericardial tamponade as a complication of invasive cardiac procedures: A review of the literature. *Advances in Interventional Cardiology/Postępy w Kardiologii Interwencyjnej, 15*(4), 394–403. https://doi.org/10.5114/aic.2019.90213

Adashek, J.J., Moran, J.A., Le, D.T., & Kurzrock, R. (2025). Lessons learned from a decade of immune checkpoint inhibition: The good, the bad, and the ugly. *Cancer and Metastasis Reviews, 44*(2), 43. https://doi.org/10.1007/s10555-025-10260-8

Agudo-Quílez, P., Martín-Moro, F., Ugalde, S.A., Blanco-Peláez, E., García-Cosío, M., Tenelanda, A., ... Gómez, J.L.Z. (2024). Primary cardiac aggressive B-cell lymphoma affecting right ventricle and acute cardiovascular events: Multidisciplinary approach. *JACC Case Reports, 29*(19), 102562. https://doi.org/10.1016/j.jaccas.2024.102562

Al-Ogaili, A., Ayoub, A., Fugar, S., Kolkailah, A., Rios, L.P., & Fuentes, H. (2018). Cardiac tamponade incidence, demographics and in-hospital outcomes: Analysis of the national inpatient sample database. *Journal of the American College of Cardiology, 71*(11, Suppl.), A1155. https://doi.org/10.1016/s0735-1097(18)31696-6

Borlaug, B.A., & DeCamp, M.M. (2024a, June 3). Pericardial disease associated with cancer: Clinical presentation and diagnosis. In S.B. Yeon & S.M. Shah (Eds.), *UpToDate*. Retrieved October 27, 2025, from https://www.uptodate.com/contents/pericardial-disease-associated-with-cancer-clinical-presentation-and-diagnosis

Borlaug, B.A., & DeCamp, M.M. (2024b, June 3). Pericardial disease associated with cancer: Management. In S.B. Yeon & S.M. Shah (Eds.), *UpToDate*. Retrieved October 27, 2025, from https://www.uptodate.com/contents/pericardial-disease-associated-with-cancer-management

Chahine, J., Shekhar, S., Mahalwar, G., Imazio, M., Collier, P., & Klein, A. (2021). Pericardial involvement in cancer. *American Journal of Cardiology, 145*, 151–159. https://doi.org/10.1016/j.amjcard.2020.12.092

Chiabrando, J.G., Bonaventura, A., Vecchié, A., Wohlford, G.F., Mauro, A.G., Jordan, J.H., ... Abbate, A. (2020). Management of acute and recurrent pericarditis: JACC state-of-the-art review. *Journal of the American College of Cardiology, 75*(1), 76–92. https://doi.org/10.1016/j.jacc.2019.11.021

Cremer, P.C., Klein, A.L., & Imazio, M. (2024). Diagnosis, risk stratification, and treatment of pericarditis: A review. *JAMA, 332*(13), 1090–1100. https://doi.org/10.1001/jama.2024.12935

Curigliano, G., Cardinale, D., Dent, S., Criscitiello, C., Aseyev, O., Lenihan, D., & Cipolla, C.M. (2016). Cardiotoxicity of anticancer treatments: Epidemiology, detection, and management. *CA: A Cancer Journal for Clinicians, 66*(4), 309–325. https://doi.org/10.3322/caac.21341

Farinde, A., Nguyen, H.C.T., Yau, S.W.F., Amanullah, A.M., & Hermelin, D. (2025, October 9). Pericardial fluid analysis. *Medscape*. http://emedicine.medscape.com/article/2123066-overview

Hatta, S.S.W.M., Mirza, A.R., Sunni, N., & Bashir, A. (2025). Heart-breaking tumours: A case series of malignant pericardial effusion. *European Heart Journal Case Reports, 9*(3), ytaf009. https://doi.org/10.1093/ehjcr/ytaf009

Hoit, B.D. (2024a, March 19). Cardiac tamponade. In S.B. Yeon (Ed.), *UpToDate*. Retrieved October 27, 2025, from http://www.uptodate.com/contents/cardiac-tamponade

Hoit, B.D. (2024b, December 3). Pericardial effusion: Approach to diagnosis. In S.B. Yeon (Ed.), *UpToDate*. Retrieved October 27, 2025, from https://www.uptodate.com/contents/pericardial-effusion-approach-to-diagnosis

Hoit, B.D. (2024c, June 3). Pericardial effusion: Approach to management. In S.B. Yeon (Ed.), *UpToDate*. Retrieved October 27, 2025, from https://www.uptodate.com/contents/pericardial-effusion-approach-to-management

Imazio, M., & De Ferrari, G.M. (2019). Cardiac tamponade: An educational review. *European Heart Journal: Acute Cardiovascular Care, 10*(1), 102–109. https://doi.org/10.1177/2048872620939341

Kaplan, M. (2018). Cardiac tamponade. In C.H. Yarbro, D. Wujcik, & B.H. Gobel (Eds.), *Cancer nursing: Principles and practice* (8th ed., pp. 1075–1093). Jones and Bartlett Learning.

Keyvanfar, A., Najafiarab, H., Ramezani, S., & Tehrani, S. (2024). Cardiac tamponade in people living with HIV: A systematic review of case reports and case series. *BMC Infectious Diseases, 24*(1), 882. https://doi.org/10.1186/s12879-024-09773-4

Koutsoukis, A., Ntalianis, A., Repasos, E., Kastritis, E., Dimopoulos, M.-A., & Paraskevaidis, I. (2018). Cardio-oncology: A focus on cardiotoxicity. *European Cardiology Review, 13*(1), 64–69. https://doi.org/10.15420/ecr.2017:17:2

Lorenzo-Esteller, L., Ramos-Polo, R., Pons Riverola, A., Morillas, H., Berdejo, J., Pernas, S., ... Moliner, P. (2024). Pericardial disease in patients with cancer: Clinical insights on diagnosis and treatment. *Cancers, 16*(20), 3466. https://doi.org/10.3390/cancers16203466

Mori, S., Bertamino, M., Guerisoli, L., Stratoti, S., Canale, C., Spallarossa, P., ... Ameri, P. (2024). Pericardial effusion in oncological patients: Current knowledge and principles of management. *Cardio-Oncology, 10*(1), 8. https://doi.org/10.1186/s40959-024-00207-3

Mudra, S.E., Rayes, D., Kumar, A.K., Li, J.Z., Njus, M., McGown, K., ... Klein, A.L. (2024). Malignant pericardial effusion: A systematic review. *CJC Open, 6*(8), 967–972. https://doi.org/10.1016/j.cjco.2024.05.003

Mueller, D.K. (2024, September 3). Pericardial window. *Medscape*. http://emedicine.medscape.com/article/1829679-overview

Nair, N. (2021, November 19). Cardiac tamponade. *Medscape*. http://emedicine.medscape.com/article/152083-overview

National Cancer Institute. (2025). *Cardiopulmonary syndromes (PDQ®)–Health professional version: Malignant pericardial effusion*. https://www.cancer.gov/about-cancer/treatment/side-effects/cardiopulmonary-hp-pdq#_40

Ning, M.S., Tang, L., Gomez, D.R., Xu, T., Luo, Y., Huo, J., ... Liao, Z. (2017). Incidence and predictors of pericardial effusion after chemoradiation therapy for locally advanced non-small cell lung cancer. *International Journal of Radiation Oncology, Biology, Physics, 99*(1), 70–79. https://doi.org/10.1016/j.ijrobp.2017.05.022

Nova-Camacho, L.M., Gomez-Dorronsoro, M., Guarch, R., Cordoba, A., Cevallos, M.I., & Panizo-Santos, A. (2023). Cardiac metastasis from solid cancers: A 35-year single-center autopsy study. *Archives of Pathology and Laboratory Medicine, 147*(2), 177–184. https://doi.org/10.5858/arpa.2021-0418-OA

Rehman, I., Nassereddin, A., & Rehman, A. (2023). Anatomy, thorax, pericardium. In *StatPearls*. In StatPearls Publishing. https://www.ncbi.nlm.nih.gov/books/NBK482256

Ripley, R.T. (2023). Malignant pleural and pericardial effusions. In V.T. DeVita Jr., T.S. Lawrence, & S.A. Rosenberg (Eds.), *DeVita, Hellman, and Rosenberg's cancer: Principles and practice of oncology* (12th ed., pp. 1681–1688). Wolters Kluwer.

Salem, J.-E., Manouchehri, A., Moey, M., Lebrun-Vignes, B., Bastarache, L., Pariente, A., ... Moslehi, J.J. (2018). Cardiovascular toxicities associated with immune checkpoint inhibitors: An observational, retrospective, pharmacovigilance study. *Lancet Oncology, 19*(12), 1579–1589. https://doi.org/10.1016/s1470-2045(18)30608-9

Shelton, B.K. (2022). Pericarditis, pericardial effusion, and pericardial tamponade. In D. Camp-Sorrell, R.A. Hawkins, & D.G. Cope (Eds.), *Clinical manual for the oncology advanced practice nurse* (4th ed., pp. 399–411). Oncology Nursing Society.

Shirakabe, A., Matsushita, M., Shibata, Y., Shighihara, S., Nishigoori, S., Sawatani, T., ... Asai, K. (2023). Organ dysfunction, injury, and failure in cardiogenic shock. *Journal of Intensive Care, 11*(1). https://doi.org/10.1186/s40560-023-00676-1

Spangler, S., & Gentlesk, P.J. (2019, April 2). Acute pericarditis. *Medscape.* http://emedicine.medscape.com/article/156951-overview

Stashko, E., & Meer, J.M. (2023). Cardiac tamponade. In *StatPearls.* StatPearls Publishing. https://www.ncbi.nlm.nih.gov/books/NBK431090

Strimel, W.J., Ayub, B., & Contractor, T. (2025, May 27). Pericardial effusions. *Medscape.* https://emedicine.medscape.com/article/157325-overview

Tyebally, S., Chen, D., Bhattacharyya, S., Mughrabi, A., Hussain, Z., Manisty, C., ... Guha, A. (2020). Cardiac tumors: *JACC CardioOncology* state-of-the-art review. *JACC CardioOncology, 2*(2), 293–311. https://doi.org/10.1016/j.jaccao.2020.05.009

Van Dam, M.N., Hashmi, M.F., & Fitzgerald, B.M. (2024). Pulsus paradoxus. In *StatPearls.* StatPearls Publishing. https://www.ncbi.nlm.nih.gov/books/NBK482292

von Kemp, B.A., & Cosyns, B. (2023). Radiation-induced pericardial disease: Mechanisms, diagnosis, and treatment. *Current Cardiology Reports, 25*(10), 1113–1121. https://doi.org/10.1007/s11886-023-01933-3

Wang, T.K.M., Klein, A.L., Cremer, P.C., Imazio, M., Kohnstamm, S., Luis, S.A., ... Wohlford, G.F. (2025). 2025 Concise Clinical Guidance: An ACC expert consensus statement on the diagnosis and management of pericarditis. *Journal of the American College of Cardiology, 86*(25), 2691–2719. https://doi.org/10.1016/j.jacc.2025.05.023

Willner, D.A., Shams, P., & Grossman, S.A. (2025). Pericardiocentesis. In *StatPearls.* StatPearls Publishing. https://www.ncbi.nlm.nih.gov/books/NBK470347

Sara Gomes, MSc, RN

CHAPTER 2

Superior Vena Cava Syndrome

FAST FACTS

- **Description:** Superior vena cava syndrome occurs when the superior vena cava is obstructed, typically due to tumor compression, tumor invasion, or internal blockage by a thrombus. This impairs venous return from the head and upper body, leading to venous congestion. The resulting decrease in blood flow to the heart subsequently diminishes cardiac output.
- **Incidence:** The syndrome is primarily associated with chest malignancies near the superior vena cava or surrounding lymph nodes (e.g., lung cancer, lymphoma, breast cancer), as well as metastatic tumors, occluding central venous catheters, and vena cava filters that capture clots.
- **Clinical Manifestations:** Common symptoms resulting from reduced cardiac output include dyspnea and cough. Additional signs may include skin mottling, decreased distal pulses, and oliguria.
- **Risk Factors and Etiology:** Four mechanisms may cause superior vena cava syndrome: occlusion by an extrinsic mass, direct tumor invasion through the vessel wall, a thrombus around a central venous catheter, and a thrombus occurring within the superior vena cava.
- **Pathophysiology and Patient Evaluation:** A complete patient history and physical examination are essential to determine the underlying cause, severity, and duration of symptoms. Early physical signs are dilated veins of the face, neck, thorax, breasts, and upper extremities, and face edema. Late physical signs are cyanosis, confusion, tachypnea, dysphagia, and stridor.
- **Advanced Practice Considerations:** Chest x-ray, magnetic resonance imaging, and contrast-enhanced computed tomography scans of the chest are the primary diagnostic methods used to evaluate superior vena cava syndrome, revealing tumor location, level of invasion, and presence of thrombus. Histopathologic diagnosis can also be necessary.
- **Treatment Modalities:** Radiation therapy is the most effective treatment for radiosensitive tumors, including Hodgkin lymphoma and non-small cell lung cancer, providing rapid symptom relief. It is also beneficial for chemosensitive tumors, such as high-grade lymphoma, small cell lung cancer, and testicular cancer. In cases involving vena cava clots, treatment with thrombolytics or anticoagulants is recommended. Endovascular stenting has also become a standard first-line intervention for managing superior vena cava syndrome over the past two decades.
- **Nursing Management:** Key priorities include maintaining airway protection, ensuring cardiovascular support, and implementing comfort measures. Patients are often anxious because of severe dyspnea and typically cannot tolerate lying flat. IV lines should be avoided in the upper chest and neck, as venous return is compromised; infusions

administered through hand veins may also be ineffective. Blood pressure may be falsely elevated when measured in the upper extremities, and notable pressure differences can occur between the right and left sides.

- **Outcomes:** Although superior vena cava syndrome is rarely fatal, it can cause significant morbidity and distress. Superior vena cava syndrome may present at initial diagnosis or during disease recurrence or progression. Management depends on a patient's individual goals of care.

Introduction

Superior vena cava syndrome (SVCS) is an uncommon condition, occurring in approximately 3%–4% of patients with cancer involving the chest (Chow et al., 2024). The superior vena cava (SVC) is the major vein that carries deoxygenated blood from the head, neck, upper extremities, and upper thorax to the right side of the heart. Obstruction or compression of the SVC may occur either acutely or gradually due to various space-occupying lesions in the mediastinum. The acuity of onset influences the severity of symptoms and whether the obstruction is located above or below the azygos vein (Azizi et al., 2020; Chow et al., 2024). Cardiac output may be reduced from diminished blood return to the heart. SVCS compromises the heart, resulting in a complex of symptoms and physical findings (Azizi et al., 2020; Chow et al., 2024).

Mediastinal malignancies are the most common cause of SVC obstruction in lung cancer, lymphoma, mediastinal tumors, and breast cancer. However, thrombosis or tumors occurring within the SVC lumen can also lead to obstruction, and such cases have been increasing in recent years (Mir et al., 2022). SVC obstruction causes venous congestion; increased venous pressure in the head, neck, upper extremities, and upper thorax; and impaired venous return to the right atrium. Symptoms of SVCS typically develop gradually, over weeks to months, but may also occur quickly depending on the proliferation rate of the malignancy (Patriarcheas et al., 2022). Although SVCS is usually not life threatening, it can become an oncologic emergency when obstruction is severe enough to cause reduced cardiac filling, cerebral edema, respiratory distress, or tracheal obstruction (Patriarcheas et al., 2022). Oncology nurses must be aware of patients at risk for SVCS and recognize early signs and symptoms. Prompt recognition and intervention may prevent SVCS from progressing to a life-threatening oncologic emergency.

Incidence

The global incidence of SVCS ranges from as high as 1 in 650 to 1 in 3,100 patients (Chow et al., 2024). Adults aged 50–70 years, particularly males, have a higher incidence of SVCS primarily due to increased rates of lung cancer in this population (Nickloes et al., 2024).

The incidence of SVCS unrelated to cancer appears to be increasing (Azizi et al., 2020). Retrospective studies indicate that nonmalignant conditions account for as many as 15%–40% of SVC obstruction cases, specifically because of an increase in thrombus formation related to vascular access devices, central venous monitoring catheters, and cardiac pacemaker electrodes. However, other less common etiologies include mediastinal fibrosis, which develops in response to the presence of fungal infections, and postradiation fibrosis (Chow et al., 2024).

Clinical Manifestations

Venous congestion may lead to laryngeal and cerebral edema, rarely progressing to stupor, convulsions, and coma (Wright et al., 2023). Elevated pressure in the collateral circulation can lead to systemic–pulmonary shunts, downhill esophageal varices, and high levels of venous congestion (Azizi et al., 2020; Chow et al., 2024). The degree of SVC obstruction may vary greatly depending on the nature of the obstruction and the rate of change. The development of collateral circulation to return blood to the right atrium correlates with the extent of SVC obstruction and the patency of the azygos pathways, which often become the most common venous collateral route. If both the SVC and azygos vein are obstructed, other interconnected venous routes become more developed, including the internal mammary, lateral thoracic, superficial thoracoabdominal veins, and the vertebral venous plexus (Chow et al., 2024). Previously, SVCS was classified based on venographic patterns, but this has been replaced with a grading system that uses clinical symptoms to more accurately reflect the severity of the disease. According to Yu et al. (2008), cited by Azizi et al. (2020), the grades are from 0 to 5:

- 0—Asymptomatic: SVC on imaging without symptoms
- 1—Mild: edema of the head or neck
- 2—Moderate: edema of the head or neck with functional impairment
- 3—Severe: mild or moderate cerebral edema/laryngeal edema or diminished cardiac reserve
- 4—Life-threatening: significant cerebral edema, laryngeal edema, and hemodynamic compromise
- 5—Fatal: death

Risk Factors and Etiology

SVCS was first recognized in 1757 in a patient with a syphilitic aneurysm of the ascending aorta (Hunter, 1957).

Four mechanisms may cause SVCS: occlusion by an extrinsic mass, direct tumor invasion through the vessel wall, a thrombus around a central venous catheter, and a thrombus occurring within the SVC (Chow et al., 2024). Risk factors for thrombus formation include a hypercoagulable state induced by malignancy, intimal damage to the vein from central venous catheters, or venous stasis resulting from external compression to the SVC. Thrombosis is more likely than tumor infiltration to result in acute and complete SVC obstruction (Chow et al., 2024). Partial or complete occlusion of the SVC increases venous pressure (venous hypertension), leading to venous stasis and vein engorgement in the areas usually drained by the SVC. The rising venous pressure leads to third spacing of fluid into adjacent tissue. Third spacing refers to the accumulation of fluid that is unavailable to support circulation but remains inside the body. Fluid accumulation can further compress the vena cava and other vital structures in the mediastinum, potentially resulting in pleural or pericardial effusions (Wright et al., 2023). If the pleural fluid is cloudy and white, obstruction of the thoracic duct and chylothorax may be suspected, but this does not typically alter treatment (Azizi et al., 2020; Chow et al., 2024).

Prior to the mid-20th century, malignancies accounted for only one-third of all SVCS cases. Most were attributed to infectious conditions, such as granulomatous infections from tuberculosis or nocardiosis, goiter, aortic aneurysms, or histoplasmosis-related mediastinal fibrosis (Azizi et al., 2020). With the development of effective treatments for these infections, mediastinal malignancies, especially right-sided lung cancer, now account for 70%–95% of SVCS cases and are the initial presenting symptom in up to 60% of those affected (McNally, 2018).

Although patients with small cell lung cancer (SCLC) represent 65%–80% of SVCS cases, an increasing number are linked to non-small cell lung cancers (NSCLCs), such as squamous cell carcinoma and adenocarcinoma, which occur more frequently and are associated with longer life expectancies (Azizi et al., 2020; Chow et al., 2024) (see Figure 2-1).

SVCS occurs as the presenting feature of malignancy in 25% of patients who have SCLC and in approximately 50% of those with NSCLC (Chow et al., 2024). Lymphoma, primarily non-Hodgkin lymphoma (NHL), is the fourth most common malignancy associated with SVCS, accounting for 10% of cases (Chow et al., 2024). SVCS is more likely to occur with the high-grade subtypes of NHL that are commonly present with mediastinal masses, such as diffuse large cell and lymphoblastic lymphoma, and is rarely seen with Hodgkin lymphoma despite the high incidence of mediastinal involvement (Chow et al., 2024). Patients with NHL often present with concomitant pleural effusion (typically involving the right lung), pericardial effusions, or tracheobronchial obstruction (McNally, 2018).

FIGURE 2-1. Etiologies of Superior Vena Cava Syndrome

Malignant: Primary or Metastatic (70%)	Nonmalignant (30%)
• Non-small cell lung cancer (50%) • Small cell lung cancer (25%) • Other cancers, including esophageal carcinoma, thyroid carcinoma, breast carcinoma, testicular cancer, thymoma, mesothelioma, leukemia, cardiac myxoma (15%) • Non-Hodgkin lymphoma, including diffuse large cell, lymphoblastic, and cardiac involvement (10%)	• Thrombosis, including indwelling central venous catheters, especially located in the subclavian vein • Cardiac, including aneurysm, arteriovenous fistula, pacemaker wires, and pericarditis (25%–30%) • Other benign causes, including benign tumor of the chest, mediastinal fibrosis (e.g., tuberculosis, prior radiation therapy, histoplasmosis), granulomatous disease (e.g., sarcoidosis, tuberculosis), infection (e.g., histoplasmosis, nocardiosis, tuberculosis), trauma, iatrogenic (1%–5%)

Note. Based on information from Azizi et al., 2020; Chow et al., 2024.

Breast cancer and testicular cancer metastatic to the mediastinum are the metastatic malignancies most often associated with SVCS. Other cancers related to SVCS include thyroid cancer, thymoma, granulocytic leukemia, melanoma, gastrointestinal malignancies, renal cancer, and Kaposi or other sarcomas (Chow et al., 2024).

Pathophysiology and Patient Evaluation

Anatomy

The SVC is the major conduit for venous drainage from the head, neck, upper extremities, and upper thorax to the right atrium of the heart. It is located in the middle third of the right anterior superior mediastinum behind the sternum. The SVC is surrounded by relatively rigid structures, such as the trachea, esophagus, right main bronchus, aorta, pulmonary artery, and vertebral bodies, as well as perihilar and paratracheal lymph nodes (see Figure 2-2). It is a thin-walled, low-pressure (< 5 mm Hg) vessel, measuring approximately 7 cm long and 1.5–2 cm wide. The SVC originates at the junction of the left and right brachiocephalic veins in the middle third of the mediastinum and terminates in the right atrium. It lies posterior and to the right of the ascending aorta and joins posteriorly by the azygos vein as it loops over the right mainstem bronchus. The mediastinal parietal pleura is lateral to the SVC, creating a confined space. Several lymph node groups on the right, including the paratracheal, azygos, right hilar, and subcarinal lymph nodes, lie adjacent to the SVC. The low pressure of the blood flow through the SVC may contribute to extrinsic compression and intraluminal thrombus formation (Azizi et al., 2020; Chow et al., 2024).

Mechanisms Contributing to Superior Vena Cava Syndrome

SVCS develops when the SVC becomes obstructed and compressed before it enters the right atrium (Azizi et al., 2020; Chow et al., 2024). Several features of the anatomy and location of the SVC render it particularly vulnerable to obstruction by any local space-occupying process. The thin walls and low-pressure hemodynamics permit the SVC to collapse readily. The location on the right side of the superior mediastinum, directly behind the sternum and adjacent to the right mainstem bronchus, does not allow much flexibility when a space-occupying mediastinal lesion is present, such as expanding bronchogenic tumors, tumors growing within the mediastinal parietal pleura, or lymph nodes enlarged with disease (Azizi et al., 2020; Chow et al., 2024). Metastatic involvement of regional lymph nodes can obstruct the SVC through direct extension or extrinsic compression, resulting in congestion of the collateral veins of the neck, anterior chest wall, face, and right arm. In unusual cases, unilateral right-sided SVCS may occur, with the inclusion of only one of the brachial plexus veins and one-sided symptoms (Azizi et al., 2020; Chow et al., 2024).

The azygos vein is a major auxiliary vessel of the SVC and returns venous blood to the heart from the compensatory collateral circulation system that develops in the upper body. The azygos system can expand easily and accommodate the shunted blood

FIGURE 2-2. Superior Vena Cava Obstruction With Azygos Venous System

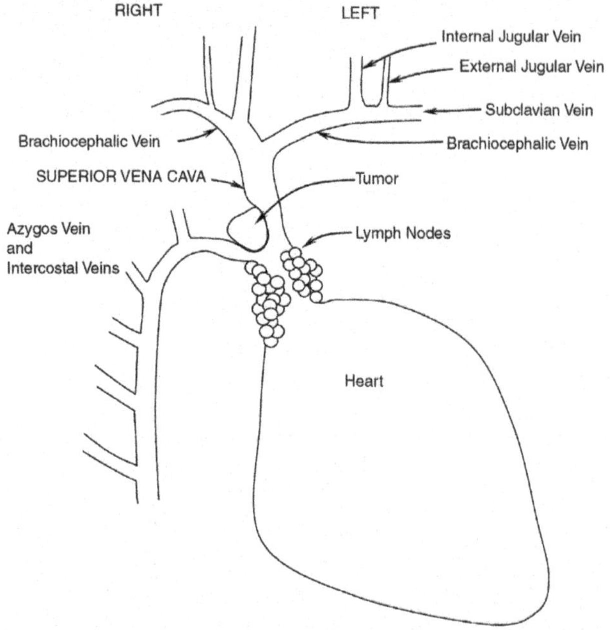

The superior vena cava is formed by the merger of the left and right brachiocephalic (or innominate) veins in the upper mediastinum. They are the major veins returning blood to the superior vena cava and are formed by the convergence of the corresponding internal jugular and subclavian veins.

Note. Based on information from Dragomir et al., 2021.

so that the venous pressure does not increase significantly in the head, arms, and upper thorax (Patriarcheas et al., 2022). If SVC obstruction occurs below the azygos vein, more severe manifestations of SVCS develop (Azizi et al., 2020; Chow et al., 2024).

Venous pressure is higher below the azygos arch, and blood flow back to the heart is more circuitous and complex. With lower SVC obstruction, the collateral circulation returns blood to the heart via the upper abdominal veins and inferior vena cava, requiring higher venous pressure.

Patient Assessment

History

SVCS may present as a sign of malignancy or may develop in patients with a known cancer history. A complete patient history and physical examination are essential to determine the underlying cause, severity, and duration of symptoms (Chow et al., 2024). Because SVC is most commonly associated with lung cancer, clinicians should question patients with no known cancer history about smoking habits or other risk factors for lung cancer, such as environmental or occupational exposure to carcinogens or previous radiation to the mediastinum. In young patients or nonsmokers, an exploration of allergies, infections (especially viral, such as HIV), autoimmune diseases, or exposure to immunosuppressive medications may reveal risk factors for NHL. Patients with previously diagnosed malignancies, such as bronchogenic cancer, lymphoma, or metastatic disease, are at increased risk for SVCS regardless of prior history of the syndrome (McNally, 2018).

Healthcare providers should assess patients for the presence of a central venous catheter, an implanted venous access port, or a pacemaker. During insertion of the vascular access device, the wall of the vena cava may have been injured, resulting in inflammation or thrombus formation, or the device may irritate chemotherapy infusions. Additionally, a cardiac history should be reviewed, as patients with coronary disease, hypertension, or heart failure may be at increased risk for SVCS due to added strain on the cardiovascular system.

Physical Examination

The classic signs and symptoms of SVCS (see Figure 2-3) are so specific to the syndrome and so uncommon to other conditions that clinicians often can make the diagnosis by clinical examination alone. Although pericardial tamponade and congestive heart failure may produce similar signs and symptoms, a focused physical examination can quickly exclude both conditions (Azizi et al., 2020).

Early Physical Signs

A prominent venous pattern with dilated veins of the face, neck, thorax, breasts, and upper extremities typically presents with SVCS. It may be accompanied by edema in those areas. Patients may exhibit facial plethora, characterized by a ruddy complexion of the face or cheeks. They also may experience jugular venous distension, periorbital edema, and edema of the conjunctivae. Although often bilateral, it may be more pronounced on the right side of the body. Blood pressure is often elevated in the upper extremities, particularly on the right, and is reduced in the legs. Compensatory tachycardia can occur. Horner syndrome may also be observed, manifested by unilateral drooping eyelid (ptosis), constricted pupil, and lack of sweating (anhidrosis) on one side of the forehead because of pressure on the cervical sympathetic nerves (Azizi et al., 2020).

FIGURE 2-3. Common Signs and Symptoms of Superior Vena Cava Syndrome

Signs	Symptoms
• Arm edema • Chest pain • Cough • Dyspnea • Facial and neck edema (Stokes sign) • Sensation of fullness in the head	• Altered level of consciousness • Cyanosis • Plethora of the face • Syncope and/or headache • Venous distension of the chest wall • Venous distension of the neck

Note. Based on information from Azizi et al., 2020.

Late Physical Signs

Late physical signs of SVCS develop in fewer than 2% of cases and appear more commonly in patients with rapidly progressing severe disease (Azizi et al., 2020). Examples of late physical signs include the following (Azizi et al., 2020):
- Cyanosis of the face and upper torso
- Decreased or absent peripheral pulses
- Congestive heart failure
- Decreased blood pressure
- Chest pain
- Mental status changes (e.g., confusion, somnolence, changes in level of consciousness, stupor, coma)
- Tachypnea, tachycardia, orthopnea
- Engorged conjunctivae, or orbital edema
- Visual disturbances (e.g., blurred vision, diplopia)
- Syncope
- Dysphagia
- Unequal swallowing
- Hoarseness caused by paralysis of the true vocal cord
- Stridor

The two potentially life-threatening manifestations are airway obstruction and cerebral edema (McNally, 2018). Stridor represents an ominous sign and indicates severe airway compromise and impending respiratory failure. Patients may have progressive cyanosis and edema of the face or upper torso, orbital edema, and engorged conjunctivae, presenting with the appearance of a purple frog. They may also experience reduction or absence of upper extremity peripheral pulses, decreased blood pressure, and syncope. Manifestations of respiratory distress, such as orthopnea, tachypnea, or tachycardia, may be present. Cerebral edema may occur, characterized by changes in mental status and vision, syncope, seizures, and coma, as well as tracheal edema. If left untreated, tracheal obstruction or brain herniation will result in death (Azizi et al., 2020).

Advanced Practice Considerations

Imaging Studies

Chest x-ray, magnetic resonance imaging (MRI), and contrast-enhanced computed tomography (CT) scans of the chest are the primary diagnostic methods used to evaluate SVCS. Although contrast venography was previously the mainstay for confirmatory diagnosis, it is now rarely needed because of the accuracy of contrast-enhanced CT scans (Sen et al., 2022). However, venography remains necessary before placement of an SVC stent or surgical bypass. Typically, a mass exists in the superior mediastinum, right hilum or perihilar region, or right upper lobe. Hilar adenopathy is present in 50% of patients with SVCS, and pleural effusion occurs in 25% of patients, which often appears as exudative and chylous (Chow et al., 2024).

More than 60% of patients with SVCS have a widening of the mediastinum, most commonly on the right side, due to a space-occupying lesion, or they present with a dilated SVC and collateral veins evident on chest x-ray (Nickloes et al., 2024). A chest x-ray is often the initial diagnostic test and may show confirmatory diagnostic changes in up to 80% of patients (Patriarcheas et al., 2022). Suspicious radiologic findings may include widened mediastinum, dilated SVC, right-sided chest mass, or dilated collateral veins, but thrombus must be confirmed with CT scans (Nickloes et al., 2024).

The most useful radiographic tools for diagnosing SVCS include the contrast-enhanced spiral or helical CT scans (Azizi et al., 2020). Advances in CT scanning technology have demonstrated its role in determining the location and extent of thrombi, vascular compression and invasion, and pathways of venous circulation, including collateral venous pathways (Dragomir et al., 2021). CT imaging allows visualization of the thoracic anatomy, specifically the size and location of the tumor relative to the SVC, trachea, and heart (Sen et al., 2022). It is also used to localize a tumor for CT-guided biopsy and to determine radiation treatment fields (Sen et al., 2022). CT venography merges a CT scan with venography and enables a more accurate diagnosis in patients with chronic abnormalities of the central veins (Dragomir et al., 2021). MRI may also function as a noninvasive diagnostic tool, particularly when CT scans are contraindicated (Sen et al., 2022). MRIs can provide greater detail than CT regarding mediastinal structures in multiple planes. Although MRI has a 96% sensitivity rate for the detection of SVC obstruction, it has a longer scanning time and an increased cost (Sen et al., 2022). Additionally, patients may be unable to tolerate lying flat for the prolonged procedure time of an MRI scan.

Venography provides valuable and accurate pathophysiologic data, such as the presence of vascular lumen filling problems associated with clots and the flow of blood through collateral vessels (Sen et al., 2022). Contrast venography involves injecting contrast material via the antecubital veins to visualize the mediastinal blood vessels. This provides detailed information regarding the patency of the vena cava, whether the obstruction is extrinsic or intrinsic, the presence and degree of thrombosis, and the adequacy of collateral circulation. However, because of its invasiveness, venography is not used on a routine basis (Azizi et al., 2020).

Tissue Diagnosis

Histopathologic diagnosis of the underlying condition causing SVCS is essential to providing optimal treatment. To obtain a tissue diagnosis, clinicians should use the least invasive method. Cytologic diagnosis of malignancy causing SVCS is a priority and should be performed before treatment unless life-threatening symptoms are present. Cells for cytologic examination can be acquired from sputum samples, bronchial brushings, or pleural fluid. A bronchoscopy with a fine biopsy or biopsy of palpable cervical or subclavian lymph nodes may also provide tissue diagnosis for these mediastinal tumors (Aung et al., 2022). Clinicians should perform mediastinoscopy when necessary to establish a histologic diagnosis when less invasive procedures have been unsuccessful (McNally, 2018). Although previously contraindicated in patients with

SVCS because of the risk of hemorrhage, mediastinoscopy has been performed safely with few complications (Aung et al., 2022; Chow et al., 2024).

Treatment Modalities

The treatment plan selected depends on the etiology of the SVCS, the severity of the symptoms, the patient's prognosis, the underlying malignancy, and the presence or absence of intraluminal thrombosis. Treatment focuses on relieving the obstruction and associated symptoms, as well as controlling the underlying disease. SVCS is considered a medical emergency when it develops acutely and requires prompt relief of the obstruction. The goal of treatment is to cure when the primary disease is SCLC, NHL, or a germ cell tumor (Sun et al., 2021). Treatment of SVCS secondary to the presence of cancer most often involves chemotherapy, radiation therapy, or both. Other treatment options include thrombolytic therapy and anticoagulation, surgical bypass, intravascular stent placement, and medical management with systemic corticosteroids and diuretics (Sen et al., 2022).

Stent Placement

In the past two decades, endovascular stenting has emerged as a standard first-line treatment for SVCS (Aung et al., 2022). Analysis of several studies on malignant SVCS reveals that the use of percutaneously placed intravascular stents was effective in reopening the occluded SVC in more than 75%–85% of patients and resulted in complete or partial symptom relief in 68%–100% (Sen et al., 2022). Stenting has shown equal symptom relief in a shorter amount of time when compared to chemotherapy and radiation therapy, especially with tumors not sensitive to those modalities (Azizi et al., 2020). The procedure has been advocated as the first choice for palliative treatment of SVCS because it does not preclude the use of subsequent chemotherapy or radiation therapy and provides immediate and dramatic relief of symptoms (Azizi et al., 2020). In clinical practice, stenting is used for patients with severe symptoms or recurrent SVCS after initial treatment (Aung et al., 2022). Following stent insertion, relief of headache is immediate, and most other symptoms, such as facial and arm edema, typically disappear within 24–72 hours (Trivedi et al., 2022). However, dyspnea has been reported to be the most difficult symptom to alleviate (Trivedi et al., 2022).

Stent placement takes approximately two hours and is generally performed by an interventional radiologist with the patient under local anesthesia. The approach for stent placement may be through the basilic or subclavian veins, the femoral vein, or others if necessary. The stents are constructed of cylindrically shaped, self-expandable polyurethane that can be compressed and introduced into the obstructed area through an 8–12 Fr catheter (Trivedi et al., 2022). Once released, the stent re-expands, dilating the SVC. If significant vessel obstruction or stenosis is present, balloon angioplasty or radiofrequency wires before or during stent insertion may enhance the success of the procedure (Trivedi et al., 2022).

Thrombus formation occurs in 30%–50% of patients with SVCS and can create confusion about the underlying cause of the syndrome. If a thrombus is exacerbating SVCS, stent placement combined with thrombolytic therapy or balloon angioplasty may help to lyse the clot (Trivedi et al., 2022). Nonmetallic stents offer less thrombosis and easier placement compared to traditional metallic stents (Trivedi et al., 2022). Blood flow in the SVC is under low pressure and may contribute to clot formation in the stented area; therefore, patients typically receive heparin during the procedure. Oral anticoagulation therapy with warfarin (1 mg/day) or low-molecular-weight heparin twice daily may follow stent placement for three to six months to prevent thrombus formation. However, this practice is controversial because of the risk of hemorrhage and the lack of evidence that anticoagulation prevents recurrence (Trivedi et al., 2022).

Other complications of SVC stenting, occurring in up to 12.8% of cases, include stent migration into the right atrium, potentially causing cardiac arrhythmias, vascular perforation, cardiac decompensation during the procedure, infection, pulmonary embolus, hematoma, and bleeding (Wright et al., 2023). Nursing care following stent placement should include monitoring for potential complications such as groin hematoma, infection, and femoral deep vein thrombosis. Nurses should check vital signs regularly and administer analgesics as ordered.

Radiation Therapy

Radiation therapy is the gold standard for treating SVCS caused by NSCLC and is also recommended for SVCS resulting from other malignancies (Sun et al., 2021). Tumor type, extent of disease, history of previous radiation in the area, and performance status determine the radiation dose and treatment plan. Radiation fields for mediastinal treatment generally include the mediastinal, hilar, and supraclavicular lymph nodes and any adjacent lung lesions. Small studies using stereotactic radiation therapy suggest equivalent efficacy with theoretical protection of healthy tissue (Park & Lee, 2023).

Before radiation therapy begins, a treatment planning session called a simulation is completed. If using three-dimensional or intensity-modulated radiation therapy, clinicians perform a planning CT scan. With the assistance of physicists and dosimetrists, the radiation oncologist outlines the treatment volume, and the treatment plan is specified. A basic treatment plan for the first few doses of radiation can be accomplished within hours, but a more comprehensive plan may require days. Patient positioning may be uncomfortable, as it usually requires that patients lie flat with their arms above their heads.

Radiation therapy may be used for local tumor control either following or concomitantly with chemotherapy in patients with large cell lymphoma and large mediastinal masses (Sen et al., 2022). An external beam linear accelerator delivers an initial boost of radiation, but definitive anticancer therapy via intensity-modulated radiation therapy is preferred for maximum antitumor effects. Lymphomas are generally very radiosensitive and may require less radiation than other tumor types. For the treatment of lymphoma with curative intent, 3,500–4,500 cGy given in fractions of 180–200 cGy over four to five weeks is commonly recommended (Sen et al., 2022).

The use of radiation to treat the underlying disease requires a different planning approach than treatment for SVCS and also depends on the type of machine. No established standards exist for radiation doses and schedules in the treatment of SVCS (Guhlich et al., 2022; Sen et al., 2022). In general, radiation therapy doses range from 3,000 cGy in 10 fractions (300 cGy/day) to 5,000 cGy in 25 fractions (200 cGy/day), but they may be as high as 6,000–7,000 cGy in six to seven weeks (Sen et al., 2022). High-dose fractions of 300–400 cGy for the initial two to four radiation treatments have been used to try to obtain faster symptom relief, followed by standard daily dose fractions of 180–200 cGy (Sun et al., 2021). However, studies have not noted greater improvement in the response of SVCS with the high doses, and conclusions regarding patient outcomes, such as response rates and survival, have been inconsistent (Sen et al., 2022).

Symptom relief from SVCS occurs in approximately 70% of patients with lung cancer and 95% of patients with lymphoma (Wright et al., 2023), with a one-year survival of 24% (Sen et al., 2022). Most patients experience symptom relief within seven days of starting radiation therapy, with maximum relief at three to four weeks. Patients demonstrating dramatic antineoplastic responses to radiation therapy may require recalculation of the radiation field midway through their treatment plan to ensure precision and safety (Sen et al., 2022).

The potential side effects of radiation delivered to the mediastinum are related to the total dose, the fraction dose, the amount of healthy tissue in the radiation field, and whether concomitant chemotherapy is part of the treatment regimen. Early side effects that may occur during or shortly after initiation of radiation therapy include fatigue, cough, nausea, dysphagia, heartburn, and skin irritation or erythema (Sen et al., 2022). More serious treatment-related complications are rare but include bleeding or SVC perforation (McNally, 2018). Delayed side effects following radiation may occur after weeks to months, including pneumonitis, pulmonary fibrosis, esophageal ulceration or stenosis, cardiac changes, spinal cord myelopathy, and brachial plexopathy (Sen et al., 2022).

Chemotherapy

Combination chemotherapy is the primary treatment for SVCS caused by highly chemosensitive malignancies, such as SCLC, NHL, and some NSCLCs and germ cell tumors (Sun et al., 2021; Wright et al., 2023). More than 80% of patients with SCLC and SVCS demonstrate a good response to treatment with chemotherapy alone (Sun et al., 2021).

In general, SVCS caused by cancers sensitive to both chemotherapy and radiation can respond quickly to either treatment modality. Patients treated with chemotherapy usually experience symptom relief within 7–14 days (Sun et al., 2021). In contrast, alleviation of symptoms takes longer for those with less sensitive solid tumors.

Patients with NSCLC who lack cytogenetic markers indicating chemosensitivity receive radiation therapy as initial treatment (Šutić et al., 2021). Selecting the specific chemotherapy agents for chemosensitive tumors is an evolving specialty practice that can be accessed and guided by resources from the National Comprehensive Cancer Network (Riely et al., 2024) or the Oncology Nursing Society. Neoadjuvant chemotherapy may be administered to shrink extensive tumors in the mediastinum before starting radiation, allowing smaller subsequent radiation fields to be used and sparing healthy lung tissue (McNally, 2018). In patients who already had prior mediastinal irradiation, chemotherapy alone may be the treatment of choice.

Routes for administering chemotherapy to patients with SVCS require careful planning. The venous stasis in the upper thorax that accompanies SVCS may cause chemotherapy drugs to become locally concentrated if they are infused into the upper extremities. A femoral approach is safer and more effective because the greater volume of blood flow dilutes the chemotherapy agents and allows them to readily enter systemic circulation (Azizi et al., 2020). Peripheral infusion into the lower extremities should be avoided because of the risk of extravasation with irritant and vesicant drugs. A long-term venous access catheter may need to be placed into the inferior vena cava through the femoral vein for safe drug administration (Azizi et al., 2020).

Combination chemotherapy with radiation may result in quicker symptomatic relief of SCLC-associated SVCS and has been linked to increased survival (Sun et al., 2021). However, when the two therapies are combined, the severity of side effects increases because the chemotherapy potentiates the radiation effects (Sen et al., 2022; Sun et al., 2021). As a result, patients undergoing concurrent chemoradiation require vigilant nursing management to monitor for myelosuppression, nausea, vomiting, infection, stomatitis, esophagitis, and skin breakdown.

Surgery

Historically, surgical interventions for malignancy-induced SVCS have been rare because of limited success and high morbidity (Chow et al., 2024). However, newer and less invasive surgical procedures, such as thrombectomy, are now available and used with some frequency (Mir et al., 2022). Surgical procedures that can effectively restore ventilation or vascular patency may enhance the efficacy of radiation therapy or chemotherapy (Mir et al., 2022). Vascular bypass surgery to create a circulatory route around the SVC obstruction to the right atrium may be performed using autologous saphenous veins, synthetic materials, or the autologous pericardium (McNally, 2018). Thrombosis of the surgically created graft continues to be a confounding clinical concern until the vena cava occlusion resolves. Postsurgical complications include atrial fibrillation, stroke, respiratory failure, myocardial infarction, and Horner syndrome (Mir et al., 2022).

Surgical bypass grafts are considered the standard of care for patients with acute cerebral or laryngeal edema, extensive SVC thrombosis, and inadequate collateral circulation. They are also indicated for patients with tumors that can be totally excised or when a tissue diagnosis cannot be obtained without surgical mediastinal exploration (Azizi et al., 2020).

Medical Management

Supportive Medical Therapies

Supportive medical management may be appropriate when SVCS symptoms are minimal and adequate collateral circulation is present, or to alleviate symptoms while the etiology of SVCS is being determined (Azizi et al., 2020). Loop diuretics, such as furosemide, may be administered to reduce edema and fluid retention. However, they may cause dehydration, which could contribute to thrombus formation, as well as cause hypovolemia, and could further compromise venous return to the heart (Chow et al., 2024). Patients may receive supplemental oxygen and bronchodilators to relieve dyspnea, while analgesics and anxiolytics help manage chest pain and anxiety associated with respiratory distress. Steroids are beneficial in cases of SVCS caused by lymphoma, which tends to respond well to corticosteroid treatment. Their use is more limited in SVCS because of lung cancer (Azizi et al., 2020; Nickloes et al., 2024). Steroids may also be used to support patients during the early phase of treatment when chemotherapy or radiation therapy causes inflammation and transient symptom worsening (Azizi et al., 2020).

Thrombolytic Therapy

Patients with cancer frequently have an indwelling central venous access device. This technology has contributed to an increased frequency of nonmalignant causes of SVCS over the past two decades (Azizi et al., 2020). Venous catheter–induced intraluminal thrombus formation is typically treated with an IV thrombolytic agent, administered either through the catheter itself or through a peripheral site to lyse the clot, followed by heparin anticoagulation to prevent reembolization (McNally, 2018). U.S. Food and Drug Administration–approved thrombolytic agents include streptokinase, urokinase, and recombinant tissue plasminogen activator, with implementation guidelines available through established oncologic protocols for the management of thromboembolic disease (Aung et al., 2022; Streiff et al., 2024). Bleeding remains the most common clinical concern for patients receiving systemic thrombolytic or anticoagulant therapy (Dragomir et al., 2021). Administration of recombinant tissue plasminogen activator is associated with increased febrile reactions and serious adverse effects, such as anaphylaxis and angioedema. Therefore, emergency equipment should be available in the event of anaphylaxis, and clinicians should monitor patients for signs of bleeding (McNally, 2018). All patients should have rapid access to blood products to treat potential hemorrhage.

Prognosis

The prognosis depends on how rapidly SVC obstruction develops, the degree of vena cava blockage, and the adequacy of collateral circulation (Trivedi et al., 2022). For patients with SVCS secondary to malignancy, survival varies depending on the tumor's histologic type. In select patients, open surgery may still be the best treatment option and can positively influence prognosis (Patriarcheas et al., 2022). The average life expectancy for patients with SVCS related to malignancy is six months, although it varies with etiology; refractory malignancy carries a poorer prognosis than thrombosis or infectious diseases. Patients with cancer who develop SVCS can die of the syndrome itself, and it can be life threatening (Park & Lee, 2023).

The presence of SVCS at diagnosis in patients with SCLC reflects the severity of the disease and is regarded as a poor prognostic marker. The median survival of patients treated with combined postoperative chemotherapy and antivascular targeted therapy is, on average, seven months (Wei et al., 2020). Given the poor overall prognosis of most patients with malignant tumors, palliation is often the primary focus of treatment (Dragomir et al., 2021).

Nursing Management

Nursing interventions for patients with SVCS focus on assessing patients' clinical condition, instituting measures to relieve symptoms, monitoring response to treatment and side effects, and providing comfort measures and reassurance while undergoing treatment (see Table 2-1). A baseline nursing assessment includes monitoring vital signs, physical appearance, level of consciousness, visual changes, tissue perfusion and edema, respiratory status, functional status, emotional status, and activity endurance level (Relf et al., 2018). Evidence of venous congestion, such as jugular venous distension or pulsation, or distended veins on the chest wall or upper extremities, indicates a prolonged prodrome prior to clinical presentation. Any symptoms of airway obstruction or cerebral edema (causing mental status and neurologic changes) require emergency intervention (Lopes et al., 2022). Patients are also monitored for the effectiveness and side effects of drugs that they may receive, such as corticosteroids, diuretics, thrombolytics, and anticoagulants (Lopes et al., 2022).

Assessment of the respiratory system includes monitoring oxygen saturation by pulse oximetry and observing for signs of respiratory distress, such as cyanosis, hoarseness, stridor, dyspnea, tachypnea, and cough (Lopes et al., 2022). Measures to relieve respiratory distress take priority over other aspects of care. The use of supplemental oxygen, bed rest with the head of the bed elevated to promote venous drainage, and activity restrictions to decrease energy expenditure may relieve dyspnea (Relf et al., 2018). Increased risk and severity of obstructive sleep apnea have been noted in SVCS patients and should be included in the nursing assessment (Karim & Laurore-Fray, 2023). Blood pressure is typically higher on the right side of the upper body, and pulses are often stronger in the upper extremities than in the lower extremities.

Assessment of the cardiac system includes monitoring for tachycardia, dysrhythmias, and hypotension (Wright et al., 2023). Nurses should monitor patients' fluid and electrolyte status. Overhydration may exacerbate symptoms of SVCS, whereas dehydration, especially in patients receiving diuretics and following a low-salt diet, may increase the risk of thrombosis (Chow et al., 2024). Blood pressure and venipunctures should be performed in the lower extremities rather than the upper extremities. IV chemotherapy agents or other drugs may need to be administered through a femoral or central venous line with the tip past the point of obstruction (Azizi et al., 2020). Rings and restrictive clothing should be removed from the upper extremities (Azizi et al., 2020; Chow et al., 2024).

Central nervous system assessment is essential. Nurses should report any changes in mental status, such as lethargy, somnolence, headache, and vomiting, as they may indicate cerebral edema caused by a lack of oxygen to the brain. They should also instruct patients to avoid the Valsalva maneuver, which is elicited by bending, stooping, lying flat, coughing, or straining at stool, as it increases intracranial pressure,

TABLE 2-1
Overview of Nursing Management of Superior Vena Cava Syndrome

Problem	Intervention
Respiratory and cardiac compromise	Assess the respiratory system, paying particular attention to the presence of cyanosis, hoarseness, stridor, orthopnea, dyspnea, tachypnea, cough, and rales/rhonchi. Assess breath sounds with special attention to tracheal stridor or high airway wheezing. Use caution with pulse oximetry in the upper extremities, as it may be inaccurate. Assess cardiac system (e.g., tachycardia, dysrhythmias, hypotension, reduced pulse quality). Monitor oxygen saturation/administer oxygen. Monitor for signs of increased respiratory distress. Maintain airway. Maintain hydration. Administer respiratory medications as needed. Check vital signs every 4 hours until stable. Situate in the Fowler or semi-Fowler position to maximize respiratory effort. Limit physical activity by assisting with activities of daily living. Administer cough medication as needed.
Neurologic compromise	Assess the central nervous system, such as altered mental status, lethargy, somnolence, headache, vomiting, and visual changes. Assess for anxiety, and administer anxiolytics or mild sedatives. Monitor for signs and symptoms of increased intracranial pressure, such as Cushing triad of hypertension, bradycardia, and sensorium changes. Maintain a calm, restful environment. Maintain low lighting to decrease the impact of blurred vision. Explain all activities to patients. Position the call bell within easy reach and provide frequent reassurance of staff availability. Administer corticosteroids for cerebral edema.
Circulatory compromise	Assess distal capillary refill. Assess skin integrity in edematous areas. Check blood pressure in both arms and note differences. Monitor for excessive bleeding after invasive procedures in areas of venous engorgement. Remove rings and restrictive clothing. Avoid the upper extremities for venipuncture and administration of IV medications. Avoid right-sided positioning that further impairs venous return.

(Continued on next page)

TABLE 2-1
Overview of Nursing Management of Superior Vena Cava Syndrome *(Continued)*

Problem	Intervention
Metabolic and electrolyte disturbances	Check for steroid-induced hyperglycemia. Evaluate for muscle weakness. Monitor for euphoria, mood swings, or other signs of central nervous system stimulation. Monitor laboratory values, such as complete blood count and arterial blood gases, and imaging, such as chest x-ray and scans. Monitor for signs and symptoms of hyponatremia, such as listlessness, mental confusion, loss of skin turgor, and postural hypotension. Monitor for signs and symptoms of hypokalemia, including muscle weakness, decreased bowel sounds, depression, cardiac arrhythmias, and tetany. Record daily weights, intake, and output. Administer diuretics and fluids.
Patient safety	Assess fall risk. Assess vision and proprioception to determine the patient's risk of falls due to cerebral congestion. Monitor for blood pressure changes, such as early hypertension and late hypotension, that can affect safe physical activity. Provide for environmental safety, such as a bed in a low position, side rails up, a call light, and personal items within reach. Assist with ambulation as needed. Implement bleeding precautions, especially if the patient is receiving thrombolytic or anticoagulant therapy for vena caval thrombosis.
Emotional and psychological concerns	Provide brief explanations of planned procedures and treatments. Provide a forum for the expression of concerns, fears, and feelings regarding the situation. Provide supportive measures to reduce fatigue, such as pacing activity, rest periods, progressive activity to allow adjustment, and assistance with activities of daily living. Administer analgesics for comfort. Reassure that alterations in appearance resolve with successful therapy.
Patient and family education	Instruct in self-care management. Educate about treatment and side effect management in clear, simple terms. Provide instruction on energy conservation techniques. Educate regarding bleeding precautions. Teach relaxation techniques. Instruct in avoidance of Valsalva maneuver (as well as bending, stooping, coughing, lying flat), which increases intracranial pressure. Instruct regarding signs and symptoms of recurrent superior vena cava syndrome.

Note. Based on information from McNally, 2018; Relf et al., 2018.

which may exacerbate SVCS symptoms (McNally, 2018). Cough suppressants and stool softeners may be indicated to minimize intracranial and intrathoracic pressure.

Nursing interventions for patients undergoing definitive therapies to treat SVCS focus on monitoring treatment effectiveness and the potential side effects of corticosteroids, thrombolytics, chemotherapy, and radiation therapy. Corticosteroid doses may be high and result in emotional lability, insomnia, and hyperglycemia. Definitive anticancer therapy may cause myelosuppression, nausea, vomiting, infection, stomatitis, esophagitis, pulmonary reactions, and skin reactions (Relf et al., 2018). Patients who have undergone stent placement should be closely monitored for signs of continued perfusion deficit or blood loss. Upper body venous engorgement in the area can contribute to excessive bleeding following invasive procedures.

Some patients may be distressed by the changes in self-image caused by facial and periorbital edema and plethora (purple frog appearance) and need reassurance that these changes disappear with effective treatment (Lopes et al., 2022). To help patients manage discomfort and cope with symptoms while awaiting treatment effects, analgesics and anxiolytics may be administered as prescribed (Lopes et al., 2022). Nurses must also provide emotional support and assist with relaxation techniques during this period, and if necessary, refer to the psychologist of the interprofessional team (McNally, 2018).

Patient and Caregiver Education

For some patients, the development of SVCS is the first sign that they have cancer. This requires education and support for patients and caregivers as they learn about the diagnosis, symptoms, and treatments. Nurses play a key role in providing tools and resources related to symptom management, along with emotional support and reassurance to both patients and caregivers. Discharge planning from the hospital or outpatient care includes educating patients and caregivers about treatment goals and self-care measures at home. Nurses should provide instructions for recognizing the signs and symptoms of recurrent SVCS and emphasize the importance of prompt reporting. They should also instruct patients on how gravity and upright positioning help to alleviate venous congestion in the upper body. Providing reassurance, emotional support, and a calm, restful environment can help to reduce anxiety and oxygen requirements. Nurses should teach strategies for managing side effects of chemotherapy and radiation therapy, as well as energy conservation measures. Patients taking anticoagulants should receive guidance on bleeding precautions, potential medication interactions, and how to schedule blood tests to monitor therapeutic levels (McNally, 2018). Patients who respond well to treatments targeting the underlying malignancy typically experience rapid resolution of SVCS symptoms. Once resolved, long-term special care is usually not required (Azizi et al., 2020).

Summary

SVCS is an obstructive vascular complication commonly associated with chest tumors, such as lung cancer, lymphoma, and various benign causes. SVCS can progress to an obstructed airway or increased intracranial pressure, which are highly distressing for patients and potentially life threatening. Nurses caring for patients with a malignant diagnosis must be aware of the increased potential for developing SVCS. Although SVCS is generally rare, its incidence may be rising due to the increased use of central venous catheters and longer survival of patients with cancer. Nurses working in diverse settings, such as infusion centers, ambulatory care, inpatient units, home care, and hospice, need to be aware of the link between venous access devices and SVCS and should be vigilant for early signs and symptoms of vena cava thrombosis. Because most cases of SVCS develop gradually, early detection and timely intervention may prevent progression to an acute emergency. Understanding the mechanisms behind the syndrome helps nurses to recognize early symptoms and support patients with SVCS.

The author would like to acknowledge Brenda K. Shelton, DNP, APRN-CNS, RN, CCRN, AOCN®, for her contribution to this chapter that remains unchanged from the previous edition of this book.

References

Aung, E.Y.-S., Khan, M., Williams, N., Raja, U., & Hamady, M. (2022). Endovascular stenting in superior vena cava syndrome: A systematic review and meta-analysis. *Cardiovascular and Interventional Radiology, 45*(9), 1236–1254. https://doi.org/10.1007/s00270-022-03178-z

Azizi, A.H., Shafi, I., Shah, N., Rosenfield, K., Schainfeld, R., Sista, A., & Bashir, R. (2020). Superior vena cava syndrome. *JACC: Cardiovascular Interventions, 13*(24), 2896–2910. https://doi.org/10.1016/j.jcin.2020.08.038

Chow, R., Simone, C.B., II, & Rimner, A. (2024). Management of malignant superior vena cava syndrome. *Annals of Palliative Medicine, 13*(3), 620–626. https://doi.org/10.21037/apm-23-573

Dragomir, L., Marina, V., Anghele, M., & Anghele, A.-D. (2021). Clinical or imaging diagnosis of the current medical practice for superior vena cava syndrome? *Diagnostics, 11*(11), 2058. https://doi.org/10.3390/diagnostics11112058

Guhlich, M., Maag, T.E., Dröge, L.H., El Shafie, R.A., Hille, A., Donath, S., ... Rieken, S. (2022). Symptom relief, prognostic factors, and outcome in patients receiving urgent radiation therapy for superior vena cava syndrome: A single-center retrospective analysis of 21 years' practice. *Strahlentherapie und Onkologie, 198*(12), 1072–1081. https://doi.org/10.1007/s00066-022-01952-z

Hunter, W. (1957). History of an aneurysm of the aorta, with some remarks on aneurysms in general. *Medical Observations and Inquiries, 1,* 323–357.

Karim, N., & Laurore-Fray, G. (2023). Uncovering the hidden threat: A case study on superior vena cava thrombosis. *Cureus, 15*(4), e37040. https://doi.org/10.7759/cureus.37040

Lopes, G.M.J., Simino, G.P.R., Rocha, P.R.S., Aguiar, B.R.L., Reis, P.E.D., & Ferreira, E.B. (2022). Cuidados de enfermagem em emergências oncológicas: Revisão integrativa. *Revista de Enfermagem Do Centro-Oeste Mineiro, 12,* 1–12. https://doi.org/10.19175/recom.v12i0.4350

McNally, G.A. (2018). Superior vena cava syndrome. In C.H. Yarbro, D. Wujcik, & B.H. Gobel (Eds.), *Cancer nursing: Principles and practice* (8th ed., pp. 1187–1196). Jones and Bartlett Learning.

Mir, T., Uddin, M., Shafi, O., Qureshi, W., Kaur, J., Zghouzi, M., ... Saydain, G. (2022). Thrombotic superior vena cava syndrome: A national emergency department database study. *Journal of Thrombosis and Thrombolysis, 53*(2), 372–379. https://doi.org/10.1007/s11239-021-02548-7

Nickloes, T.A., Kallab, A.M., & Dunlap, A.B. (2024, February 5). Superior vena cava syndrome (SVCS). *Medscape.* https://emedicine.medscape.com/article/460865-overview

Park, J., & Lee, J.E. (2023). Comparison between 1-week and 2-week palliative radiotherapy courses for superior vena cava syndrome. *Radiation Oncology Journal, 41*(3), 178–185. https://doi.org/10.3857/roj.2023.00626

Patriarcheas, V., Grammoustianou, M., Ptohis, N., Thanou, I., Kostis, M., Gkiozos, I., ... Dimakakos, E. (2022). Malignant superior vena cava syndrome: State of the art. *Cureus, 14*(1), e20924. https://doi.org/10.7759/cureus.20924

Relf, M.V., Shelton, B.K., & Jones, K.M. (2018). Common immunological disorders. In P.G. Morton & D.K. Fontaine (Eds.), *Critical care nursing: A holistic approach* (11th ed., pp. 1140–1178). Wolters Kluwer.

Riely, G.J., Wood, D.E., Ettinger, D.S., Aisner, D.L., Akerley, W., Bauman, J.R., ... Hang, L. (2024). Non-small cell lung cancer, version 4.2024, NCCN Clinical Practice Guidelines in Oncology. *Journal of the National Comprehensive Cancer Network, 22*(4), 249–274. https://doi.org/10.6004/jnccn.2204.0023

Sen, I., Kalra, M., & Gloviczki, P. (2022). Interventions for superior vena cava syndrome. *Journal of Cardiovascular Surgery, 63*(6), 674–681. https://doi.org/10.23736/S0021-9509.22.12448-1

Streiff, M.B., Holmstrom, B., Angelini, D., Ashrani, A., Buckner, T., Diep, R., ... Sliker, B. (2024). Cancer-associated venous thromboembolic disease, version 2.2024, NCCN Clinical Practice Guidelines in Oncology. *Journal of the National Comprehensive Cancer Network, 22*(7), 483–506. https://doi.org/10.6004/jnccn.2024.0046

Sun, M., Chen, X., Li, H., Zhang, X., Wang, X., Zheng, R., ... Li, D. (2021). Clinical analysis of 48 cases of malignant superior vena cava syndrome. *World Journal of Surgical Oncology, 19*(1), 1–7. https://doi.org/10.1186/s12957-021-02300-8

Šutić, M., Vukić, A., Baranašić, J., Försti, A., Džubur, F., Samaržija, M., ... Knežević, J. (2021). Diagnostic, predictive, and prognostic biomarkers in non-small cell lung cancer (NSCLC) management. *Journal of Personalized Medicine, 11*(11), 1102. https://doi.org/10.3390/jpm11111102

Trivedi, S.B., Ray, C., Chadalavada, S., Makramalla, A., & Kord, A. (2022). Superior vena cava syndrome: An update and literature review of percutaneous endovascular treatments. *Seminars in Interventional Radiology, 39*(4), 446–453. https://doi.org/10.1055/s-0042-1757344

Wei, S., Liu, J., Li, X., Song, Z., Dong, M., Zhao, H., ... Chen, J. (2020). A retrospective stenting study on superior vena cava syndrome caused by lung cancer. *Thoracic Cancer, 11*(7), 1835–1839. https://doi.org/10.1111/1759-7714.13461

Wright, K., Digby, G.C., Gyawali, B., Jad, R., Menard, A., Moraes, F.Y., & Wijeratne, D.T. (2023). Malignant superior vena cava syndrome: A scoping review. *Journal of Thoracic Oncology, 18*(10), 1268–1276. https://doi.org/10.1016/j.jtho.2023.04.019

Yu, J.B., Wilson, L.D., & Detterbeck, F.C. (2008). Superior vena cava syndrome—A proposed classification system and algorithm for management. *Journal of Thoracic Oncology,* 3(8), 811–814. https://doi.org/10.1097/JTO.0b013e3181804791

Kelli Thoele, PhD, RN, and Patryk Madrid, DNP, FNP-C

CHAPTER 3

Pleural Effusion

FAST FACTS

- **Description:** Pleural effusion is the abnormal collection of fluid in the pleural space, and malignant pleural effusion is characterized by malignant cells in the pleural fluid. It is a common complication of advanced cancer, most often seen with lung cancer, breast cancer, lymphoma, cancers of the gastrointestinal tract and ovary, and mesothelioma.
- **Incidence:** Approximately 150,000 cases of malignant pleural effusion are diagnosed in the United States each year, primarily in patients with breast and lung cancers.
- **Clinical Manifestations:** Patients with pleural effusion can be asymptomatic or can present with dyspnea, cough, generalized fatigue, or pleuritic chest pain.
- **Risk Factors and Etiology:** Pleural effusion is associated with more than 50 identified etiologies, such as underlying pleural and lung diseases, systemic conditions, and organ dysfunction, as well as some medications. Lung and breast cancers account for the largest percentage of malignant pleural effusion, and the most common causes of nonmalignant pleural effusion include congestive heart failure, cancer, pneumonia, and pulmonary embolism.
- **Pathophysiology and Patient Evaluation:** Pleural effusion is the pathologic accumulation of fluid in the pleural space when fluid production exceeds removal. Chest radiography can confirm the diagnosis of effusion. Thoracentesis under ultrasound guidance may be indicated to diagnose the presence of effusion and obtain pleural fluid for evaluation and definitive diagnosis. The Light criteria are used to differentiate exudative from transudative effusions. Computed tomography scans can help identify small effusions and distinguish between benign and malignant disease.
- **Advanced Practice Considerations:** The multiple possible etiologies of pleural effusion necessitate a systematic approach in diagnostic investigation to reduce the number of invasive procedures required to make a definitive diagnosis. Several scientific groups have established evidence-based recommendations for the diagnosis and management of pleural effusions to guide and inform clinical practice.
- **Treatment Modalities:** Interventions are directed at treating the underlying disorder, draining pleural fluid, and preventing reaccumulation. Treatment options may include thoracentesis, indwelling pleural catheters, pleurodesis to obliterate the pleural space, and surgery, such as video-assisted thoracoscopic surgery, lung resection, or pleuroperitoneal shunt and pump placement.
- **Nursing Management:** Supportive symptom management, along with the provision of comfort care and emotional support at the end of life, are primary nursing responsibilities aimed at ensuring optimal relief from dyspnea, chest pain, distress, and anxiety.
- **Outcomes:** Prompt recognition and intervention are essential. Malignant pleural effusion is associated with late-stage disease, but treatment may alleviate symptoms and enhance quality of life in patients.

Introduction

Pleural effusion develops when fluid accumulates abnormally in the space between the visceral and parietal pleura surrounding the lungs (Gayen, 2022; Jany & Welte, 2019; Josan, 2025) (see Figure 3-1). The presence of a pleural effusion is associated with significant morbidity and diminishing quality of life (QoL) because of debilitating symptoms, including breathlessness, cough, chest pain, and activity intolerance (Josan, 2025; Mishra & Stanton, 2024). Malignant pleural effusion (MPE) is confirmed by the presence of malignant cells in the pleural fluid. Tumor cells metastasize to the pleural cavity via the bloodstream or by tumor invasion into the pleural cavity (Dipper et al., 2020; Gayen, 2022). Approximately 15%–20% of patients with cancer develop MPE, which is associated with advanced malignancy and reduced life expectancy ranging from 3–12 months (Dipper et al., 2020; Gayen, 2022; Gonnelli et al., 2024). Therefore, treatment goals shift from aggressive invasive measures aimed at preventing pleural fluid reaccumulation to a focus on symptom relief and patient needs at the end of life. These goals include palliating symptoms effectively, restoring the ability to perform activities of daily living, enhancing QoL, minimizing the number of interventions, and reducing the time spent in the hospital (Feller-Kopman et al., 2018; Jacobs et al., 2022; Orlandi et al., 2024).

FIGURE 3-1. Pleural Effusion

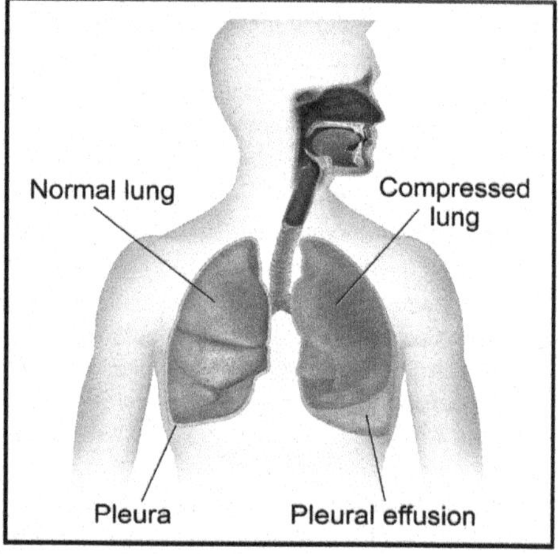

Note. Image courtesy of BruceBlaus, 2015 (https://commons.wikimedia.org/wiki/File:Blausen_0993_Pleural Effusion.png). Licensed under CC BY-SA 4.0 (https://creativecommons.org/licenses/by-sa/4.0/deed.en).

Incidence

In the United States, approximately 1.5 million cases of pleural effusion and 150,000 cases of MPE are diagnosed each year (Josan, 2025). Malignancies commonly associated with MPE are lung cancer, breast cancer, lymphoma, mesothelioma, gastrointestinal cancer, and ovarian cancer (Gayen, 2022; Gonnelli et al., 2024; Jany & Welte, 2019; Roberts et al., 2023). Lung and breast cancers account for 50%–65% of MPE cases (Gayen, 2022; Jacobs et al., 2022; Jany & Welte, 2019; Roberts et al., 2023).

Clinical Manifestations

The clinical presentation of MPE varies and depends on the rate and amount of pleural fluid accumulation. Patients with small pleural effusions may be asymptomatic.

However, dyspnea, cough, pleuritic chest pain, generalized fatigue, or weight loss are common symptoms (Gayen, 2022; Jany & Welte, 2019; Josan, 2025; Orlandi et al., 2024; Roberts et al., 2023). Dyspnea at rest or with exertion is the most common presenting symptom and results from restricted lung expansion and decreased lung volume (Josan, 2025). Dyspnea is also the most common indication for intervention (Gayen, 2022). Patients may have sharp pleuritic chest pain caused by the friction between the pleural spaces and irritation of sensory fibers. The pain usually worsens with coughing, sneezing, and deep breathing (Josan, 2025). Pain may also be attributed to malignant infiltration of the chest (Roberts et al., 2023). Dull, constant pain characterizes the discomfort associated with malignant tumors in contrast with the sharp, intermittent pain associated with an inflammatory process (Krishna et al., 2024).

Risk Factors and Etiology

Pleural effusion is associated with more than 50 identified etiologies, such as underlying pleural and lung diseases, systemic conditions, and organ dysfunction, as well as some medications (Bashour et al., 2022; Gayen, 2022; Josan, 2025). Two categories of pleural effusions related to cancer exist: malignant and paramalignant. MPE results from tumor metastasis to the pleural cavity, demonstrated by the presence of malignant cells in pleural fluid and confirmed via cytologic examination of pleural fluid. In contrast, metastatic invasion of the pleural space does not occur in paramalignant pleural effusion; that is, malignant cells are not recovered during fluid analysis. Paramalignant pleural effusion arises from side effects of cancer treatments, tumor-related obstruction of the airway with lung collapse, lymphatic obstruction, pneumonia, or pulmonary emboli (Bashour et al., 2022; Gayen, 2022; Josan, 2025). The most common causes of nonmalignant pleural effusion are congestive heart failure, cancer, pneumonia, and pulmonary embolism (Jany & Welte, 2019) (see Table 3-1).

Pathophysiology and Patient Evaluation

The pleura is a membrane covering the lungs and chest walls and is divided into two layers: visceral and parietal. The visceral pleura lines the entire surface of the lungs, and the parietal pleura lines the chest wall, including the mediastinum and diaphragm. The pleural space lies between the two layers of pleura. It contains a thin layer of pleural fluid (approximately 0.1 ml/kg body weight), which has a low protein concentration and acts as a lubricant enabling the lungs to glide smoothly against the chest wall during respiration (D'Agostino & Edens, 2023; Josan, 2025). The pleural fluid is normally produced by the pleura and resorbed by lymphatic vessels continually, with dynamic equilibrium between production and resorption to maintain homeostasis (Ferreiro et al., 2024; Jany & Welte, 2019).

Pleural effusion is the pathologic accumulation of fluid in the pleural space when fluid production exceeds removal. Decreased resorption of pleural fluid can occur

TABLE 3-1
Differential Diagnosis by Mechanisms Causing Pleural Effusion

Classification	Mechanism	Underlying Etiology
Increased volume of pleural fluid	Increased pulmonary capillary pressure	Renal failure Heart failure
	Increased pulmonary capillary permeability	Pneumonia
	Increased pleural permeability	Infection Inflammation
	Decreased intrapleural pressure	Atelectasis
	Increased venous pressure	Airway obstruction Congestive heart failure Superior vena cava syndrome
	Decreased plasma oncotic pressure	Cachexia Hypoalbuminemia Malnutrition Nephrotic syndrome
	Obstruction of pleural lymphatic drainage	Malignancy
	Rupture of thoracic vessels	Chylothorax Hemothorax
Decreased outflow of pleural fluid	Impaired lymphatic drainage	Lymphatic dysfunction Malignancy

Note. Based on information from Ferreiro et al., 2024; Jacobs et al., 2022; Krishna et al., 2024.

with increased resistance to lymphatic flow, such as with obstruction due to tumor infiltration (Josan, 2025). Excessive fluid in the pleural space can be attributed to increased pulmonary capillary pressures (e.g., heart failure, superior vena cava syndrome), increased pulmonary capillary permeability (e.g., inflammation, infection, malignancy), reduced intravascular pressure (e.g., hypoalbuminemia), decreased intrapleural pressure (e.g., atelectasis), and ineffective lymphatic drainage from the pleura or lungs due to obstruction by tumor deposits (D'Agostino & Edens, 2023; Gonnelli et al., 2024; Jany & Welte, 2019; Josan, 2025).

Pleural effusions are classified as either transudative or exudative based on the mechanism of fluid formation and composition of pleural fluid. Differentiating between them is important in determining the origin of effusions and subsequent management. Table 3-2 lists the types of pleural effusion and underlying diseases, differentiating exudates from transudates.

Transudative and Exudative Effusions

Transudative effusions manifest with clear fluids and are usually not associated with malignancy (D'Agostino & Edens, 2023; Jany & Welte, 2019). They result from increased hydrostatic pressure or decreased osmotic pressure across an intact capillary barrier. Congestive heart failure and cirrhosis are the primary causes of transudative pleural effusions, with nephrotic syndrome and pulmonary embolism as other potential causes (D'Agostino & Edens, 2023; Jany & Welte, 2019; Josan, 2025; Roberts et al., 2023). Transudative pleural effusions usually resolve with effective treatment of the underlying disease; therefore, they do not always necessitate invasive diagnostic and therapeutic procedures, such as aspirations (D'Agostino & Edens, 2023).

Exudative effusions present with a cloudy fluid and are typically associated with malignancy or inflammatory conditions (D'Agostino & Edens, 2023; Jany & Welte, 2019; Roberts et al., 2023). Exudative effusions develop from the leakage of protein and fluid across an injured capillary barrier rendered highly permeable from damage caused by infectious or inflammatory conditions. Exudates have higher protein and

TABLE 3-2
Types of Pleural Effusion Based on Causative Condition

Type	Pathophysiology	Diagnostic Criteria	Conditions
Exudative	Results from various pleural pathologic conditions leading to increased vascular permeability or impaired fluid resorption	One or more of the following: • Pleural protein to serum protein ratio > 0.5 • Pleural LDH to serum LDH ratio > 0.6 • Pleural fluid LDH > two-thirds of the upper limit of normal LDH serum value	After cardiac surgery Chylothorax Hemothorax Infections—bacterial, viral, parasitic Inflammation—pancreatitis, lupus, rheumatoid arthritis Lymphatic obstruction Malignancy—primary or metastatic Pancreatitis Pulmonary embolism Trauma Tuberculosis
Transudative	Results from increased hydrostatic pressure or a reduction in plasma oncotic pressure with a normal pleura	Criteria for exudative effusion not met	Atelectasis Cirrhosis Congestive heart failure Hypoalbuminemia Nephrotic syndrome Peritoneal dialysis Superior vena cava syndrome Urinothorax

LDH—lactate dehydrogenase

Note. Based on information from Jacobs et al., 2022; Josan, 2025; Krishna et al., 2024; Roberts et al., 2023; Shen-Wagner et al., 2023.

lactate dehydrogenase (LDH) levels than transudates (D'Agostino & Edens, 2023; Jany & Welte, 2019; Josan, 2025). Malignancy, pleural infection pneumonia, and pulmonary emboli account for most exudative effusions. The fluid from an MPE is almost always an exudate (Jany & Welte, 2019; Orlandi et al., 2024; Roberts et al., 2023).

The Light criteria are commonly used to differentiate between exudative and transudative effusions. The determination is based on laboratory measurements of protein and LDH levels in the serum and pleural fluid (Jany & Welte, 2019; Josan, 2025; Light et al., 1972). The pleural effusion is considered an exudate if it meets at least one of the following three elements of the Light criteria; if no criteria are met, the fluid is classified as a transudate (Light et al., 1972):

- Ratio of pleural fluid to serum protein > 0.5
- Ratio of pleural fluid to serum LDH > 0.6
- Pleural fluid > two-thirds of the upper limit of normal for serum LDH

Although the Light criteria are considered highly accurate, with a sensitivity of nearly 100% for the detection of an exudate, the criteria may miscategorize transudative effusion as exudative in some patients, particularly those with congestive heart failure receiving diuretic therapy (Jany & Welte, 2019; Sharma et al., 2023).

Vascular endothelial growth factor is a protein that stimulates the growth of new blood vessels. It may play a significant role in the development of exudative MPEs because tumor cells may increase its production or affect the vascular endothelial growth factor pathway, resulting in increased vascular permeability (Zhao et al., 2022).

Prognosis

MPE is a prognostic indicator of advanced disease and is associated with a median overall survival of 3–12 months; however, survival varies by patient and tumor characteristics (Dipper et al., 2020; Gayen, 2022; Gonnelli et al., 2024). In patients with MPE, the following are associated with a worse prognosis:

- Poor Eastern Cooperative Oncology Group (ECOG) performance status
- Breathlessness
- Weight loss
- Hypoxia
- Systemic markers of inflammation associated with a worse prognosis

Additionally, overall survival in patients with MPE is generally shorter in those with lung or gastrointestinal cancers compared to those with hematologic or breast cancers (Jacobs et al., 2022). To identify key prognostic indicators and develop a clinical risk score, Clive et al. (2014) investigated various indicators of overall survival for patients with MPE. They identified four factors as having prognostic significance:

- L—pleural fluid LDH
- E—ECOG performance status
- N—neutrophil-to-lymphocyte ratio
- T—tumor type

Based on their findings, they subsequently developed and validated the LENT prognostic scoring system. The LENT system assigns scores to variables, and risk categories are defined based on total scores: 0–1 indicates low risk, 2–4 indicates moderate risk, and 5–7 indicates high risk. Applying the LENT prognostic score, the researchers determined a median survival of 319 days for patients at low risk, 130 days for patients at moderate risk, and 44 days for patients at high risk (Clive et al., 2014). Table 3-3 describes the LENT scoring system, risk categories, and median survival data.

Psallidas et al. (2018) developed the pleurodesis response markers in malignant pleural effusion (PROMISE) score to predict three-month mortality in patients with MPE. They identified seven factors as having prognostic significance in the clinical PROMISE score:

- History of chemotherapy
- History of radiation therapy
- Hemoglobin
- White blood cell count
- C-reactive protein
- ECOG performance status
- Cancer type

TABLE 3-3

Scoring System Calculations, Risk Categories, and Predicted Median Survival

LENT Score Calculation

Variable	Value	Score
L—lactate dehydrogenase level in pleural fluid	< 1,500 IU/L	0
	> 1,500 IU/L	1
E—Eastern Cooperative Oncology Group performance status	0	0
	1	1
	2	2
	3–4	3
N—neutrophil-to-lymphocyte ratio	< 9	0
	> 9	1
T—tumor type	Lowest risk tumor types • Hematologic malignancy • Mesothelioma	0
	Moderate risk tumor types • Breast cancer • Gynecologic cancer • Renal cell cancer	1
	Highest risk tumor types • Lung cancer • Other tumor types	2

(Continued on next page)

TABLE 3-3
Scoring System Calculations, Risk Categories, and Predicted Median Survival *(Continued)*

LENT Risk Categories and Median Survival

Risk Category	Total LENT Score	Predicted Median Survival
Low risk	0–1	319 days (n = 43) 1 month: 100% 3 months: 98% 6 months: 86%
Moderate risk	2–4	130 days (n = 129) 1 month: 81% 3 months: 59% 6 months: 47%
High risk	5–7	44 days (n = 31) 1 month: 65% 3 months: 13% 6 months: 3%

Clinical PROMISE Score Calculation

Variable	Value	Score
Prior chemotherapy	Yes	4
	No	0
Prior radiation therapy	Yes	2
	No	0
Hemoglobin (g/dl)	> 16	0
	14–16	1
	12–14	2
	10–12	3
	< 10	4
Serum white blood cell count (109 cells/L)	< 4	0
	4–6.3	2
	6.3–10	4
	10–15.8	7
	≥ 15.8	10
C-reactive protein (IU/L)	< 3	0
	3–10	3

(Continued on next page)

TABLE 3-3
Scoring System Calculations, Risk Categories, and Predicted Median Survival *(Continued)*

Clinical PROMISE Score Calculation *(Cont.)*

Variable	Value	Score
C-reactive protein (IU/L) *(Cont.)*	10–32	5
	32–100	8
	> 100	11
Eastern Cooperative Oncology Group performance status	0–1	0
	2–4	7
Cancer type	Mesothelioma	0
	All other types of cancer	4
	Lung	5

PROMISE Categories and Risk of 3-Month Mortality

Category	Clinical PROMISE Score	Risk of 3-Month Mortality
A	0–20	< 25%
B	21–27	25% to < 50%
C	28–35	50% to < 75%
D	> 35	≥ 75%

Note. Based on information from Clive et al., 2014; Psallidas et al., 2018.

The PROMISE system assigns scores to variables, and risk categories are defined based on total scores: Category A (0–20 points), Category B (21–27 points), Category C (28–35 points), and Category D (> 35 points). The lowest risk category, Category A, is associated with a 25% risk of three-month mortality, whereas the highest risk category, Category D, is associated with a 75% or greater risk. Table 3-3 describes the PROMISE scoring system, risk categories, and risk of three-month mortality.

Understanding the prognosis and life expectancy of patients plays an important role in determining their optimal treatment plan. Although tools such as the LENT and PROMISE scoring systems provide information on the survival of patients with MPE, data on their impact on clinical practice and their ability to improve outcomes remain limited (Gonnelli et al., 2024; Roberts et al., 2023).

Patient Assessment

Initial assessment should include the history of the present illness and the chief complaint. Patients' subjective reports may include shortness of breath, cough, hemoptysis, and chest pain. Nurses should assess the severity and characteristics of reported symptoms. A detailed medical history should include information on any past or current acute or chronic illnesses, such as cancer, liver disease, respiratory infections, cardiovascular disease, tuberculosis or potential exposure, and chest surgery or trauma, which all may be possible causes of the pleural effusion. It can also provide guidance in differentiating among etiologies. Exposure to asbestos should be assessed, as it is a risk factor for mesothelioma (Josan, 2025; Krishna et al., 2024; Shen-Wagner et al., 2023). Nurses should also obtain any information about the history of respiratory or cardiac conditions that could relate to patient reports of dyspnea and cough, including chronic obstructive pulmonary disease, pulmonary embolus, interstitial lung disease, congestive heart failure, or treatment-induced cardiac toxicities secondary to chemotherapy or radiation therapy. Medication history is also important to obtain, as some pleural effusions may be drug induced (Josan, 2025; Krishna et al., 2024; Shen-Wagner et al., 2023).

Objective data collection includes physical examination of patients' general appearance, level of consciousness, behavior, and affect. Patients with effusions less than 300 ml may not manifest any symptoms, and physical examination may yield no relevant findings (Josan, 2025). For patients who are symptomatic, the severity of symptoms does not closely correlate with the size of the effusion (Gayen, 2022; Jany & Welte, 2019; Krishna et al., 2024). On auscultation, breath sounds may be unilaterally or bilaterally diminished over the area of effusion. Egophony (*ee* sounding like *ay* during auscultation) is also apparently superior to the area of effusion. Other findings include dullness to percussion, tactile fremitus, and pleural friction rub (Josan, 2025; Shen-Wagner et al., 2023). A larger-volume effusion causes compression and overdistension of the lung, resulting in intercostal space fullness, percussion dullness, and mediastinal shift away from the effusion (Josan, 2025; Krishna et al., 2024). Additionally, patients may present with findings resulting from the underlying cause of the pleural effusion (Shen-Wagner et al., 2023). The following are other clinical manifestations observed with pleural effusion (Josan, 2025; Krishna et al., 2024; Shen-Wagner et al., 2023):

- Absent tactile fremitus (vibration of the chest wall during speaking) over the effusion
- Asymmetric chest expansion
- Bulging intercostal margins
- Dry nonproductive cough
- Dyspnea
- Hyperresonance on percussion above the fluid level
- Increased use of accessory muscles
- Pleuritic chest pain
- Reduced tactile vocal fremitus (vibration intensity heard upon auscultation)
- Weight loss

The physical examination will focus not only on respiratory status but also on assessing any signs of acute or systemic illnesses that need to be ruled out as the cause of the effusion.

Advanced Practice Considerations

The multiple possible etiologies of pleural effusion necessitate a systematic approach in diagnostic investigation to reduce the number of invasive procedures required to make a definitive diagnosis. Several scientific groups have established evidence-based recommendations for the diagnosis and management of pleural effusions to guide and inform clinical practice. Guidelines available include the following:

- British Thoracic Society Guideline for pleural disease (Roberts et al., 2023)
- American Thoracic Society/Society of Thoracic Surgeons/Society of Thoracic Radiology: clinical practice guideline for management of MPEs (Feller-Kopman et al., 2018)
- American College of Radiology: workup of pleural effusion or pleural disease (Morris et al., 2023)

Table 3-4 summarizes the rationale for diagnostic testing for pleural effusion. Table 3-5 summarizes pertinent history and clinical findings essential in an MPE differential diagnosis.

TABLE 3-4
Rationale for Diagnostic Tests for Pleural Effusion

Test	Rationale
Chest radiography	A lateral upright chest radiography can detect an effusion as small as 50 ml, and a lateral decubitus view may detect effusions as small as 10–25 ml. Pleural effusions ≥ 200 ml are revealed in an abnormal posterior-anterior chest radiography.
Ultrasound-guided pleural fluid aspiration	Ultrasound guidance during pleural fluid aspiration provides for a more precise technique and reduces the risk of pneumothorax and other complications.
Pleural fluid analysis	Pleural fluid analysis guides the differential diagnosis of pleural effusion etiology. Pleural fluid should be evaluated for protein, LDH, pH, cell count, cytology, and culture.
Light criteria	Light criteria categorize pleural effusions into transudates and exudates based on evaluation of total pleural and serum fluid protein and LDH levels. Exudates manifest: • Ratio of pleural fluid to serum protein > 0.5 • Ratio of pleural fluid to serum LDH > 0.6 Pleural fluid > two-thirds of the upper limit of normal for serum LDH
Fluid analysis	LDH level serves as an indicator of vascular permeability, reveals the degree of cellular turnover, and reflects the degree of inflammation in pleural space.
	Protein level serves as an indicator of vascular permeability; very high protein levels may be caused by tuberculosis and very low protein levels may be a result of dural leak, urinothorax, or entrapped lung.

(Continued on next page)

TABLE 3-4
Rationale for Diagnostic Tests for Pleural Effusion *(Continued)*

Test	Rationale
Fluid analysis *(Cont.)*	Pleural pH: • Pleural pH is measured in nonpurulent effusions. • Pleural fluid acidosis (pH < 7.2) could indicate an infectious etiology. Pleural fluid acidosis (pH < 7.3) occurs in MPEs.
	Glucose < 60 mg/dl is common in MPE.
	Gram stain and culture identify the causative organisms and can guide therapy.
	Cell count and differential: • Pleural fluid differential cell counts are helpful in narrowing diagnosis but are not disease specific. • White blood cell count > 10,000 cells/mcl suggests empyemas, or pancreatitis – Lymphocyte predominance could be caused by tuberculosis, lymphoma, liver or renal failure, or rheumatoid arthritis. – Neutrophil predominance could be caused by parapneumonic effusion, pulmonary embolism, or pancreatitis. Eosinophil predominance may be caused by malignant pleural effusion and parapneumonic effusion.
	Cytology may confirm primary site of metastasis in MPE.
	Creatinine level aids in identifying urinothorax.
	Amylase level is elevated in patients with pleural effusions secondary to esophageal perforation, pancreatic disease, or malignant disease.
	Triglyceride level indicates chylothorax.
	N-terminal pro-brain natriuretic peptide > 1,500 pg/ml indicates transudate from cardiac etiology.
CT scans	A contrast-enhanced CT scan should be performed before complete drainage of pleural fluid. A CT scan is performed in an undiagnosed exudative pleural effusion to distinguish between malignant and benign thickening of the pleura.
Thoracoscopy	Thoracoscopy is recommended as a minimally invasive diagnostic examination in exudative pleural effusion when the diagnostic pleural aspiration is inconclusive and malignancy is suspected.
Pleuroscopy	Insertion of a pleuroscope visualizes the pleural space for tissue biopsy or diagnosis.

CT—computed tomography; LDH—lactate dehydrogenase; MPE—malignant pleural effusion

Note. Based on information from Gayen, 2022; Jacobs et al., 2022; Jany & Welte, 2019; Josan, 2025; Mercer et al., 2016; Orlandi et al., 2024; Shen-Wagner et al., 2023.

TABLE 3-5
Differential Diagnosis of Pleural Effusions

Potential Etiology of Pleural Effusion	Pertinent History or Clinical Findings
Cirrhosis	Ascites
Drug-induced pleural effusion	Recent use of amiodarone, beta-blockers, clozapine, methotrexate, nitrofurantoin, phenytoin, procarbazine
Empyema	Frank pus in the pleural fluid
Esophageal rupture	Recent esophageal procedure, alcohol bingeing
Heart failure	Elevated jugular venous pressure, cardiomegaly, bilateral leg swelling, N-terminal (amino-terminal) pro-brain natriuretic peptide in pleural fluid, orthopnea
Hemothorax	Trauma
Hepatic hydrothorax	History of cirrhosis, alcohol abuse, ascites, jaundice
Malignancy	Past history of cancer, new cancer diagnosis, significant unexplained weight loss, hepatosplenomegaly, lymphadenopathy, exposure to risk factors for cancer (e.g., smoking, asbestos)
Pancreatic disease	History of alcohol abuse, pancreatitis
Parapneumonic pleural effusion	Recent pulmonary infection, pneumonia, infected bronchiectasis, fever
Postcardiac injury syndrome	Recent history of cardiac surgery
Pulmonary embolism	Recent leg swelling or deep vein thrombosis, unilateral leg swelling
Tuberculosis	Acute or subacute presentation of cough, chest pain, fever, body malaise, weight loss, sweating, being a young adult
Urinothorax	Ammonia-like smell of pleural fluid, increased fluid to serum creatinine level

Note. Based on information from Jacobs et al., 2022; Jany & Welte, 2019; Josan, 2025; Krishna et al., 2024; Roberts et al., 2023.

Laboratory Studies

Several blood tests can assist in establishing a diagnosis. A complete blood count with differential can demonstrate any signs of infection, inflammation, or hematologic malignancy. A complete metabolic panel can indicate any renal impairment. Liver enzymes can suggest any hepatic causes, and B-type natriuretic peptide may indicate congestive heart failure (Josan, 2025; Krishna et al., 2024; Shen-Wagner et al., 2023).

Pleural Fluid Analysis

Pleural fluid analysis results guide the selection of the optimal therapeutic modality for patients and are obtained during a thoracentesis. Pleural fluid should be evaluated for LDH, pH, color, protein, glucose, cell count, culture, and cytology (Gayen, 2022; Shen-Wagner et al., 2023). The gross appearance and odor of pleural fluid are noted on examination. Black fluid suggests *Aspergillus* or *Rhizopus* infection, malignant melanoma, or non-small cell lung cancer. Milky fluid indicates chylothorax due to lymphatic obstruction, whereas purulent fluid suggests empyema (Jany & Welte, 2019; Josan, 2025; Shen-Wagner et al., 2023). A blood-tinged or hemorrhagic appearance heightens suspicion of malignancy or trauma (Jany & Welte, 2019; Josan, 2025; Shen-Wagner et al., 2023).

Evaluation of pleural fluid protein and LDH in comparison to serum protein and LDH can distinguish between exudative and transudative effusions using the Light criteria (Light, 1972). In patients with MPE, the pleural fluid LDH level can be used along with the serum neutrophil to lymphocyte ratio, performance status, and tumor type to predict survival, with an LDH level greater than 1,500 IU/L indicating poorer survival (Clive et al., 2014). In an evaluation of pleural fluid, glucose and pH are often low in patients with MPE, with pH less than 7.3 and glucose less than 60 mg/dl (Gayen, 2022; Jacobs et al., 2022; Jany & Welte, 2019; Orlandi et al., 2024).

Pleural fluid cytology is a standard diagnostic test for malignant effusions; however, distinguishing between cell types may be challenging. Results indicating the absence of malignant cells do not exclude malignancy (Shen-Wagner et al., 2023).

Immunohistochemical tests and identification of biomarkers can further assist in MPE diagnosis. Biomarkers that may be evaluated during the MPE diagnostic process include carcinoembryonic antigen, CYFRA 21-1, carbohydrate antigen 19-9, cancer antigen 15-3, and cancer antigen 72-4 (Roberts et al., 2023). The diagnostic accuracy of these biomarkers shows a specificity of 0.88–1 but a sensitivity of 0.38–0.58, demonstrating that they are strong indicators of MPE but insufficient for excluding nonmalignant pleural effusion (Roberts et al., 2023).

Imaging Studies

Radiographic studies are performed to confirm the clinical suspicion of pleural effusion and may suggest a possible underlying etiology. The most frequently ordered studies are chest radiography, ultrasonography, and computed tomography (CT) scans, with thoracoscopy and pleuroscopy used in some instances as well.

Radiography

Chest radiography is performed to visualize the location and determine the size of the pleural effusion. Figure 3-2 shows a chest radiograph of a left-sided pleural effusion. Pleural effusion is seen as an opacity where the fluid accumulates, usually between the diaphragm and the lower lobe. Posteroanterior, lateral, and lateral decubitus radiography can provide visualization of the effusion, with the lateral decubitus view providing the highest sensitivity for smaller effusions (Josan, 2025; Shen-Wagner et al., 2023).

FIGURE 3-2. Chest Radiograph of a Left-Sided Pleural Effusion

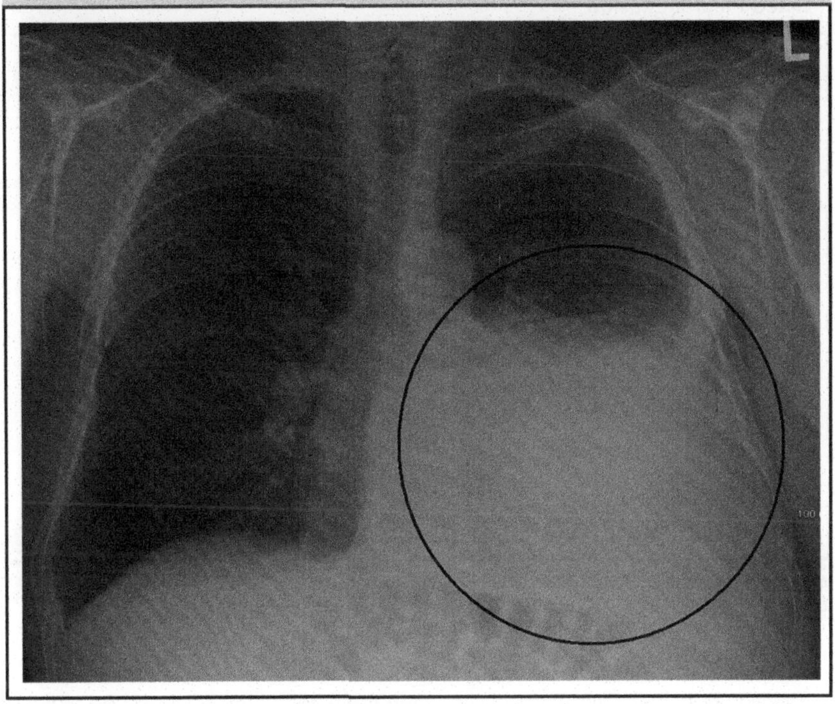

Note. Image courtesy of James Heilman, 2011 (https://commons.wikimedia.org/w/index.php?curid=14634441). Licensed under CC BY-SA 3.0 (https://creativecommons.org/licenses/by-sa/3.0/deed.en).

Ultrasonography

Thoracic ultrasonography can confirm the presence, characteristics, and volume of pleural fluid; identify areas of loculation; and detect abnormalities suggestive of malignancy, such as pleural or diaphragmatic thickening. Ultrasound allows visualization of the optimal site for thoracentesis and biopsies (Gayen, 2022; Gonnelli et al., 2024; Krishna et al., 2024; Orlandi et al., 2024; Roberts et al., 2023). At initial presentation of an undiagnosed unilateral pleural effusion, a thoracic ultrasound should be used to assess the size and character of the effusion. Additionally, the use of ultrasound to guide diagnostic and therapeutic thoracentesis improves patient safety by reducing the risk of pneumothorax and other complications (Feller-Kopman et al., 2018; Roberts et al., 2023).

Computed Tomography

A CT scan should be conducted when malignancy is suspected, although a negative scan does not exclude malignancy (Roberts et al., 2023; Shen-Wagner et al., 2023). It is helpful in determining the location and size of an effusion or potential malignancy and identifying other causes of dyspnea, such as pulmonary embolism or esophageal rupture (Shen-Wagner et al., 2023). Figure 3-3 shows a chest CT image indicating a

FIGURE 3-3. Computed Tomography Scan of the Chest Showing a Left-Sided Pleural Effusion

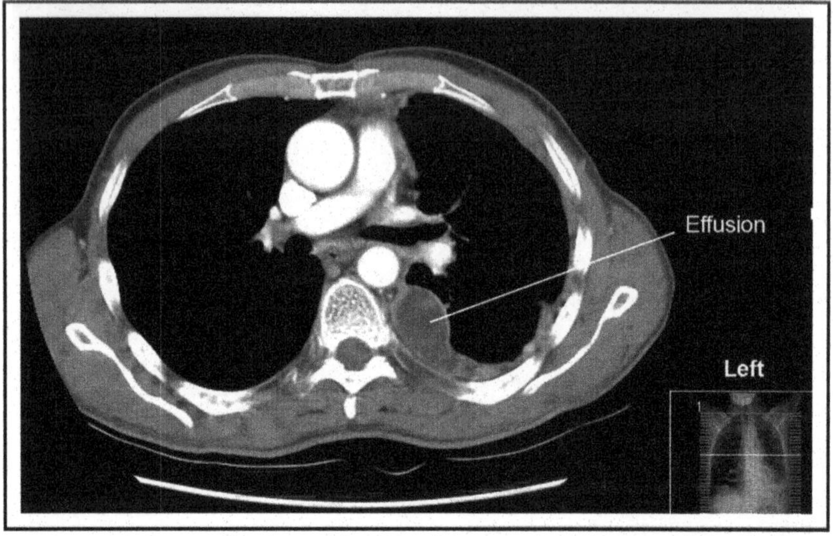

Note. Image courtesy of Drriad, 2009 (https://commons.wikimedia.org/w/index.php?curid=2262905). Licensed under CC BY-SA 3.0 (https://creativecommons.org/licenses/by-sa/3.0/deed.en).

left-sided pleural effusion. Positron-emission tomography imaging can lead to false-positive or false-negative results and is not routinely recommended for the diagnosis of MPE but may be considered in the presence of a suspicious CT scan or clinical features (Gonnelli et al., 2024; Orlandi et al., 2024; Roberts et al., 2023).

Thoracoscopy

Thoracoscopy is a minimally invasive procedure that may be used to aid in the diagnosis of pleural effusion. Often conducted with local anesthesia and moderate sedation, it involves the insertion of a camera into the chest cavity through a small incision in the chest wall to visualize the pleural cavity. Additionally, a biopsy may be obtained during the procedure. Thoracoscopy is most frequently indicated for an undiagnosed exudative pleural effusion. However, it may also be used for patients who are not surgical candidates or who are at high risk of complications related to more invasive procedures. Although the procedure is safe and well tolerated, complications may still occur, including infection, bleeding, pneumothorax, fever, and subcutaneous emphysema (Bashour et al., 2022; Jacobs et al., 2022; Orlandi et al., 2024).

Treatment Modalities

The main treatment goal of pleural effusions is to improve patient QoL by reducing distressing and debilitating symptoms (Gayen, 2022). Multiple options are often considered because no single treatment method has shown sustained superior control of these symptoms (Feller-Kopman et al., 2018). To avoid unnecessary invasive procedures, costs, or hospitalization, an individualized treatment plan considers patient performance status and preferences, severity of symptoms, expected survival, comorbidities (e.g., cardiac or respiratory conditions), effusion size, rate of fluid accumulation and recurrence, cancer type, and tumor characteristics (Orlandi et al., 2024). Although treatment of the underlying condition (e.g., via systemic cancer therapy) may successfully resolve MPE, pleural interventions should not be deferred (Roberts et al., 2023).

Pleural interventions include serial thoracentesis or definitive interventions, such as an indwelling pleural catheter (IPC) placement, chemical pleurodesis, pleuroperitoneal shunting, pleurectomy, and decortication. The term *definitive* indicates a procedure intended to produce long-term relief of symptoms (Bibby et al., 2018). It is recommended to treat pleural effusions as they present, rather than deferring until after systemic anticancer therapy (Roberts et al., 2023). Additionally, for asymptomatic MPEs, therapeutic pleural interventions are not recommended because the risks of the procedure outweigh the clinical benefits (Feller-Kopman et al., 2018). In these asymptomatic cases, if interventions are otherwise indicated (e.g., fluid or tissue sampling), draining the asymptomatic effusion would be appropriate. Table 3-6 summarizes the recommended treatment modalities for the management of MPE.

TABLE 3-6
Treatment Modalities for Management of Malignant Pleural Effusion

Treatment Modality	Description	Indication	Possible Complications
Thoracentesis	Diagnostic procedure to obtain pleural fluid for initial analysis; therapeutic drainage of effusion for immediate symptom relief	Patients who are symptomatic with advanced malignancies, survival limited to weeks or months, poor functional status, and slowly reaccumulating or chemotherapy-responsive effusions	Abdominal hemorrhage Air embolism Catheter fragment in the pleural space Cough Diaphragmatic injury Empyema Hemothorax Infection Intercostal damage Internal mammary vessel damage Internal organ damage Liver injury Lung laceration Pain Pneumothorax Splenic injury

(Continued on next page)

TABLE 3-6
Treatment Modalities for Management of Malignant Pleural Effusion *(Continued)*

Treatment Modality	Description	Indication	Possible Complications
Indwelling pleural catheter	Insertion of a catheter to intermittently drain malignant effusion; performed on an outpatient or inpatient basis	Recurrent effusions in patients with trapped lung, good performance status, good lung reexpansion, and longer survival period	Bleeding Catheter malfunction Cellulitis Dislocated catheter Empyema Infection Obstructed catheter Pain pneumothorax Tract metastasis
Pleurodesis	Installation of a sclerosing agent into the pleural space to cause pleural fibrosis	Patients with survival beyond 3 months and near-complete lung expansion	Acute respiratory distress syndrome Arrhythmias Cardiac arrest Chest pain Empyema Fever Hypotension Local site infection Longer hospital stays Myocardial infarction
Pleuroperitoneal shunt	Drainage of pleural fluid from the pleural space into the peritoneal cavity using a subcutaneous pumping chamber	Patients with recurrent malignant pleural effusion who failed pleurodesis, have trapped lung, or are poor surgical candidates	Shunt blockage
Video-assisted thoracoscopic surgery	Minimally invasive surgery providing adequate visualization of the procedure using a small camera inserted via small chest wall incisions	Patients with longer life expectancy and adequate cardiopulmonary function	Bleeding Infection Intercostal nerve damage Respiratory
Decortication	Removal of fibrous tissue adhesions restricting lung expansion	Patients with tumors limiting lung expansion who are good surgical candidates; macroscopic complete resection must be feasible.	Bronchopleural fistulae Empyema Hemorrhage Subcutaneous emphysema

Note. Based on information from Bibby et al., 2018; Brauner & Bailey, 2020; Feller-Kopman et al., 2018; Gayen, 2022; Gonnelli et al., 2024; Jacobs et al., 2022; Orlandi et al., 2024; Roberts et al., 2023.

Therapeutic Thoracentesis

Large-volume thoracenteses are commonly performed as initial pleural interventions for diagnostic or therapeutic purposes to relieve symptoms by draining accumulated fluid (Feller-Kopman et al., 2018; Gonnelli et al., 2024; Jacobs et al., 2022). Although not considered a definitive intervention, serial thoracentesis is practical and less expensive; it can occur in inpatient or outpatient settings (Orlandi et al., 2024). Large-volume thoracentesis (> 1 L) is not meant to prevent reaccumulation of fluid, but instead allows for assessment of lung expansion, symptomatic response following pleural fluid drainage, and rate of reaccumulation, which further guides management (Feller-Kopman et al., 2018; Jacobs et al., 2022). Lung expandability (i.e., expandable vs. nonexpandable) assists with therapeutic recommendations; a nonexpandable lung (NEL) is seen in at least 30% of MPEs (Feller-Kopman et al., 2018).

Complications that may occur related to thoracentesis include iatrogenic pneumothorax, solid organ puncture, hemothorax, air embolism, diaphragmatic injury, empyema, infection, pain at the site, and, more rarely, reexpansion pulmonary edema (Brauner & Bailey, 2020; Feller-Kopman et al., 2018; Orlandi et al., 2024). Iatrogenic pneumothorax (secondary to medical intervention) is a common complication of thoracentesis, leading to increased hospital length of stay (Feller-Kopman et al., 2018). Pneumothorax has been reported as high as 39%, although studies have shown reduced rates, especially with ultrasound guidance to identify intercostal vessels and improve the accuracy of needle site insertion (Feller-Kopman et al., 2018; Roberts et al., 2023). Ultrasound guidance during thoracentesis is strongly recommended to reduce the risk of lung puncture (Feller-Kopman et al., 2018; Roberts et al., 2023).

Based on institutional policy, patient considerations, and provider preferences, a pleural thoracentesis can be performed with or without sedation. After inserting a soft catheter in the optimal intercostal space, the pleural effusion is drained (usually < 1.5 L) by gravity, syringe, or vacuum bottle drainage. Results, however, are not sustained with thoracentesis; more than 50%–60% of MPEs reaccumulate after initial drainage (e.g., within nine days), prompting the need for definitive pleural interventions (Bibby et al., 2018; Feller-Kopman et al., 2018).

Indwelling Pleural Catheter

An IPC is considered a first-line treatment for MPE, allowing for intermittent drainage of fluid without hospitalization, offering immediate symptom relief in an ambulatory setting (Jacobs et al., 2022; Orlandi et al., 2024). Soft silicone tubes (15.5 Fr) are inserted into the pleural space with imaging guidance, following IV sedation and local anesthesia. Up to 1.5 L of pleural fluid may be drained initially. The IPC has a one-way safety valve that prevents air or fluid flow into the pleural cavity. Sutures in the thorax secure the IPC. A chest radiograph is performed to evaluate for pneumothorax or trapped lung and is repeated at two weeks, then monthly thereafter while the IPC is in place (University of Texas MD Anderson Cancer Center, 2023). For outpatient or in-home intermittent drainage, the IPC is connected to a vacuum bottle and often drained on a regimen- or symptom-guided basis (Roberts et al., 2023). For symptom control, pleural fluid should be drained at least every two to three days. If removal of the IPC is a priority, daily drainage is recommended to increase rates of autopleurodesis, which is seen in up to 37.3% of patients (Gonnelli et al., 2024; Roberts et al., 2023).

To minimize the risk of reexpansion pulmonary edema, patients and caregivers are instructed to drain a maximum of 1 L of fluid at home. The recommendations on IPC drainage frequency vary between institutions. Although standard practice in the United States and Canada involves daily drainage, symptom-guided fluid drainage is also observed (Muruganandan et al., 2018).

The Australasian Malignant Pleural Effusion-2 (AMPLE-2) trial was a multicenter randomized study that compared aggressive daily IPC drainage to symptom-guided drainage to determine which method was superior for improving patient-relevant clinical outcomes, specifically degree of breathlessness, physical activity patterns, rate of spontaneous pleurodesis, adverse events, and healthcare costs (Muruganandan et al., 2018). The study demonstrated the superiority of daily IPC over symptom-guided drainage regimens to promote spontaneous pleurodesis (Muruganandan et al., 2018).

Once the drainage amount is less than 50 ml on three or more occasions, the IPC is removed. The reduced volume of drainage indicates that spontaneous pleurodesis has potentially occurred, a commonality within six weeks of IPC placement. The prolonged contact of the catheter with the pleural surfaces causes inflammation and adhesions over time, leading to spontaneous pleurodesis (Gayen, 2022; Gonnelli et al., 2024).

Although IPC complications are low, they may include pain requiring catheter removal, drain or catheter fracture during removal (10%), pneumothorax, catheter blockage or loculations (about 10%), cellulitis (five-fold increased risk compared to pleurodesis), catheter-related pleural infection (e.g., empyema; about 5% of patients), bleeding, and rare cases of catheter tract metastasis (< 1%) (Feller-Kopman et al., 2018; Jacobs et al., 2022; Roberts et al., 2023). In patients with IPC-associated infections, guidelines recommend first treating the infection (e.g., oral or IV antibiotics) without catheter removal (Feller-Kopman et al., 2018). If the infection does not improve with treatment, catheter removal should be considered; however, treatment decisions should be individualized based on the clinical status of the patient (e.g., pleural sepsis), infection type (e.g., tunnel infection vs. cellulitis), and the risks associated with removing the IPC (Feller-Kopman et al., 2018). These patients should be closely monitored to ensure clinical improvement, with the potential to escalate interventions as needed.

Pleurodesis

With more than 50% of MPEs reaccumulating after an initial thoracentesis, definitive intervention using an individualized, patient-centered approach is a priority (Feller-Kopman et al., 2018; Gayen, 2022). Pleurodesis is a definitive procedure aimed at preventing reaccumulation of MPE by inducing diffuse inflammation in the pleura, resulting in pleural damage, fibrin deposition, and extensive adhesions between the visceral and parietal pleura, ultimately leading to obliteration of the pleural space (Jacobs et al., 2022; Orlandi et al., 2024). Not only does pleurodesis improve dyspnea, but it has also been shown to improve survival (Orlandi et al., 2024). Historically, pleurodesis was the treatment of choice for MPE management, although guidelines recommend either pleurodesis or IPC, depending on the specific case (e.g., considering lung expandability) (Feller-Kopman et al., 2018).

Pleurodesis can be achieved mechanically via manual abrasion of the pleura by thoracoscopy or chemically via instillation of a sclerosing agent. Because chemical pleurodesis requires pleural apposition (e.g., through a chest tube) with the use of sclerosing agents, this treatment is not indicated in patients with a NEL (Jacobs et al., 2022). See Table 3-7 for a list of sclerosing agents.

Chemical pleurodesis is a standard treatment option for MPE in patients with good performance status and a life expectancy greater than three months (Feller-Kopman et al., 2018; Jacobs et al., 2022; Roberts et al., 2023). A variety of drugs have been used as sclerosing agents, including tetracycline, doxycycline, and bleomycin. However, talc poudrage or talc slurry are the most commonly effective agents for managing MPE because of their lower pleurodesis failure rates in comparison to other agents (Dipper et al., 2020; Feller-Kopman et al., 2018; Jacobs et al., 2022; Roberts et al., 2023).

When comparing talc poudrage via video-assisted thoracoscopic surgery to talc slurry via chest tube, the guidelines do not recommend one over the other. The decision on the agent should be made based on factors such as local expertise or if patients have a chest tube already in place (Feller-Kopman et al., 2018; Roberts et al., 2023). With longer hospital length of stay, higher complication rates, healthcare costs, and increased

TABLE 3-7
Chemical Sclerosing Agents

Agent	Dose	Success Rate
Bleomycin	60–120 U	63%–85%
Corynebacterium parvum (no longer available)	7 mg in 20 ml saline	76%–100%
Doxycycline	500 mg in 100–200 ml of 0.9% normal saline	59%–100%
Interferon-beta	5–20 million units, maximum of 3 administrations	30% if used alone 56%–76% if used with immunotherapy, interleukin-2, and interferon alpha
Talc	2–5 g	80%–95%
Tetracycline (discontinued for this use in the United States in 1992)	20 mg/kg	33%–48%
Tumor necrosis factor	0.15–1.01 mg	87%

Note. Based on information from Ali et al., 2025; Kaifi et al., 2012; Ripley, 2023; Yendamuri et al., 2016.

hospital mortality (up to 8%), chemical pleurodesis or IPC may be preferred over video-assisted thoracoscopic surgery pleurodesis (Gayen, 2022; Gonnelli et al., 2024).

Pleurodesis is initiated after drainage of pleural fluid with a patent chest tube in situ and full lung expansion to the chest wall (Ali et al., 2025). Consent is obtained prior to the procedure, and education is provided to reduce patients' anxiety. A chest tube is inserted following IV sedation and local anesthetics. A sclerosing agent is administered via a 24–32-Fr chest tube. Following agent instillation, the chest catheter is clamped for one to four hours, following institutional protocol, allowing the chemical agent to dwell in the pleural space to induce an intense inflammatory response. After the desired time has elapsed, the chest tube is unclamped and connected to negative water suction (–20 cm). It remains in place until there is no further fluid output and a chest radiograph confirms lung expansion (Ali et al., 2025). Successful pleurodesis requires apposition, or close contact, of the visceral and parietal pleura (Feller-Kopman et al., 2018). Incomplete lung expansion, as seen in trapped lung, prevents pleural apposition and will render pleurodesis unsuccessful.

Considerations for Management

Effective management of MPE centers on symptom palliation and QoL, allowing patients to spend less time in the hospital, reducing costs for the patients, and saving healthcare resources. In patients who are symptomatic with recurrent effusions with a known or suspected expandable lung, guidelines recommend either IPC placement or pleurodesis (e.g., talc slurry, talc poudrage) as the first-line definitive treatment for MPE management (Bibby et al., 2018; Feller-Kopman et al., 2018; Roberts et al., 2023). Conversely, in patients with a NEL (> 25% radiologically), loculated effusion, or failed pleurodesis, guidelines recommend IPC over pleurodesis for MPE management (Feller-Kopman et al., 2018; Roberts et al., 2023). IPC is favored in this population because of the increased hospital length of stay and healthcare costs associated with pleurodesis (Feller-Kopman et al., 2018). In symptomatic MPEs with a NEL (< 25% radiologically), talc slurry pleurodesis may be considered to improve symptoms (Roberts et al., 2023). Other considerations when choosing a definitive pleural intervention may include possible altered body image with IPCs, increased hospital length of stay with pleurodesis, and the ability for patients and their caregivers to perform IPC drainage at home (Roberts et al., 2023).

Surgical Options

When conservative options do not relieve patient symptoms, surgical options may be considered for select patients with refractory MPE after failed IPC and pleurodesis. These procedures may include a pleuroperitoneal shunt or pleurectomy. Although rarely recommended, pleuroperitoneal shunting may be an option in patients with malignant chylothorax and high volumes of pleural fluid drainage. Pleuroperitoneal shunting is associated with a complication rate of 15%–25%, primarily due to shunt fracture, occlusion, and infection (Karadayı & Şahin, 2021). Shunt placement requires general anesthesia and thoracoscopy or the use of interventional radiology. An example of a shunt catheter is the Denver pleuroperitoneal shunt that allows for unidirectional flow away from the pleural space and into the peritoneum. Evidence suggests that pleuroperitoneal shunting may provide palliation in up to 95% of patients (Karadayı & Şahin, 2021).

Total or partial pleurectomy involves the resection of the visceral and parietal pleura with decortication (or fibrous pleural rind removal). Decortication surgery may be considered to improve pleurodesis success in patients with NEL (Roberts et al., 2023). A pleurectomy is regarded as a last resort because it is highly invasive. Surgical candidates must have a reasonably long expected survival of more than 12 months.

Medical Management

Systemic chemotherapy and radiation therapy are indicated for the treatment of the underlying disease causing MPE (Roberts et al., 2023). In specifically selected symptomatic patients with MPE, intrapleural fibrinolytics may be considered to improve breathlessness. It is not recommended to routinely use intrapleural chemotherapy specifically for MPE treatment (Roberts et al., 2023).

Nursing Management

Nurses play a key role in the care of patients with pleural effusions, including managing symptoms, monitoring response to treatments, assessing side effects, and providing education and emotional support. Care of patients with pleural effusions includes periodic assessment of increased dyspnea and shortness of breath, which may indicate fluid reaccumulation or recurrence of effusion. Administering supplemental oxygen helps improve hypoxemia. To allow for maximum lung expansion, nurses can assist in patient positioning. Instructing patients in pursed-lip breathing can reduce breathlessness. Another strategy that may help reduce feelings of breathlessness is placing a fan to blow on the side of the patient's face (Sato et al., 2023). Emotional support and reassurance may help reduce the anxiety about feelings of breathlessness. It is important for nurses to assess patients for the presence of pain and response to current pain management regimens, which may include nonsteroidal anti-inflammatory drugs or narcotic medications, depending on the severity of pain.

Extensive patient and caregiver education on device management and routine self-drainage is essential (Jacobs et al., 2022). An IPC drainage educational video is typically available from vacuum bottle manufacturers. Nurses should also provide primary and secondary preventive education, including exercising regularly and as tolerated, having a healthy diet, limiting or avoiding alcohol, abstaining from smoking, receiving vaccinations to prevent respiratory infections, and knowing occupational safety measures (e.g., respiratory protection) (Krishna et al., 2024). Additionally, it is important for nurses to provide education to assist with the early detection of complications from disease or treatments (Krishna et al., 2024).

MPE is often associated with a poor prognosis. Nurses should provide emotional support and explain to patients and caregivers the various resources and options to enhance their QoL. The decision to decline further aggressive therapies and receive end-of-life palliative care with symptom control, pain relief, and comfort measures should be supported by nurses. They should also assist with referrals to specialists in palliative care, home care, hospice, pain management, and social work, as well as psychologists and clergy, as appropriate (Kaplan, 2017). As patients near the end of life, nurses can help them achieve optimal control of cough, anorexia, pain, distress, and anxiety with medication management (Albert, 2017). Table 3-8 summarizes nursing care interventions for patients with MPE.

TABLE 3-8
Nursing Care of Patients With Malignant Pleural Effusion

Nursing Problems	Interventions	Expected Outcomes
Ineffective breathing pattern Impaired gas exchange	Provide oxygen supplementation as needed. Position the patient for maximum lung expansion. Teach the patient how to do pursed-lip breathing.	The patient will have effective breathing as evidenced by: • Respirations with regular rate, depth, and pattern • Absence of cyanosis • Pulse oximetry within normal limits Patient maintains optimal gas exchange.
Activity intolerance	Pace activities (e.g., avoid strenuous activities)	Patient maintains an adequate level of activity within their capability.
Risk for falls Risk for injury	Provide patient education. Reinforce the need to call for assistance, especially when connected to a drainage system. Keep essential items within easy reach. Institute fall precautions.	Patient will be free from falls or injury.
Acute or chronic pain	Administer pain medication as needed.	Patient will have lessening or absence of pain as manifested by verbalization of pain relief.
Impaired skin integrity	Assess the chest tube or indwelling pleural catheter insertion site periodically. Cleanse the insertion site as ordered. Change dressing as appropriate.	Patient will maintain skin integrity around the chest tube or the indwelling pleural catheter site as evidenced by: • Absence of skin irritation • Absence of erythema
Anxiety	Provide reassurance. Support verbalization of anxiety.	Patient will demonstrate increased psychological functioning as evidenced by verbalization of reduced anxiety.

(Continued on next page)

TABLE 3-8
Nursing Care of Patients With Malignant Pleural Effusion *(Continued)*

Nursing Problems	Interventions	Expected Outcomes
Risk for ineffective coping (patient or caregiver)	Encourage verbalization of feelings. Provide patient and caregiver education about available support resources. Provide referrals to specialists.	Patient and caregiver will demonstrate effective coping skills. Patient and caregiver will be able to demonstrate goals of care.
Knowledge deficit	Provide explanations and instructions related to diagnostic and surgical procedures and drain care (if indicated). Ensure the patient and caregiver are able to teach-back or demonstrate care.	The patient and caregiver will demonstrate adequate knowledge of care for an indwelling pleural catheter, as evidenced by: • Accurate verbalization of instructions • Accurate demonstration of the technique to drain an indwelling pleural catheter

Note. Based on information from Matthews, 2023.

Patient and caregiver education is structured to meet individualized needs. In general, core content should include an explanation of the various diagnostic tests patients must undergo. It is important for nurses to provide patients and caregivers with information about any planned invasive procedures, including thoracentesis, pleurodesis, or other surgical interventions. Consent should be obtained from patients or their surrogates prior to any testing or treatment, and discussions must outline the reasons for the procedure, its risks and benefits, any available alternatives, and the option to forgo the procedure. Nurses should provide instructions to patients and their caregivers about how to manage drainage systems at home and record drainage amounts. They must also teach patients and caregivers to recognize and report signs and symptoms of fluid reaccumulation. Education should include relief measures for dyspnea and pain. Fatigue can be a concern for patients with MPE and their caregivers, and nurses should teach them energy-conserving measures, such as avoiding strenuous activities and pacing activities of daily living to minimize exertion.

Nurses should also educate patients and caregivers on the implications of MPE as a sign of advanced disease. They should facilitate patient–provider discussions or caregiver–healthcare team conferences regarding the prognosis. As the treatment goals are established based on the patient's overall health condition, general prognosis, and personal preferences, it is important for nurses to assess patients' and caregivers' understanding of the goals of care and their coping abilities and to make referrals to specialists as needed.

Summary

MPE is an oncologic emergency that can lead to life-threatening respiratory impairment. Its occurrence typically heralds advanced disease and is associated with a significantly impaired QoL and limited survival. A thorough, systematic evaluation of the effusion is critical in establishing etiology and determining the course of treatment. Given the limited life expectancy of patients with MPE, management is individualized and focused on functional status, comorbidities, prognosis, and personal preferences. The objectives of treatment are to achieve symptom palliation and enhanced QOL, and minimize inpatient hospitalization and aggressive interventions.

Kelli Thoele's authorship of this chapter is in no manner affiliated with Lilly.

The authors would like to acknowledge Anna Liza Rodriguez, MSN, MHA, RN, OCN®, for her contribution to this chapter that remains unchanged from the previous edition of this book.

References

Albert, R.H. (2017). End-of-life care: Managing common symptoms. *American Family Physician, 95*(6), 356–361. https://www.aafp.org/pubs/afp/issues/2017/0315/p356.html

Ali, M., Sharma, S., & Surani, S. (2025). Pleurodesis. In *StatPearls*. StatPearls Publishing. https://www.ncbi.nlm.nih.gov/books/NBK560685

Bashour, S.I., Mankidy, B.J., & Lazarus, D.R. (2022). Update on the diagnosis and management of malignant pleural effusions. *Respiratory Medicine, 196*, 106802. https://doi.org/10.1016/j.rmed.2022.106802

Bibby, A.C., Dorn, P., Psallidas, I., Porcel, J.M., Janssen, J., Froudarakis, M., ... Maskell, N.A. (2018). ERS/EACTS statement on the management of malignant pleural effusions. *European Respiratory Journal, 52*(1), 1800349. https://doi.org/10.1183/13993003.00349-2018

Brauner, M.E., & Bailey, R.A. (2020, September 11). Thoracentesis. *Medscape*. https://emedicine.medscape.com/article/80640-overview

Clive, A.O., Kahan, B.C., Hooper, C.E., Bhatnagar, R., Morley, A.J., Zahan-Evans, N., ... Maskell, N.A. (2014). Predicting survival in malignant pleural effusion: Development and validation of the LENT prognostic score. *Thorax, 69*(12), 1098–1104. https://doi.org/10.1136/thoraxjnl-2014-205285

D'Agostino, H.P., & Edens, M.A. (2023). Physiology, pleural fluid. In *StatPearls*. StatPearls Publishing. https://www.ncbi.nlm.nih.gov/books/NBK513353

Dipper, A., Jones, H.E., Bhatnagar, R., Preston, N.J., Maskell, N., & Clive, A.O. (2020). Interventions for the management of malignant pleural effusions: A network meta-analysis. *Cochrane Database of Systematic Reviews, 4*(4), CD010529. https://doi.org/10.1002/14651858.CD010529.pub3

Feller-Kopman, D.J., Chakravarthy, B.R., DeCamp, M.M., Diekemper, R.L., Gould, M.K., Henry, T., ... Balekian, A.A. (2018). Management of malignant pleural effusions: An official ATS/STS/STR clinical practice guideline. *American Journal of Respiratory and Clinical Care Medicine, 198*(7), 839–849. https://doi.org/10.1164/rccm.201807-1415ST

Ferreiro, L., Toubes, M.E., Suárez-Antelo, J., Rodríguez-Núñez, N., & Valdés, L. (2024). Clinical overview of the physiology and pathophysiology of pleural fluid movement: A narrative review. *ERJ Open Research, 10*(5), 00050–2024. https://doi.org/10.1183/23120541.00050-2024

Gayen, S. (2022). Malignant pleural effusion: Presentation, diagnosis, and management. *American Journal of Medicine, 135*(10), 1188–1192. https://doi.org/10.1016/j.amjmed.2022.04.017

Gonnelli, F., Hasan, W., Bonifazi, M., Pinelli, V., Bedawi, E.O., Porcel, J.M., ... Mei, F. (2024). Malignant pleural effusion: Current approach and therapeutic approach. *Respiratory Research, 25*(1), 47. https://doi.org/10.1186/s12931-024-02684-7

Jacobs, B., Sheikh, G., Youness, H.A., Keddissi, J.I., & Abdo, T. (2022). Diagnosis and management of malignant pleural effusion: A decade in review. *Diagnostics, 12*(4), 1016. https://doi.org/10.3390/diagnostics1204101

Jany, B., & Welte, T. (2019). Pleural effusion in adults: Etiology, diagnosis, and treatment. *Deutsches Arzleblatt International, 116*(21), 377–386. https://doi.org/10.3238/arztebl.2019.0377

Josan, E.S. (2025, April 3). Pleural effusion. *Medscape.* https://emedicine.medscape.com/article/299959overview

Kaifi, J.T., Toth, J.W., Gusani, N.J., Kimchi, E.T., Staveley-O'Carroll, K.F., Belani, C.P., & Reed, M.F. (2012). Multidisciplinary management of malignant pleural effusion. *Journal of Surgical Oncology, 105*(7), 731–738. https://doi.org/10.1002/jso.22100

Kaplan, M. (2017). Malignant pleural effusion. In K. Kuebler (Ed.), *Integration of palliative care in chronic conditions: An interdisciplinary approach* (pp. 327–338). Oncology Nursing Society.

Karadayı, Ş., & Şahin, E. (2021). Surgical treatment in malignant pleural effusion. *Turkish Journal of Thoracic and Cardiovascular Surgery, 29*(4), 577–585. https://doi.org/10.5606/tgkdc.dergisi.2021.20580

Krishna, R., Antoine, M.H., Alahmadi, M.H., & Rudrappa, M. (2024). Pleural effusion. In *StatPearls.* StatPearls Publishing. https://www.ncbi.nlm.nih.gov/books/NBK448189

Light, R.W., MacGregor, M.I., Luchsinger, P.C., & Ball, W.C., Jr. (1972). Pleural effusions: The diagnostic separation of transudates and exudates. *Annals of Internal Medicine, 77*(4), 507–513. https://doi.org/10.7326/0003-4819-77-4-507

Matthews, L. (2024). Respiratory symptoms. In J.M. Brant, D.G. Cope, & M.G. Saría (Eds.), *Core curriculum for oncology nursing* (7th ed., pp. 454–461). Elsevier.

Mercer, R.M., Corcoran, J.P., & Rahman, N.M. (2016). Modern management of malignant pleural effusions. *Clinical Pulmonary Medicine, 23*(6), 265–272. https://doi.org/10.1097/CPM.0000000000000174

Mishra, E.K., & Stanton, A. (2024). Patient-reported outcomes in pleural effusions: A systematic review. *Cureus, 16*(1), e52430. https://doi.org/10.7759/cureus.52430

Morris, M.F., Henry, T.S., Raptis, C.A., Amin, A.N., Auffermann, W.F., Hatten, B.W., ... Chung, J.H. (2023). ACR Appropriateness Criteria®: Workup of plural effusion or pleural disease. *Journal of the American College of Radiology, 21*(6, Suppl.), S342–S352. https://doi.org/10.1016/j.jacr.2024.02.013

Muruganandan, S., Azzopardi, M., Fitzgerald, D.B., Shrestha, R., Kwan, B.C.H., Lam, D.C.L., ... Lee, Y.C.G. (2018). Aggressive versus symptom-guided drainage of malignant pleural effusion via indwelling pleural catheters (AMPLE-2): An open-label randomized trial. *Lancet Respiratory Medicine, 6*(9), 671–680. https://doi.org/10.1016/S2213-2600(18)30288-1

Orlandi, R., Cara, A., Cassina, E.M., Degiovanni, S., Libretti, L., Raveglia, F., ... Patrella, F. (2024). Malignant pleural effusion: Diagnosis and treatment—Up-to-date perspective. *Current Oncology, 31*(11), 6867–6878. https://doi.org/10.1164/rccm.201807-1415ST

Psallidas, I., Kanellakis, N.I., Gerry, S., Thézénas, M.L., Charles, P.D., Samsonova, A., ... Rahman, N.M. (2018). Development and validation of response markers to predict survival and pleurodesis success in patients with malignant pleural effusion (PROMISE): A multicohort analysis. *Lancet Oncology, 19*(7), 930–939. https://doi.org/10.1016/S1470-2045(18)30294-8

Ripley, R.T. (2023). Malignant pleural and pericardial effusions. In V.T. DeVita Jr., T.S. Lawrence, & S.A. Rosenberg (Eds.), *DeVita, Hellman, and Rosenberg's cancer: Principles and practice of oncology* (12th ed., pp. 1681–1688). Wolters Kluwer.

Roberts, M.E., Rahman, N.M., Maskell, N.A., Bibby, A.C., Blyth, K.G., Corcoran, J.P., ... Walker, S. (2023). British Thoracic Society Guideline for pleural disease. *Thorax, 78*(3, Suppl.), s1–s42. https://doi.org/10.1136/thorax-2022-219784

Sato, T., Taito, S., Nakashima, Y., Sakai, K., & Kako, J. (2023). Safety and feasibility of fan therapy for dyspnea: A scoping review. *Cureus, 15*(8), e43668. https://doi.org/10.7759/cureus.43668

Sharma, K., Fultariya, L., Mallimala, P.R., Shah, K., & Sharma, V. (2023). Comparison of the efficacy of Light's criteria with serum-effusion albumin gradient and pleural effusion glucose. *Cureus, 15*(8), e43319. https://doi.org/10.7759/cureus.43319

Shen-Wagner, J., Gamble, C., & MacGilvray, P. (2023). Pleural effusion: Diagnostic approach in adults. *American Family Physician, 108*(5), 464–475. https://pubmed.ncbi.nlm.nih.gov/37983698

University of Texas MD Anderson Cancer Center. (2023). *Intrapleural catheter (IPC) management* [v.4]. https://www.mdanderson.org/content/dam/mdanderson/documents/for-physicians/algorithms/clinical-management/clin-management-intrapleural-catheters-web-algorithm.pdf

Yendamuri, S., Nwogu, C., & Demmy, T.L. (2016). Malignant pleural and pericardial effusions. In F.W. Sellke, P.J. del Nido, & S.J. Swanson (Eds.), *Sabiston and Spencer surgery of the chest* (9th ed., pp. 481–498). Elsevier.

Zhao, J., Liu, B., Liu, N., Zhang, B., He, X., Ma, Q., & Wang, Y. (2022). The role of angiogenesis in malignant pleural effusion: From basic research to clinical application. *American Journal of Cancer Research, 12*(11), 4879–4891.

Brenda S. Nettles, DNP, MS, ACNP-BC, AOCNP®, CNE,
and Allison Mitchell, BSN, RN, OCN®

CHAPTER 4

Bowel Obstruction

FAST FACTS

- **Description:** A bowel obstruction is a serious impairment of healthy gastrointestinal function associated with benign and malignant conditions. Although symptoms may have a gradual onset, a timely diagnosis and early intervention are key to minimizing life-threatening complications, such as ischemia, perforation, and sepsis.
- **Incidence:** Approximately 15% of hospital admissions for acute abdominal pain in the United States are caused by bowel obstructions, and 20% of these patients require emergency surgical evaluations. A malignant bowel obstruction is a common complication seen in 10%–28% of patients presenting with an advanced stage of gastrointestinal cancer and 51% of those with advanced ovarian cancer.
- **Clinical Manifestations:** Abdominal pain, nausea, vomiting, and bloating, along with the absence of flatus or bowel movements, are the most common symptoms reported with a bowel obstruction. However, the severity of the symptoms will vary based on the degree and the anatomical location of the obstruction in the gastrointestinal system.
- **Risk Factors and Etiology:** Patients with a history of having undergone an extensive oncologic surgical resection of the abdomen or pelvis or radiation therapy are also at an increased risk for developing adhesions and strictures that limit regular bowel motility. A malignant bowel obstruction develops from the presence of a large primary tumor in the gastrointestinal tract, malignant ascites, or advanced peritoneal disease.
- **Pathophysiology and Patient Evaluation:** The physiologic changes associated with a malignant bowel obstruction include a reduction or the complete absence of movement through the intestine and an accumulation of gastrointestinal secretions. The progressive dilation of the affected bowel increases the risk of perforations and tissue necrosis proximal to the site of obstruction.
- **Advanced Practice Considerations:** Serial laboratory testing is recommended to evaluate for possible electrolyte imbalances, impaired renal function, systemic signs of infection, and ischemia, as well as to monitor patient response to treatment. Diagnostic imaging is used to identify the site of the obstruction and rule out potential life-threatening conditions, such as ischemic bowel, perforations, and signs of peritonitis.
- **Treatment Modalities:** Goals of treatment will vary based on the degree of obstruction (partial vs. complete) and the patient's level of health. The initial treatment of a partial bowel obstruction includes conservative measures such as the use of isotonic IV fluids for fluid resuscitation, bowel rest to allow for a reduction in pressure, and the possible clearing of the blockage.
- **Nursing Management:** The goals of nursing care are to alleviate symptoms and provide guidance for patients at an increased risk for developing a bowel obstruction. Nurses should actively triage patient symptoms and work with the clinical team to refer patients to the appropriate level of care.

- **Outcomes:** The response to treatment for malignant bowel obstructions is often unpredictable; however, shared decision-making, clear communication about prognosis, and a comprehensive review of the risks and benefits associated with treatment are key to ensuring that the plan of care aligns with patient values and goals of care.

Introduction

A bowel obstruction is a serious impairment of healthy gastrointestinal (GI) function that negatively affects a patient's quality of life and can result in an oncologic emergency. An obstruction of the intestine can occur in any segment (see Figure 4-1); however, it more commonly occurs in the small bowel (60%–75% of cases) rather than the large bowel (Jackson & Vigiola Cruz, 2018). The underlying causes of an obstruction are associated with both benign and malignant conditions and may present as an acute or chronic health concern. Although symptoms may have a gradual onset, a timely diagnosis and early intervention are key to minimizing life-threatening complications, such as ischemia, perforation, and sepsis.

Incidence

Approximately 15% of hospital admissions for acute abdominal pain in the United States are caused by bowel obstructions, and 20% of these patients require emergency surgical evaluations (Demarest et al., 2023). Obstructions account for nearly 30,000 deaths per year and contribute to more than $3 billion in direct medical costs (Catena et al., 2019). A malignant bowel obstruction (MBO) is a common complication seen in an estimated 10%–28% of patients presenting with advanced-stage GI cancer and 51% with advanced ovarian cancer (Shariff et al., 2022).

FIGURE 4-1. Etiology of Gastrointestinal Obstructions

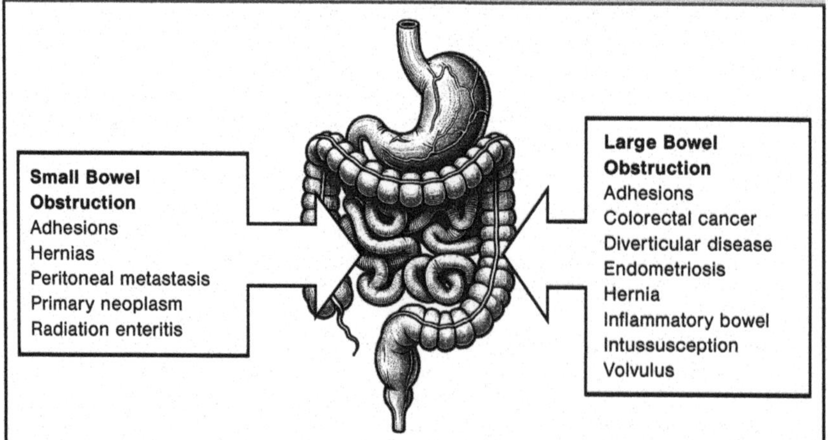

Clinical Manifestations

Abdominal pain, nausea, vomiting, and bloating, along with the absence of flatus or bowel movements for more than 72 hours, are the most common symptoms reported with a bowel obstruction (Demarest et al., 2023). However, the severity of these symptoms will vary based on the degree and the anatomical location of the obstruction in the GI system. During the acute phase of obstruction, patients may present with hemodynamic instability (e.g., tachycardia, hypotension), electrolyte imbalances, metabolic abnormalities, and malnutrition (Nelms & Kann, 2021; Sullivan et al., 2024).

Risk Factors and Etiology

Mechanical bowel obstructions are caused by external compression, an invasion of the intestinal wall, or a reduction in healthy bowel motility, which results in a partial or complete blockage of the bowel. Functional obstructions occur when motility is impaired by a tumor infiltrating the mesentery or the celiac and enteric plexus (Madariaga et al., 2022). Some common benign causes of obstruction are adhesions, hernia, chronic constipation, inflammatory bowel disease, and drug-induced ileus. The most common etiologies for bowel obstructions in the small intestine are adhesions, hernias, peritoneal metastasis, radiation enteritis, and primary neoplasm. In the large intestine, bowel obstruction is most often caused by colorectal cancer, diverticular disease, volvulus, inflammatory bowel disease, hernia, adhesions, endometriosis, and intussusception. Patients who have undergone an extensive oncologic surgical resection of the abdomen or pelvis or radiation therapy are also at an increased risk for developing adhesions and strictures that limit regular bowel motility (Yu et al., 2020).

An obstruction associated with a malignancy may develop from the presence of a large primary tumor in the GI tract, malignant ascites, or advanced peritoneal disease. Common cancers associated with bowel obstruction are gastric, pancreatic, gallbladder, cholangiocarcinoma, colon, and ovarian (see Figure 4-2). About 80% of bowel obstructions from colorectal cancer involve the sigmoid and left colon distal to the splenic flexure (Sullivan et al., 2024).

FIGURE 4-2. Malignant Bowel Obstructions and Associated Cancers

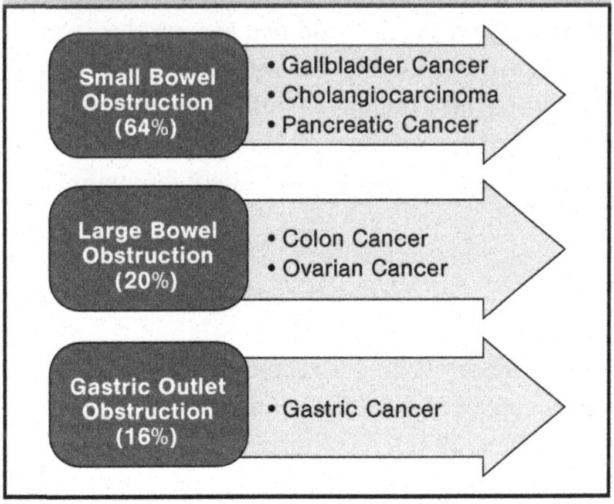

Note. Based on information from Demarest et al., 2023.

Pathophysiology and Patient Evaluation

Healthy bowel motility requires synchronous wave-like contractions of the muscles along the digestive tract to move nutrients and eliminate waste from the body. The physiologic changes associated with an MBO include a reduction or the complete absence of movement through the intestine, an accumulation of GI secretions, and a progressive dilation of the affected loops of bowel. A decrease in motility due to obstruction leads to an imbalance of fluids and electrolytes, an increase in luminal pressure, and a reduction in bowel perfusion (Jackson & Vigiola Cruz, 2018). The bowel often becomes dilated proximal to the site of obstruction, with a decompression of the bowel distal to the area of obstruction. Perforations may occur as a result of increased wall stress and tissue necrosis proximal to the site of obstruction or at the site of a tumor that has eroded into the colonic wall (Sullivan et al., 2024).

A comprehensive patient evaluation is key to diagnosing and initiating the appropriate level of treatment. A detailed review of past medical and surgical history helps in identifying possible contributing factors for the development of obstruction (e.g., cancer, inflammatory bowel disease, radiation treatment, previous abdominal surgery). A patient may be considered a poor surgical candidate based on their comorbidities (e.g., cardiopulmonary, renal, liver impairment), clinical staging consistent with metastatic or advanced disease (e.g., ascites, carcinomatosis, palpable intra-abdominal masses), or the presence of multiple obstructions (Krouse, 2019).

Early signs of obstruction may include vague symptoms of nausea, bloating, increased belching, and abdominal discomfort that may later progress to nausea with vomiting, fever, chills, cramping, abdominal pain, and weakness (Johnson & Hawkins, 2021). Findings on physical examination will vary depending on the location, duration, and degree of the obstruction.

A comprehensive approach includes the inspection, auscultation, percussion, and palpation of the abdomen as tolerated by the patient. The inspection of the abdomen may be significant for distension and bloating (Jackson & Vigiola Cruz, 2018). On auscultation, the bowel sounds (borborygmi) will range from hyperactive to hypoactive, or the absence of sound is noted due to a lack of intestinal activity (Fahim et al., 2021). The percussion of the abdomen may produce a tympanic sound, which is consistent with gas trapped within the intestine. However, a dullness noted on examination is concerning for a buildup of fluid or the presence of a solid mass in the abdomen. The final step of the examination is palpation, and any areas of reported tenderness should be evaluated last to minimize patient discomfort.

Advanced Practice Considerations

Laboratory testing is recommended to evaluate for possible electrolyte imbalances, impaired renal function, systemic signs of infection, and ischemia (Johnson & Hawkins, 2021). A complete blood count, comprehensive metabolic panel, and serum lactate levels should be ordered to monitor for signs of leukocytosis, anemia, dehydration, metabolic alkalosis, and acidosis (Jackson & Vigiola Cruz, 2018).

Serial laboratory testing is required to evaluate the patient's response to medical management and monitor for signs of clinical decline during a colorectal oncologic emergency (see Table 4-1).

The selection of the appropriate imaging technique is key to identifying the site of the obstruction and ruling out a potential life-threatening condition, such as ischemic bowel, perforations, and signs of peritonitis. Abdominal x-rays are readily available in most clinical settings and were historically recommended as the initial imaging modality to assess for bowel distension, the presence of air-fluid levels, and identify the location of obstruction (Jackson & Vigiola Cruz, 2018). These x-rays are noted to have a sensitivity of 70%–86% and specificity of 72% for detecting large bowel obstructions (Demarest et al., 2023). However, approximately 75% of small bowel obstructions are caused by adhesions, which cannot be visualized on a plain abdominal x-ray (Nelms & Kann, 2021).

A computed tomography scan is recommended for the initial evaluation of patients with a clinical presentation concerning acute bowel obstruction or perforation (see Figure 4-3). These scans have a sensitivity of 80%–90% and a specificity of 70%–100% for identifying the cause, level of obstruction, and the transition point noted as a dilation proximal to the site of obstruction and a decompression of the distal bowel

TABLE 4-1
Laboratory Tests for the Evaluation of Malignant Bowel Obstruction

Laboratory Testing	Abnormal Results	Clinical Significance
Complete blood count • White blood cell (WBC) • Red blood cell (RBC) • Hemoglobin (Hgb) • Hematocrit (Hct) • Platelets (Plts)	Leukocytosis (increased WBC)	Inflammation, infection, bowel ischemia, and perforation
	Anemia (decreased Hgb/Hct)	Occult blood loss, malignancy, and chronic disease
	Dehydration (increased Hgb/Hct)	Reduced oral intake, emesis
Comprehensive metabolic panel (CMP) • Creatinine (Cr) • Blood urea nitrogen (BUN) • Sodium (Na^+) • Potassium (K^+) • Chloride (Cl^-) • Bicarbonate ($HC0_3^-$) • Serum lactate level	Hypokalemia (decreased K^+)	Reduced oral intake, emesis, nasogastric tube suctioning
	Hypochloremia (decreased Cl^-)	Reduced oral intake, impaired absorption, emesis, metabolic alkalosis
	Dehydration (increased BUN/Cr)	Reduced oral intake and impaired renal function
	Hyperlactatemia (increased serum lactate level)	Bowel ischemia and metabolic acidosis

Note. Based on information from Jackson & Vigiola Cruz, 2018.

FIGURE 4-3. Computed Tomography Scan of the Abdomen and Pelvis Showing a Partial Intestinal Obstruction

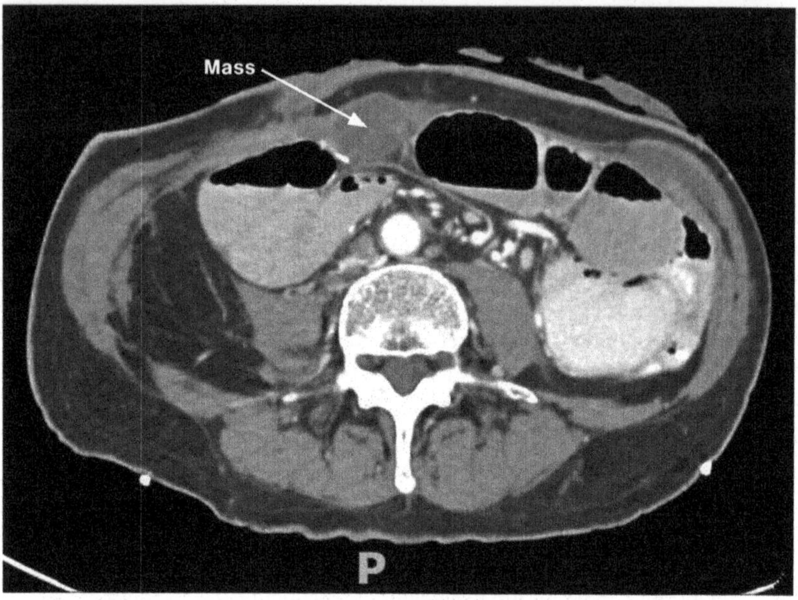

Axial computed tomography scan showing a colonic obstruction with an arrow noting a mass

(Demarest et al., 2023; Jackson & Vigiola Cruz, 2018). Computed tomography scans are also used for oncologic staging to assess for the progression or recurrence of disease. Oral contrast is not required to confirm a diagnosis of small bowel obstruction due to the presence of intraluminal fluid and gas in the bowel. However, a water-soluble rectal contrast is recommended to more effectively visualize large bowel obstructions (Catena et al., 2019).

The distension of the proximal bowel loop with the confirmation of an air-fluid level is a common finding noted on imaging (Yu et al., 2020). The 3-6-9 rule for radiography provides a clinical standard for the normal diameter of the small intestine (< 3 cm), large intestine (< 6 cm), and cecum (< 9 cm) (Nelms & Kann, 2021). A dilation of the bowel by an additional 3 cm at any of these levels is concerning for an increased risk of rupture of the bowel.

Treatment Modalities

Goals of treatment will vary based on the degree of obstruction (partial vs. complete) and the patient's level of health. Figure 4-4 provides a summary of treatment recommendations based on the stage of obstruction. The initial treatment of a partial bowel obstruction includes conservative measures, such as the use of isotonic IV fluids for fluid resuscitation and bowel rest to allow for a reduction in pressure and possible clearing of the blockage (Krouse, 2019). Patients experiencing persistent nausea and vomiting (> 250 ml in 24 hours) or radiographic evidence of a complete obstruction will require the placement of a nasogastric tube to promote the removal of gastric fluid and air (Demarest et al., 2023).

Antiemetics, corticosteroids, antisecretory agents, or pain medications can be initiated to promote patient comfort (Madariaga et al., 2022). A bowel regimen of osmotic laxatives can also be used to reduce stool volume and eliminate distention of the bowel wall (Fahim et al., 2021). Antibiotics are indicated during the initial phase of treatment if the patient presents with a temperature of 100.4°F (38°C) or higher and leukocytosis. The antibiotic regimen should provide coverage against both Gram-negative and anaerobic organisms (Jackson & Vigiola Cruz, 2018).

Oral intake is limited until the restoration of bowel motility is confirmed by the movement of flatus through the GI tract. MBOs cause intestinal failure that limits or completely restricts healthy intestinal movement, digestion, and absorption of nutrients passing through the bowel (Patel et al., 2024). Nutritional screenings are performed to assess possible signs of malnutrition and include the patient's baseline weight, body mass index, and total percentage of weight loss in the past three months (Fahim et al., 2021). Parenteral nutrition is recommended as a source of supplemental

FIGURE 4-4. Stages and Treatment of Bowel Obstruction

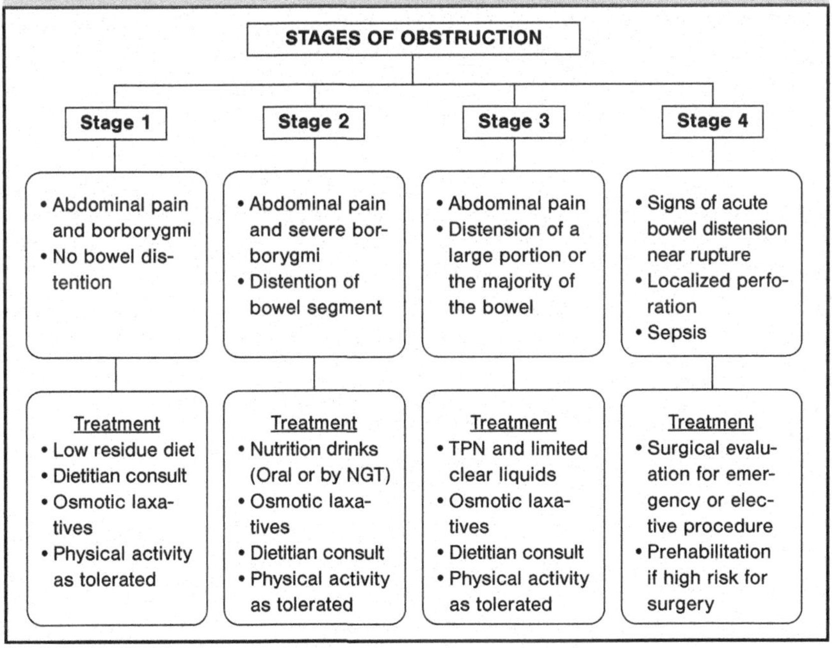

NGT—nasogastric tube; TPN—total parenteral nutrition

Note. Based on information from Fahim et al., 2021.

nutrition during periods of reduced oral intake or as a total nutritional replacement for patients unable to tolerate oral intake. However, parenteral nutrition has been shown to provide no benefit to patients living with advanced disease and should be avoided in individuals with a limited life expectancy (Patel et al., 2024).

The management of complete bowel obstructions begins with conservative measures. However, more invasive techniques, such as endoscopy or surgery, may be required to address the underlying cause of the identified obstruction. The placement of venting gastrostomy tubes is recommended to reduce the risk of aspiration in individuals who are not candidates for surgery or have not responded to medical treatment. This palliative measure relieves symptoms of nausea and vomiting in 80%–90% of patients, allows for earlier discharge to home, and leads to fewer hospital readmissions (Demarest et al., 2023). Endoscopy procedures are performed to dilate and stent segments of the bowel narrowed by stricture and obstructed by tumor (Johnson & Hawkins, 2021). It is also important to consider the risks associated with this procedure, including stent migration, bowel perforation, bleeding, and the need for repeat procedures.

MBOs can resolve without any surgical intervention in 36% of cases; however, the rate for recurrent obstruction is more than 60% (Demarest et al., 2023). Unfortunately, there are no consistent algorithms used to guide the selection of intervention for MBO, or the duration of medical treatment required before a patient should be referred for a surgical evaluation. It is noteworthy that the timing of surgical procedures significantly influences patient outcomes, as evidenced by a 30-day morbidity (33% vs. 20%) and 30-day mortality (9% vs. 3%) when comparing the outcomes of emergent versus elective surgical procedures (Fahim et al., 2021). The surgeon's clinical specialty (e.g., general surgeon, acute care surgeon, surgical oncologist) and previous experience managing colorectal emergencies may play a significant role in determining which patients are selected for surgical intervention and how MBOs are surgically managed (Shariff et al., 2022). The optimal surgical procedure is quick, safe, and effective in resolving the underlying cause of the obstruction (e.g., lysis of adhesions, hernia repair, detorsion) (Krouse, 2019). A common surgical approach is a diverting loop colostomy, which provides relief from the obstruction and time for the medical optimization of high-risk patients before proceeding with a definitive colon resection (Catena et al., 2019; Sullivan et al., 2024).

Nursing Management

The goals of nursing care are to alleviate symptoms (e.g., nausea, vomiting, pain) and guide patients who are at an increased risk for developing recurrent bowel obstruction. Proactive calls to patients can serve as an opportunity to review treatment plans for maintaining regular bowel function and allow nurses to identify patients presenting with possible early signs of obstruction (Jivraj et al., 2023). Nurses should actively triage patient symptoms and work with the clinical team to refer patients to the appropriate level of care (hospital admission vs. outpatient evaluation). Detailed nursing documentation provides the members of the clinical team with a clear timeline that tracks the progression of symptoms, prescribed medications, dietary intake, and the patient's response to treatment.

Nurses should also provide ongoing education for caregivers and patients at an increased risk for developing MBOs. The delivery of timely educational resources prepares them for self-management of persistent GI symptoms and provides a plan of treatment for maintaining regular bowel function. Patients and caregivers need clear information about the stage of the patient's disease, prognosis, and how it impacts the patient's risk of developing a recurrent MBO (Fackche & Johnston, 2021). Patients should avoid high-residue foods, such as raw fruits or vegetables, whole grains, seeds, and corn. Daily hydration goals with water should be established with modifications for patients with a history of heart failure and renal impairment to avoid fluid overload. Daily physical activity should also be encouraged, as tolerated, to enhance healthy bowel motility. The clinical team should be notified immediately if patients experience any difficulty passing gas or stool, severe abdominal pain or cramping, persistent nausea and vomiting, swelling of the abdomen, a decrease in appetite, fever and chills, or general weakness.

Summary

Acute bowel obstructions are life-threatening emergencies that require an interprofessional approach and timely intervention to restore healthy bowel motility and minimize the risk for complications across the trajectory of patient care. When developing a plan of treatment, oncology nurses must consider the patient's level of health at the time of diagnosis, interventions available to alleviate patient distress, and the patient's predicted life expectancy. Although the response to treatment for MBOs is often unpredictable, shared decision-making, clear communication about prognosis, and a comprehensive review of potential risks and benefits of all aspects of treatment are key to ensuring that the plan of care aligns with patient values and goals of care.

References

Catena, F., De Simone, B., Coccolini, F., Di Saverio, S., Sartelli, M., & Ansaloni, L. (2019). Bowel obstruction: A narrative review for all physicians. *World Journal of Emergency Surgery, 14,* 20. https://doi.org/10.1186/s13017-019-0240-7

Demarest, K., Lavu, H., Collins, E., & Batra, V. (2023). Comprehensive diagnosis and management of malignant bowel obstruction: A review. *Journal of Pain and Palliative Care Pharmacotherapy, 37*(1), 91–105. https://doi.org/10.1080/15360288.2022.2106012

Fackche, N.T., & Johnston, F.M. (2021). Malignant bowel obstruction. *Advances in Surgery, 55,* 35–48. https://doi.org/10.1016/j.yasu.2021.05.003

Fahim, M., Dijksman, L.M., Derksen, W.J.M., Bloemen, J.G., Biesma, D.H., & Smits, A.B. (2021). Prospective multicenter study of a new bowel obstruction treatment in colorectal surgery: Reduced morbidity and mortality. *European Journal of Surgical Oncology, 47*(9), 2414–2420. https://doi.org/10.1016/j.ejso.2021.05.010

Jackson, P., & Vigiola Cruz, M. (2018). Intestinal obstruction: Evaluation and management. *American Family Physician, 98*(6), 362–367. https://pubmed.ncbi.nlm.nih.gov/30215917

Jivraj, N., Lee, Y.C., Tinker, L., Bowering, V., Ferguson, S.E., Croke, J., ... Lheureux, S. (2023). Management of malignant bowel obstruction: An innovative proactive outpatient nurse-led model of care for patients with advanced gynecologic cancer. *Journal of Nursing Care Quality, 38*(1), 69–75. https://doi.org/10.1097/NCQ.0000000000000661

Johnson, W.R., & Hawkins, A.T. (2021). Large bowel obstruction. *Clinics in Colon and Rectal Surgery, 34*(4), 233–241. https://doi.org/10.1055/s-0041-1729927

Krouse, R.S. (2019). Malignant bowel obstruction. *Journal of Surgical Oncology, 120*(1), 74–77. https://doi.org/10.1002/jso.25451

Madariaga, A., Lau, J., Ghoshal, A., Dzierżanowski, T., Larkin, P., Sobocki, J., ... Lheureux, S. (2022). MASCC multidisciplinary evidence-based recommendations for the management of malignant bowel obstruction in advanced cancer. *Supportive Care in Cancer, 30*(6), 4711–4728. https://doi.org/10.1007/s00520-022-06889-8

Nelms, D.W., & Kann, B.R. (2021). Imaging modalities for evaluation of intestinal obstruction. *Clinics in Colon and Rectal Surgery, 34*(4), 205–218. https://doi.org/10.1055/s-0041-1729737

Patel, P.S., Fragkos, K., Keane, N., Wilkinson, D., Johnson, A., Chan, D., ... Di Caro, S. (2024). Nutritional care pathways in cancer patients with malignant bowel obstruction: A retrospective multicentre study. *Clinical Nutrition ESPEN, 59*, 118–125. https://doi.org/10.1016/j.clnesp.2023.11.018

Shariff, F., Bogach, J., Guidolin, K., & Nadler, A. (2022). Malignant bowel obstruction management over time: Are we doing anything new? A current narrative review. *Annals of Surgical Oncology, 29*(3), 1995–2005. https://doi.org/10.1245/s10434-021-10922-1

Sullivan, J., Donohue, A., & Brown, S. (2024). Colorectal oncologic emergencies: Recognition, management, and outcomes. *Surgical Clinics of North America, 104*(3), 631–646. https://doi.org/10.1016/j.suc.2023.12.003

Yu, K., Liu, L., Zhang, X., Zhang, Z., Rao, B., Chen, Y., ... Shi, H. (2020). Surgical and conservative management of malignant bowel obstruction: Outcome and prognostic factors. *Cancer Management and Research, 12*, 7797–7803. https://doi.org/10.2147/CMAR.S256219

Allison Mitchell, BSN, RN, OCN®,
and Brenda S. Nettles, DNP, MS, ACNP-BC, AOCNP®, CNE

CHAPTER 5

Urinary Obstruction

FAST FACTS

- **Description:** A urinary obstruction is a structural or functional disorder that negatively impacts the urinary system's ability to function properly. The most common causes of obstructive uropathy are tumors, stones, strictures, and clots. Early identification of the underlying cause and timely intervention are key to minimizing the risk of long-term effects on the urinary system.
- **Incidence:** Prostate and bladder cancers are the most common malignancies to cause urinary obstructions. Acute kidney injuries are a frequent complication of cancer-related obstructions and affect up to 50% of patients during the course of cancer treatment.
- **Clinical Manifestations:** The severity of symptoms associated with obstructive uropathy will depend on the location of the obstruction in the urinary tract. The clinical presentation may include signs of infection, pain, electrolyte imbalances, and changes in kidney or cardiac function.
- **Risk Factors and Etiology:** Risk factors include known kidney or cardiac disorders, increased age, prior radiation treatments, blockage, kidney tumors, and blood clots. The etiology depends on the location of the urinary obstruction.
- **Pathophysiology and Patient Evaluation:** An evaluation of kidney function includes a complete metabolic panel, complete blood count, and urinalysis. Diagnostic testing consists of a renal ultrasound, computed tomography scan of the abdomen and pelvis, magnetic resonance imaging of the abdomen, and retrograde or antegrade pyelography. The disease process of urinary obstructions disrupts normal physiology, leading to hemodynamic alterations and functional impairment.
- **Advanced Practice Considerations:** A comprehensive evaluation of urinary obstructions includes executing proper diagnostic imaging to determine the location of obstruction, laboratory testing, treating the cause of obstruction, and monitoring associated symptoms with the specific obstruction.
- **Treatment Modalities:** Treatment depends on the level of obstruction or urinary damage, symptoms associated with obstruction, and whether kidney and urinary tract function can be preserved.
- **Nursing Management:** Nurses should notify the clinical team of signs of infection, monitor electrolytes, and report signs of decline in renal function. They should also provide support as patients cope with the complex care required to manage urologic obstructions.
- **Outcomes:** The outcomes of treatment will vary based on the underlying cause of obstruction, the patient's level of health, and overall prognosis. Oncology care team members and patients must collaborate to develop a plan that includes treatments aligned with the patient's preferences and goals for care.

Introduction

The primary function of the genitourinary system is to transport urine from the kidneys through the ureters and into the bladder and urethra. The kidneys play a vital role in regulating blood pressure, eliminating toxins, and helping with electrolyte balance. The most common causes of obstructive uropathy are tumors, stones, strictures, and clots. Additional contributing factors may include prostate enlargement from cancer and functional disorders such as neurogenic bladder. If left untreated, genitourinary obstructions can become life threatening. Treatment strategies depend on the underlying cause of the obstruction and should be tailored accordingly.

Urinary tract obstructions can happen at any point along the genitourinary tract (see Figure 5-1) and are categorized as upper or lower urinary tract obstructions. Upper urinary tract obstructions involve the kidneys and ureters and can lead to acute or chronic renal failure, depending on the location. In contrast, lower urinary tract obstructions affect the bladder, bladder neck, prostate, or urethra. These obstructions are commonly associated with acute urinary retention and lower abdominal pain, and they may present as a sudden or complete inability to void.

FIGURE 5-1. Anatomy of the Genitourinary System

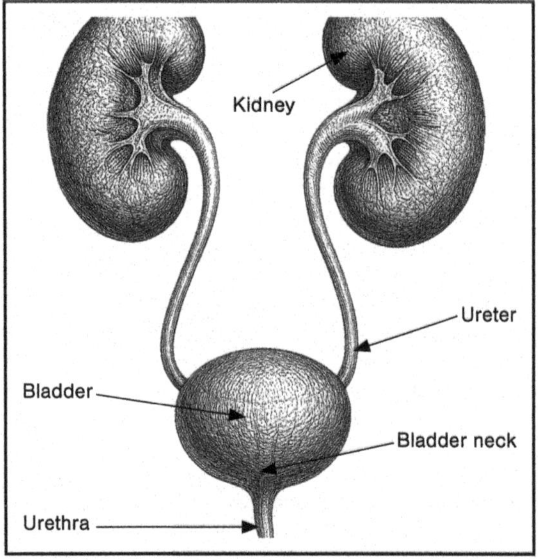

Incidence

Prostate and bladder cancers are the two most common malignancies associated with the development of urinary tract obstructions. Obstructions caused by advanced bladder cancer are associated with a poor prognosis (Habas et al., 2023). Acute kidney injury (AKI) is a significant complication associated with the development of urinary obstructions and has an estimated global incidence of 13.3 million annually (Habas et al., 2023). Older adult patients diagnosed with cancer have an increased risk of developing AKI within the first year following diagnosis (Habas et al., 2023). Despite the high prevalence of AKI in both the hospital and the outpatient settings, the exact incidence of urinary tract obstruction as a primary cause remains uncertain (Pérez-Aizpurua et al., 2024). Overall, AKI is a common complication in patients with cancer, affecting up to 50% during their illness (Habas et al., 2023).

Clinical Manifestations

It can be challenging to diagnose urinary tract obstructions because symptoms may mirror the clinical presentation of other oncologic emergencies. Clinical manifestations depend on the location of the obstruction and commonly include flank pain, nausea, vomiting, hematuria, and painful urination. Additional symptoms may include frequency and urgency of the urine stream, weak or interrupted stream, and incomplete emptying in the bladder and urethra. Flank pain and dysuria are common but may not always be present with the gradual onset of obstruction. Other manifestations can include blood pressure fluctuations (high vs. low), electrolyte imbalances, decreased urinary output, changes in the ability to void, decreased kidney function, and signs of infection. Urine output may present as normal in a partial obstruction. Ongoing surveillance of patient symptoms throughout their clinical course can assist the clinical team in identifying the type of obstruction and monitoring for progression in renal impairment.

Risk Factors and Etiology

The risk factors for urinary obstructions are blockage, blood clots, compression, kidney tumors, crystallization in renal tubules, and strictures (Habas et al., 2023). These factors can also increase AKI risk and may manifest as sinusoidal obstruction syndrome, tumor lysis syndrome, or thrombotic microangiopathy (Cosmai et al., 2021). Additional risk factors for urinary obstructions are increased age, hypotension, congestive heart failure, vascular disease, chronic kidney disease, sepsis, hypovolemia, prior surgeries, and previous radiation therapy. Radiation can cause scar tissue, which increases the risk of obstructions. Adverse side effects, such as diarrhea and vomiting caused by malignancies and specific chemotherapy agents, also increase risks for dehydration and AKI (Habas et al., 2023). Kidney tumors, calculi, and upper tract bleeding can cause some upper urinary tract obstructions. Lower urinary tract obstructions can be caused by prostatitis, benign prostatic hyperplasia, tumors, and neurogenic bladder (Yaxley & Yaxley, 2023).

Pathophysiology and Patient Evaluation

The primary role of the urinary tract is to excrete urine and toxins from the body. The urinary tract system comprises the kidneys, ureters, and bladder. The kidneys play a vital role in urine formation. Their function is to ensure an optimal environment for tissue and cell metabolism (Huether et al., 2026). The kidneys eliminate metabolic waste products, balance water and electrolytes in the blood, maintain acid-base balance, and conserve nutrients. These organs also contribute critically to blood pressure regulation and erythrocyte production. The bladder stores the urine by way of the ureters until the urine is ready to be expelled from the bladder through the urethra (Huether et al., 2026).

Mechanisms Contributing to Urinary Tract Obstructions

Urinary obstructions can affect multiple organ systems, leading to hemodynamic, structural, and functional changes (Pérez-Aizpurua et al., 2024). Hemodynamic changes may vary depending on the location of the obstruction. In response to elevated intratubular pressure, the kidneys increase renal blood flow through the release of intrinsic prostaglandin E2 to help maintain an adequate glomerular filtration rate (Pérez-Aizpurua et al., 2024). Upper urinary tract obstructions cause dilation of the ureter, renal pelvis, and renal parenchyma next to the site of blocked urine from urine backflow (Huether et al., 2026). As the pressure increases, this leads to hydronephrosis and further dilation of the urinary tract. Elevated intratubular pressure causes interstitial expansion of the kidney's extracellular matrix, triggering inflammation and cellular apoptosis (Pérez-Aizpurua et al., 2024).

Urinary obstruction also impacts aquaporin tubular channels responsible for water transport. In this context, water transport is downregulated, leading to post-obstructive polyuria and impairing the kidney to reabsorb water and concentrate urine (Pérez-Aizpurua et al., 2024). Sodium levels are similarly disrupted. Kidney function can begin to decline within just one day of obstruction onset, resulting in increased natriuresis or salt-wasting due to the kidney's inability to reabsorb sodium (Pérez-Aizpurua et al., 2024). Additionally, hyperkalemia may develop as a result of decreased glomerular filtration rate from impaired blood flow, which reduces potassium filtration and excretion. Hyperkalemia is one of the most critical electrolyte imbalances and can be life threatening. Early identification is essential to preventing severe outcomes.

Clinical Assessment

Nurses are instrumental in gathering pertinent medical information and reviewing the patient's previous medical history to help the clinical team gain deeper insight into the current health concerns. Review of past medical history may include a positive history of previous renal or urinary tract obstructions, cancer, active kidney disease, or cardiac symptoms. Additional pertinent history may consist of recent urinary tract infections, prior history of Foley catheter insertion, current use of nephrostomy tubes, stent placements, previous kidney stones, and a record of chemotherapy or radiation therapy during cancer treatment. When evaluating a male patient, it is also important to rule out a previous history of benign prostate disease, such as an enlarged prostate, which may also impact the patient's ability to empty their bladder. The clinical team then uses this information to develop a comprehensive treatment plan that aligns with the patient's values and goals during this oncologic emergency.

Patients with upper urinary tract obstructions typically present with flank pain associated with renal colic (Pérez-Aizpurua et al., 2024). Obstructions leading to bacterial overgrowth in retained urine can increase infectious complications often associated with fever and other signs of infection (Pérez-Aizpurua et al., 2024). In bladder outlet obstruction, acute urinary retention is common and may present as a palpable, tender suprapubic mass. Anuria is more frequently observed in cases involving trigonal invasion by pelvic malignancies, particularly prostate and bladder cancers, and, less commonly, in bilateral obstruction or obstruction in a solitary kidney (Pérez-Aizpurua et al., 2024). Nurses must also assess for signs of Foley catheter malfunction, including patient discomfort, irritation, inflammation at the insertion site, and decreased urine output.

Physical assessment should include an evaluation of both cardiac and renal function. As part of a general assessment, nurses should monitor for signs of decreased cardiac output, such as fluid retention, hypotension, tachycardia, or chest discomfort. Cardiac symptoms often influence renal and urinary function, potentially contributing to obstructions. Areas of concern include fluid retention in the extremities, abdomen, or distended jugular veins. Nurses and caregivers should monitor for any signs of urinary retention, decreased urine output, or hematuria. Nurses should also ask patients about feelings of urinary retention despite voiding. In cases where urinary obstruction is suspected, monitoring potassium levels is essential.

Advanced Practice Considerations

A comprehensive physical examination, laboratory testing, and diagnostic imaging are essential for identifying the type of urinary tract obstruction. A complete metabolic panel should be ordered to monitor for shifts in potassium and sodium levels, which are commonly associated with this oncologic emergency. Detecting electrolyte imbalances can help nurses and providers assess for other potential signs of impaired renal function, such as changes in blood urea nitrogen, creatinine, and glomerular filtration rate. A complete blood count is used to screen for possible leukocytosis, which may indicate infection, and for reduced hemoglobin levels that could suggest blood loss or anemia. Figure 5-2 summarizes specific signs and symptoms associated with hyperkalemia and hyponatremia.

Renal ultrasounds are a less invasive imaging technique and are commonly used for imaging during the initial evaluation of a suspected urinary tract obstruction (Pérez-Aizpurua et al., 2024). Following ultrasonography, a noncontrast computed tomography (CT) scan is the most important diagnostic tool for confirming obstructive uropathy (Pérez-Aizpurua et al., 2024). A CT scan of the abdomen and pelvis with IV contrast may be used; however, it is contraindicated in patients with elevated creatinine levels because of the risks associated with iodinated contrast material (Yaxley & Yaxley, 2023). Although noncontrast CT scans are helpful, they may not detect common causes of obstruction, including urinary stones. In these cases, additional imaging may be warranted, such as multidetector CT scans (Pérez-Aizpurua et al., 2024). Figure 5-3 provides a detailed summary of the additional laboratory tests and diagnostic imaging recommended for the clinical evaluation of urinary obstructions.

FIGURE 5-2. Patient Evaluation for Urinary Tract Obstructions

Review of Patient History	Laboratory Testing	Signs of Infection	Cardiac Symptoms Associated With Fluid Retention
• Current or previous history of heart disease • Current or prior history of kidney disease • Recent placement of urinary catheter, nephrostomy placement, trauma • Recent urinary tract infection • Medications that may cause electrolyte abnormalities • Medications that can elevate potassium – Beta-blockers – Nonsteroidal anti-inflammatory drugs – Anti-mineralocorticoids	• Monitor kidney function trends. – Elevated creatinine levels that occur in chronic kidney disease or in individuals with one kidney – Decreased glomerular filtration rate or patients taking potassium-sparing medications • Monitor for concerning electrolyte trends and notify the provider. – Elevated potassium levels (hyperkalemia) * Nausea and vomiting * Fatigue * Irritability * Confusion * Irregular pulse * Heart palpitations * Muscle weakness * Muscle cramps * Loss of muscle tone * Tetany – Low sodium levels (hyponatremia): urinary sodium and fractional excretion of sodium (Urine sodium < 20 mEq/mol and fractional excretion of sodium < 1% are markers of prerenal cause of acute kidney injury.) * Dry mucous membranes * Signs of increased intracranial pressure * Muscle cramps * Muscle twitching * Dyspnea on exertion * Diminished turgor * Tachycardia * Hypotension	• Monitor for signs of infection. – Fever – Chills – Foul-smelling urine – Cloudy urine – Painful urination – Flank pain – Confusion • If the patient has a urinary catheter, monitor for the following: – Redness, warmth, or irritation near the catheter site – Yellow, green, bloody, or cloudy urinary output	• Hypertension • Reduced cardiac output • Severe shortness of breath • Decreased urine output • Abdominal swelling • Swelling in extremities

Note. Based on information from Cavusoglu et al., 2019; Harding et al., 2023; Pérez-Aizpurua et al., 2024.

FIGURE 5-3. Evaluation of Urinary Obstruction

Laboratory Testing	Diagnostic Imaging
• Complete blood count (CBC) – White blood cell (WBC) – Red blood cell (RBC) – Hemoglobin (Hgb) – Hematocrit (Hct) – Platelets (Plts) • Comprehensive metabolic panel (CMP) – Creatinine (Cr) – Blood urea nitrogen (BUN) – Sodium (Na+) – Potassium (K+) – Chloride (Cl) – Bicarbonate (HC03-) – Lactate level • Urinalysis – Color – Clarity – pH – Specific gravity – Glucose – Blood – Ketones – Nitrites – Leukocytes – Erythrocytes • Urine culture – Detection of bacteria and other organisms in the urine – Sensitivity testing to test susceptibility to antibiotics	• Renal ultrasound • Computed tomography (CT) scan • Magnetic resonance imaging (MRI) • IV urography • Voiding cystourethrogram (VCUG) • Cystoscopy

Note. Based on information from Pérez-Aizpurua et al., 2024.

Treatment Modalities

The primary goal in treating urinary obstructions is to restore healthy urine flow. Early detection is essential to preserve renal function and minimize the risk for complications, such as AKI and urinary sepsis. Renal ultrasounds and CT scans assist clinicians in identifying the location (upper vs. lower) and the severity (complete vs. partial) of the obstruction (Pérez-Aizpurua et al., 2024). The placement of percutaneous nephrostomy tubes or retrograde ureteral stents is recommended for the management of upper urinary obstructions and bladder outlet obstructions that cannot be effectively managed by directly draining the bladder (Lipe et al., 2021). Figure 5-4 shows a CT scan of the abdomen and pelvis following placement of a nephrostomy tube into the right kidney. Post-procedure complications may include catheter displacement, bleeding, urinary tract infections, and skin infections at the insertion site. Maintaining percutaneous

FIGURE 5-4. Placement of Nephrostomy Tube for Ureteral Obstruction

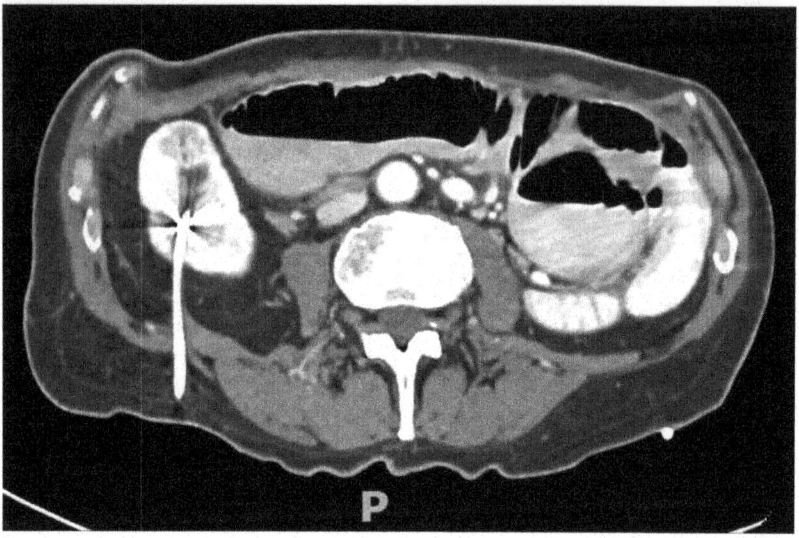

Axial computed tomography scan showing a nephrostomy tube inserted into the right kidney

nephrostomy tube patency involves flushing the catheter with sterile saline. Exchange is indicated if the patient develops signs of infection or recurrent obstruction. Although the placement of a retrograde ureteral stent is an equally effective intervention for addressing ureteral obstruction, post-procedure hematuria and dysuria may negatively affect the quality of life of patients with a limited life expectancy (Zul Khairul Azwadi et al., 2021).

Lower urinary tract obstructions are associated with incomplete bladder emptying due to bladder dysfunction or structural narrowing that limits urinary outflow. These acute obstructions require prompt bladder decompression and are commonly managed with intermittent sterile catheterization, indwelling urinary catheters, or the placement of an indwelling suprapubic cystostomy (Billet & Windsor, 2019). Potential complications of this procedure include catheter-associated urinary tract infections and hematuria. Referrals for a formal urologic surgery evaluation are recommended to address chronic conditions, such as benign prostatic hypertrophy, atrophic vaginitis, or pelvic organ prolapse (Billet & Windsor, 2019).

Nursing Management

Reviewing Symptoms

Nurses must monitor patients with urinary tract obstructions through general assessments, laboratory evaluations, and vital sign recording. A general assessment is essential for detecting signs of hemodynamic instability, symptoms related to urosepsis, or the rapid onset of complications related to obstruction (Pérez-Aizpurua et al., 2024). Assessments should include close monitoring of cardiac, respiratory, and renal function. Key cardiac indicators include hypertension or hypotension, shortness of breath, peripheral edema, and heart palpitations resulting from fluid overload due to impaired renal filtration. Peripheral edema, abdominal ascites, and distended jugular veins should be closely observed during cardiac assessments. Rapid progression of swelling and fluid retention is concerning and warrants notification of the clinical team.

Nurses should also report any changes in respiratory status, including worsening shortness of breath, oxygen saturation below 95%, shallow breathing, or respiratory complications associated with ascites. Patients should be educated on when to report worsening respiratory function to their care team. Any alteration in breathing should be treated as an emergency, and patients should be advised to seek immediate care. If temporary respiratory treatments or medications are given and fail to provide relief, further evaluation is necessary to identify the underlying cause. Respiratory symptoms may be caused by multiple factors, such as impaired cardiac function or AKI related to fluid retention.

A fever and associated symptoms must be monitored throughout the clinical course. Classic indicators of infection are fever, malaise, and chills. Nurses should promptly notify the provider of any concerning fever trends. If urosepsis is determined, immediate antibiotic treatment should be initiated, either through broad-spectrum or pathogen-directed coverage in cases of previous positive cultures (Pérez-Aizpurua et al., 2024). Regular catheter site assessments are required for proactive measures to minimize infection risk complications, as catheters increase the likelihood of infection.

Monitoring for Laboratory Abnormalities

Electrolyte imbalances must be closely monitored because of alterations in kidney function. Potassium and sodium levels are key areas of concern. Hyperkalemia can be life threatening if not identified and treated promptly. Critical signs to monitor are muscle weakness, nausea, flaccid muscle paralysis, and heart palpitations (Ellison & Farrar, 2018). Life-threatening cardiac complications, such as cardiac arrest, can be caused by serum potassium levels less than 2.5 mEq/L or greater than 7 mEq/L (Ellison & Farrar, 2018). Hyperkalemia may also result from oncologic emergencies, such as tumor lysis syndrome. Nurses should carefully review patients' current medication list to identify drug classes that may cause potassium-sparing effects, including anti-mineralocorticoids, beta-blockers, and nonsteroidal anti-inflammatory drugs (Pérez-Aizpurua et al., 2024). Hyponatremia is another critical electrolyte disturbance to monitor carefully, often associated with fluid retention. Signs and symptoms may include headaches, confusion, increased intracranial pressure, seizures, atrial fibrillation, tachycardia, and hypotension (Ellison & Farrar, 2018). In the event of seizures, it is essential to implement seizure precautions and treat the underlying cause. Overall, nurses are key in communicating detailed observations and providing timely updates to the clinical team regarding any changes in the patient's condition.

Patient and Caregiver Education

Nurses are responsible for educating patients and caregivers about the signs and symptoms of urinary tract obstructions. The symptoms may be challenging to identify, as they are often associated with other common medical conditions. Still, patients and caregivers should be advised to promptly notify their care team of any changes in clinical status. Although it may be overwhelming for patients to understand the various roles within the healthcare team, having a basic awareness of whom to contact will facilitate timely access to care when health concerns arise. For this reason, patients and their caregivers must know how to contact their healthcare team during the day and how to access care outside of regular hours. Immediate evaluation may be necessary if patients are suddenly unable to void or experience other complications associated with their catheters, stents, or nephrostomy tubes. It is important to ensure that they are well prepared to maintain these devices at home and that they know when to seek emergency care for further evaluation. Figure 5-5 provides a summary of important details that patients and caregivers should report to the clinical care team and instruction to use the teach-back method to ensure patient understanding.

FIGURE 5-5. Patient and Caregiver Education

Important Details to Report to Clinical Care Team	Progression of Clinical Symptoms	Education on How to Contact Clinical Care Team
• Previous history of cardiac and kidney disease • Recent urinary tract infections • Previous Foley catheter, stent, or nephrostomy tube • Medication history	• Worsening of swelling during a 24-hour period • Reduction in total urinary output • Urine retention despite voiding • Changes in urine appearance • Worsening of pain symptoms • Increasing shortness of breath • Signs and symptoms of urinary tract infection • Patients with long-term Foley catheter, stents, or nephrostomy tubes should be monitored for the following: – New onset or persistent abdominal or back pain – Malfunctioning of device – Signs and symptoms of infection – Reduced or lack of urinary output • Signs and symptoms associated with hyperkalemia and hyponatremia	• Advise patients and caregivers on how to contact the clinical care team, including information on office hours, office contact numbers, and the process for contacting the on-call provider. • Contact information should be posted in a convenient location. • Educate about which signs and symptoms require urgent evaluation and when to proceed to the emergency department. • Use the teach-back method to confirm understanding.

Note. Based on information from Pérez-Aizpurua et al., 2024.

Summary

A urinary obstruction is a condition that causes a blockage or interruption in the healthy flow of urine. It is a common clinical problem encountered by all medical specialties. However, as more individuals are diagnosed with cancer, clinical teams must be especially prepared to offer timely interventions for this potentially life-threatening emergency. Significant health risks associated with urinary obstruction include electrolyte imbalances, renal and cardiac dysfunction, urosepsis, and complications related to the underlying cause of the obstruction. Early symptom recognition is critical to reducing the risk of long-term renal impairment. Nurses, advanced practice providers, and physicians are responsible for educating patients about their medical condition and providing clear explanations about the available treatment options. Educating patients and caregivers about the common symptoms of urinary obstruction empowers them to access timely and appropriate care.

References

Billet, M., & Windsor, T.A. (2019). Urinary retention. *Emergency Medicine Clinics of North America, 37*(4), 649–660. https://doi.org/10.1016/j.emc.2019.07.005

Cavusoglu, Y., Kaya, H., Eraslan, S., & Yilmaz, M.B. (2019). Hyponatremia is associated with occurrence of atrial fibrillation in outpatients with heart failure and reduced ejection fraction. *Hellenic Journal of Cardiology, 60*(2), 117–121. https://doi.org/10.1016/j.hjc.2018.03.006

Cosmai, L., Porta, C., Foramitti, M., Perrone, V., Mollica, L., Gallieni, M., & Capasso, G. (2021). Preventive strategies for acute kidney injury in cancer patients. *Clinical Kidney Journal, 14*(1), 70–83. https://doi.org/10.1093/ckj/sfaa127

Ellison, D., & Farrar, F.C. (2018). Kidney influence on fluid and electrolyte balance. *Nursing Clinics of North America, 53*(4), 469–480. https://doi.org/10.1016/j.cnur.2018.05.004

Habas, E., Akbar, R., Farfar, K., Arrayes, N., Habas, A., Rayani, A., ... Elzouki, A.-N. (2023). Malignancy diseases and kidneys: A nephrologist prospect and updated review. *Medicine, 102*(15). https://doi.org/10.1097/md.0000000000033505

Harding, M.M., Kwong, J., Hagler, D., & Reinisch, C. (2023). *Lewis's medical-surgical nursing: Assessment and management of clinical problems* (12th ed.). Elsevier.

Huether, S.E., McCance, K.L., & Brashers, V.L. (2026). *Understanding pathophysiology* (8th ed.). Elsevier.

Lipe, D.N., Mann, P.B., Babakhanlou, R., Cruz Carreras, M.T., Guido Hita, A., & Wattana, M.K. (2021). Evaluation and management of genitourinary emergencies in patients with cancer. *Emergency Medicine International, 2021*(1), 4511968. https://doi.org/10.1155/2021/4511968

Pérez-Aizpurua, X., Benavente, R.C., Serrano, G.B., Peral, J.M.A., Mañas, B.G.-J., Jaumot, J.T., ... Gonzalez-Enguita, C. (2024). Obstructive uropathy: Overview of the pathogenesis, etiology and management of a prevalent cause of acute kidney injury. *World Journal of Nephrology, 13*(2), 93322. https://doi.org/10.5527/wjn.v13.i2.93322

Yaxley, J., & Yaxley, W. (2023). Obstructive uropathy – Acute and chronic medical management. *World Journal of Nephrology, 12*(1), 1–9. https://doi.org/10.5527/wjn.v12.i1.1

Zul Khairul Azwadi, I., Norhayati, M.N., & Abdullah, M.S. (2021). Percutaneous nephrostomy versus retrograde ureteral stenting for acute upper obstructive uropathy: A systematic review and meta-analysis. *Scientific Reports, 11*(1), 6613. https://doi.org/10.1038/s41598-021-86136-y

Jennifer C. Myers, DNP, MSN, RN, ANP-BC,
and Lisa Feldsien, BSN, RN, OCN®

CHAPTER 6

Spinal Cord Compression

FAST FACTS

- **Description:** Spinal cord compression occurs when a tumor invades or extends into the epidural space or pathologically collapsed vertebral bone fragments impinge on the spinal cord.
- **Incidence:** This complication is most often associated with solid tumors that metastasize—including lung, breast, and prostate cancers—as well as with multiple myeloma and lymphoma. Up to 15% of patients with cancer experience spinal cord compression during their disease process.
- **Clinical Manifestations:** Back pain is the earliest symptom, often presenting weeks before the diagnosis. It is often aggravated and potentially worsened by standing, sitting, moving, or any activity that causes straining of the back muscles (e.g., coughing, sneezing, bowel movements). If left untreated, the symptoms may progress to increasing neurologic injury and loss of functional independence, resulting in motor weakness, sensory loss, autonomic dysfunction (i.e., incontinence), and permanent paralysis.
- **Risk Factors and Etiology:** Risk factors in the development of spinal cord compression include a history of breast, prostate, or lung cancer; multiple myeloma; or non-Hodgkin lymphoma.
- **Pathophysiology and Patient Evaluation:** Spinal cord compression occurs when a malignant mass or a pathologically collapsed vertebra compresses the spinal cord or its extension, the cauda equina, resulting in a loss of sensation or motor function.
- **Advanced Practice Considerations:** Advanced practice providers should consider spinal cord compression in any patient presenting with new-onset back or radicular pain and who manifests high-risk factors (e.g., long-time smokers) or those with a prior history of cancer. Magnetic resonance imaging of the entire spine is the preferred imaging modality.
- **Treatment Modalities:** Corticosteroids are the initial treatment for all patients who are symptomatic. Definitive therapy follows decompressive surgery and spinal stabilization or radiation therapy, as indicated.
- **Nursing Management:** Nurses must coordinate care related to pain relief, prevention of injuries, mobility and safety issues, bladder and bowel dysfunction, and rehabilitation to maximize and restore function. They should also provide patient and caregiver education, give emotional support, and prepare patients for discharge to home or hospice care.
- **Outcomes:** Prompt recognition, diagnosis, and treatment are essential to preventing irreversible loss of function and paralysis. Nurses must maintain a high index of suspicion for this complication, especially following reports of new-onset back pain.

Introduction

The World Health Organization estimates that by the year 2040, approximately 29.4 million new cases of cancer will be diagnosed (Van den Brande et al., 2022).

Metastatic spinal cord compression (MSCC), a devastating consequence of cancer progression, was first described in 1925 by Spiller et al. as "rapidly progressive paralysis associated with carcinoma" (Crommett, 2019). It is considered a true oncologic emergency because, without early recognition and intervention, it can progress to intractable pain, irreversible loss of neurologic function, and death. Metastases to the spine occur in 3%–5% of all patients who have cancer and are common with breast, prostate, and lung malignancies, with the latter demonstrating an incidence rate of approximately 19% (Hawkins et al., 2023). MSCC occurs when a malignant mass or a pathologically collapsed vertebra compresses the spinal cord or its extension, the cauda equina. It traditionally presents as progressive pain followed by the development of neurologic deficits as the nerve roots or spinal cord become more compressed by the tumor (Weber-Levine et al., 2025). Although metastatic bone involvement can occur late in the course of the disease process, it can also be an initial manifestation of malignancy (Esperança-Martins et al., 2023). Survival rates for MSCC are poor, with 10% of patients surviving 18 months after initial diagnosis (Vassiliou et al., 2023).

Back pain is an early and sensitive indicator of MSCC and occurs in approximately 95% of patients (Crommett, 2019). However, acute back pain is a common and nonspecific symptom, and its significance is often missed. The connection between back pain and previous cancer history or the realization that back pain may represent the initial manifestation of cancer may not be realized until neurologic function has been irreparably compromised (Esperança-Martins et al., 2023). The more time that elapses without appropriate treatment for MSCC, the lower the likelihood of neurologic recovery (Esperança-Martins et al., 2023).

The natural course of untreated MSCC is one of increasing neurologic injury and loss of functional independence that typically occurs along a continuum, beginning with back pain and progressing to motor weakness, sensory loss, autonomic dysfunction, and, ultimately, permanent paralysis (Esperança-Martins et al., 2023; Kaplow & Webster, 2022). The prevalence of MSCC has increased due to treatment advances that have extended the survival of patients with cancer. The goals of treatment are palliative pain relief, local tumor control, treatment of spinal cord instability, and prevention of irreversible neurologic deficits (Weber-Levine et al., 2025).

Incidence

An estimated 20,000 new cases of MSCC are diagnosed annually in the United States, with peak incidence occurring among adults with a median age of 50–65 years (Shah et al., 2021; Vavourakis et al., 2024). The incidence rate of spinal cord compression may be as high as 15%–20% of all cancer cases, with spinal metastases found in up to 40% of patients with terminal cancer (Weber-Levine et al., 2025). MSCC occurs with lung cancer (31%), breast cancer (24%), gastrointestinal tract cancer (9%), prostate cancer (8%), lymphoma (6%), melanoma (4%), and kidney cancer (1%) (Vavourakis et al., 2024). Cancers associated with lower or rare incidences of MSCC are colorectal cancer, soft tissue sarcoma, head and neck cancers, and cancers of the esophagus, thyroid, or bladder.

Clinical Manifestations

Clinical manifestations of MSCC follow a similar sequence in all patients regardless of the origin of the malignancy. The earliest symptom is typically back pain, which often precedes the diagnosis of MSCC by two to five months (Crommett, 2019; Narang et al., 2020). Back pain will progress to severe and unremitting; often aggravated by standing, sitting, moving, or participating in an activity that causes straining of the back muscles (e.g., coughing, sneezing, bowel movements). Symptoms will progress sequentially to motor weakness resulting in gait disturbances and limb weakness, sensory loss (e.g., paraesthesia, numbness), autonomic dysfunction (e.g., sphincter disturbance, loss of bladder and bowel control), and finally, irreversible paralysis (Hawkins et al., 2023). Early recognition and intervention are crucial to preventing progression to permanent and devastating disability, loss of functional independence, and death. Table 6-1 outlines the clinical manifestations and types of cancers associated with the various levels of spinal involvement.

Back Pain

Back pain is the hallmark manifestation of MSCC, and it is often the presenting symptom in 80%–95% of diagnosed patients (Crommett, 2019; Lawton et al., 2019). When associated with MSCC, back pain can take several forms: local (near the site of compression), radicular (radiating along dermatomes), or referred (in a nonradicular distribution), or a combination of these features (Marino & Kaplow, 2025). The most common spinal level of MSCC is in the thoracic spine (60%–80%), followed by the lumbar spine (15%–30%), and then the cervical spine (< 10%), with multilevel involvement seen in up to 50% of all patients (Narang et al., 2020).

New-onset back pain in patients with a history of cancer is highly specific, and spinal metastasis should be considered until proven otherwise (Crommett, 2019). A careful history, coupled with a comprehensive neurologic examination and spinal imaging procedures, is essential to ensure an early diagnosis. A timely assessment is compulsory, as the median time from pain onset to diagnosis of MSCC is two months (Crommett, 2019).

Local Pain

Local pain may be described as aching, burning, or shooting, and it may be accompanied by progressive numbness, which increases in severity with time (Kaplow & Webster, 2022). This distribution of pain may also extend to the arms, legs, lower back, or buttocks. Many patients experience the greatest pain intensity when waking in the morning and report that sleeping in a sitting position provides some relief (Lawton et al., 2019). This is a unique identifier that may help to distinguish the pain of MSCC from the pain of degenerative disc disease.

If the spinal cord becomes unstable from bone destruction or a compression fracture, the back pain becomes more severe (Kaplow & Webster, 2022). Tenderness in the affected area upon percussion may also be reported.

TABLE 6-1
Etiology and Clinical Manifestations of Spinal Cord Compression by Spinal Level

Spinal Level and Incidence	Malignancy	Pain Characteristics	Potential Clinical Manifestations
Cervical spine (10%)	Head and neck Melanoma Lung (Pancoast tumor) Lymphoma	Occipital headache Radicular pain in the neck, shoulder, or arm May be exacerbated by neck flexion Neck stiffness	Lesion at or above C4: diaphragmatic weakness/paralysis (unilateral or bilateral) and respiratory insufficiency Weakness, spasticity, and wasting of neck, shoulder, and arm muscles; in time progressing to opposite arm and legs Neurogenic shock: hypotension, bradycardia, peripheral vasodilation Quadriplegia Paresthesias and sensory loss for position, vibration, and temperature in areas of weakness Lhermitte sign: electric tingling sensation down the back and upper/lower extremities on neck flexion/extension Horner syndrome: constricted pupil, upper eyelid droop, loss of sweating on affected side of face (with C8 involvement) Reflexes: hyperactive deep tendon reflexes, extensor plantar response (positive Babinski sign) Autonomic effects: late onset; bladder, bowel, and sexual dysfunction; risk of autonomic hyperreflexia; hypertension, bradycardia, pounding headache, profuse sweating; autoregulation mechanisms interrupted by spinal lesion

(Continued on next page)

TABLE 6-1
Etiology and Clinical Manifestations of Spinal Cord Compression by Spinal Level *(Continued)*

Spinal Level and Incidence	Malignancy	Pain Characteristics	Potential Clinical Manifestations
Thoracic spine (70%)	Breast Lung Lymphoma Multiple myeloma Pancreas Esophagus	Local or radicular pain, or both, in the chest and back	Weakness of abdominal muscles; arm muscles spared Lower extremity weakness or paralysis (low T-spine lesion) Band-like paresthesia around the waist Decreased sensation below the level of the lesion, increased above Reflexes: increased deep tendon reflexes distal to the lesion, extensor plantar response, Beevor sign Autonomic effects: late onset; bladder, bowel, and sexual dysfunction; risk of autonomic hyperreflexia with lesion at or above T6
Lower thoracic spine levels	Prostate Colon Renal		
Lumbosacral spine (20%)	Prostate Renal cell Ovarian	Local or radicular pain, or both, in the groin region or sciatic distribution in legs	Weakness in pelvic muscles Weakness to paralysis in lower extremities, with muscle atrophy; ataxic gait Numbness, paresthesia, sensory loss in the lower extremities Reflexes: decreased to absent knee and ankle reflexes; extensor plantar response Autonomic effects: bladder, bowel, and sexual dysfunction

(Continued on next page)

TABLE 6-1
Etiology and Clinical Manifestations of Spinal Cord Compression by Spinal Level *(Continued)*

Spinal Level and Incidence	Malignancy	Pain Characteristics	Potential Clinical Manifestations
Lower lumbrosacral spine levels	Colon Uterine Cervix	Pain on straight leg raising	Conus medullaris syndrome • Muscle weakness; fasciculations in lower extremities; spasticity possible • Saddle anesthesia: numbness in the buttocks, thighs, and perineum • Reflexes: preserved knee jerk; decreased or absent ankle and plantar reflexes; preservation of bulbocavernosus and anal reflexes • Autonomic effects: early onset; urinary retention and overflow incontinence; bowel incontinence; impotence
Cauda equina	Prostate Bladder Renal Colorectal Uterine Cervical	Local, radicular, or referred pain in the back and legs	Cauda equina syndrome • Muscle weakness, flaccidity (foot drop)/paralysis in lower extremities • Saddle anesthesia: numbness in the buttocks, thighs, and perineum • Reflexes: decreased to absent knee, ankle, plantar, bulbocavernosus, and anal reflexes • Autonomic effects: early onset; urinary retention and overflow incontinence; constipation; impotence

Note. Based on information from Laufer et al., 2024; Vavourakis et al., 2024.

Radicular Pain

Radicular pain, as an initial symptom of MSCC, can be seen in approximately 50% of cases and progresses to 80% at the time of diagnosis (Van den Brande et al., 2022). It occurs when the metastatic tumor extends into the neural foramina, resulting in nerve root compression, or when the neural foramina become narrowed due to vertebral body collapse (Fridley et al., 2020). Radicular pain can advance from a constant, dull ache to an intermittent, burning, shooting pain. It often increases with movement and with increased intra-abdominal pressure. Pain is worse at night and when patients are in the supine position because of lengthening of the spine and distension of the spinal epidural venous plexus (Fridley et al., 2020).

A lesion in the thoracic spine produces pain that radiates bilaterally across the chest or abdomen from back to front and feels like a tight or girdling band of pain (Lawton et al., 2019). An upper cervical spine lesion may produce neuropathic facial pain and midscapular pain (Dzhafarov et al., 2020; Lawton et al., 2019).

Patients with MSCC may also experience nonradicular pain that is referred to other areas, obscuring the site of cord compression (Lawton et al., 2019). A lesion confined to the vertebral body may produce referred pain that is poorly localized because of the involvement of multiple dermatomes (Fridley et al., 2020).

Motor Weakness

Neurologic dysfunction is the second most common presenting symptom of MSCC. Motor deficits are found in 35%–75% of patients with spinal metastases at the time of diagnosis (Lawton et al., 2019). Weaknesses are seen in 61%–91% of all MSCC cases, followed by sensory deficits (46%–90%), and then autonomic dysfunction (40%–57%) (Narang et al., 2020).

Motor dysfunction typically begins with weakness in the legs regardless of the level of cord compression. Early in the disease course, the weakness primarily affects the proximal muscles in the lower extremities, often manifested by difficulty in rising from a seated position or climbing stairs (Kaplow & Webster, 2022). Patients may report heaviness, spasticity, or stiffness in the legs, indicating increased muscle tone, with upper motor neuron weakness typically being symmetric.

Lower motor neuron involvement usually causes asymmetric weakness that affects the distal portions of the extremities and is accompanied by muscle flaccidity, atrophy, fasciculations, and hyporeflexia (Lawton et al., 2019). Occasionally, paralysis develops abruptly without prior clinical signs. Involvement of the cervical spine may cause weakness, impaired dexterity, and paresthesia of only one hand or, in cases of the high cervical spine region, paralysis of the diaphragm (Lawton et al., 2019). Ataxia may be the most confusing sign of MSCC and can be mistaken for alcoholism or cerebellar metastases, even when patients also report back pain (Lawton et al., 2019).

Sensory Loss

Approximately 46%–90% of patients have sensory changes (e.g., paresthesia, sensory loss) at diagnosis of MSCC (Narang et al., 2020). Although commonly seen in MSCC, patients are less likely to report sensory changes, and the level of sensory deficit on examination may correlate poorly with the level of the spine lesion (Lawton et al., 2019).

Patients may experience numbness of the fingers or toes, or paresthesia, and loss of proprioception and vibratory sense that progresses to loss of sensation for touch, pain, and temperature (Kaplow & Webster, 2022). Sensory ataxia is common with involvement of the dorsal columns.

Reflex Changes

Reflexes may be hyperactive or hypoactive depending on the level of cord compression. In general, reflex responses decrease at the level of compression and reflexes become hyperactive (Vavourakis et al., 2024). A lesion in the cervical spine can produce segmental (distributed along a dermatome) hyporeflexia in one or both arms and increased reflexes below arm level (Ko, 2022). Involvement of nerve roots in the thoracic spine may produce asymmetric abdominal muscle contraction and loss of abdominal reflexes. Lesions of the upper lumbar plexus roots produce hip flexion weakness and loss of the knee jerk reflex. Those of the lower lumbar plexus nerve roots produce foot drop and diminished ankle jerk reflex (Ko, 2022). Involvement of the conus medullaris or cauda equina is associated with diminished or lost reflexes, including loss of deep tendon reflexes, and anal and bulbocavernosus reflexes (perineal muscles), resulting in changes in the function of the bladder, rectum, and genitalia (Rider & Marra, 2023).

Autonomic Dysfunction

Autonomic symptoms are late findings in patients with MSCC and include changes in bladder, bowel, and sexual function, loss of sweating below the lesion, and orthostatic hypotension (Kaplow & Webster, 2022). Urinary or bowel incontinence, diminished urine flow, urinary retention, and new or worsening constipation should alert healthcare providers to possible MSCC (Kaplow & Webster, 2022). Compression of the conus medullaris or cauda equina can result in bilateral sensory loss in the buttocks, perineal area, posterior thigh, and lateral leg—the area of the body that would encounter a saddle, hence the term *saddle anesthesia* (Rider & Marra, 2023). Urinary retention with overflow incontinence is an important predictor of cauda equina syndrome. Male impotence or female sexual dysfunction may also be present.

Autonomic dysreflexia is a potentially life-threatening syndrome with symptoms that include a pounding headache, extreme hypertension, bradycardia, nasal congestion, facial flushing, profuse sweating, and pilomotor erection (goosebumps) above the level of the lesion (Lin & Avila, 2017; Stephenson & Berliner, 2024). Horner syndrome, which is a combination of drooping eyelid, constricted pupil, and decreased sweating on the affected side of the face, can also occur in autonomic dysreflexia (Coon, 2025).

Prognosis

Survival rates after a diagnosis of MSCC are poor, with 10% of patients still surviving 18 months after initial diagnosis (Vassiliou et al., 2023). Ambulatory and neurologic status at the time of MSCC presentation are the two most reliable prognostic indicators for functional outcome (Phillips & Schiff, 2022).

Approximately 80% of patients who were ambulatory at the time of MSCC diagnosis remain so following treatment, with 30%–45% of patients who are nonambulatory regaining full function (Phillips & Schiff, 2022). Early diagnosis and initiation of therapy for MSCC are crucial to maximizing good outcomes and survival.

The rapidity of the onset of symptoms is another important predictive factor. Faster neurologic deficit development correlates with a lower chance for recovery of motor function after treatment (Phillips & Schiff, 2022).

Radiosensitive tumors, which include breast, prostate, multiple myeloma, lymphoma, and testicular seminomas, are associated with the best prognosis based on histology. The presence of visceral metastases, tumor type, length of time to the development of motor deficits, ambulatory status at presentation, and performance score all influence eventual functional outcomes (Rades et al., 2017).

Risk Factors and Etiology

The most common risk factor in the development of MSCC is a history of breast cancer, prostate cancer, multiple myeloma, non-Hodgkin lymphoma, or lung cancer. MSCC should be considered in patients presenting with new-onset back or radicular pain and in those who manifest high-risk factors, such as long-time smokers (Narang et al., 2020).

Pathophysiology and Patient Evaluation

Spinal Column Anatomy

The spinal column comprises 33 vertebrae—7 cervical, 12 thoracic, 5 lumbar, 5 sacral, and 4 coccygeal (Singleton & Hefner, 2023) (see Figure 6-1). Except for the fused sacrum and coccyx, intervertebral discs separate each vertebra and cushion shocks. Spaces formed between adjacent vertebrae are called intervertebral foramina and serve as openings through which the spinal nerves emerge. The vertebrae form the spinal canal, which encloses and protects the spinal cord. The spinal cord extends from the foramen magnum to the L1–L2 vertebrae. The cervical and lumbar portions of the spinal cord are responsible for the innervation of the upper and lower extremities, which span from C5–T1 and L2–L3 (Singleton & Hefner, 2023). The spinal cord then narrows as it extends downward to the caudal tip, where it terminates in the cone-shaped conus medullaris, between T10–L1. A bundle of lumbar and sacral spinal nerve roots called the cauda equina (Latin for horse's tail, which it resembles) extends below the level of the cord (Berg & Ashurst, 2023).

The spinal cord is divided into 31 segments, each of which has a pair of anterior (motor) and posterior (sensory) spinal nerve roots, which merge to form a mixed spinal nerve as they exit the vertebral column through the intervertebral foramina (Lavignolle, 2020).

The skin segment that sends sensory signals into a given spinal cord segment is called a dermatome. These vary in size and shape and are mapped on the surface of the skin, loosely corresponding with the spinal cord segments. The nerve roots of the cauda equina fill the lower part of the spinal canal to the level of the second sacral vertebra and are arranged according to the spinal segments from which they originate (Sassack

FIGURE 6-1. Diagram of the Spinal Cord

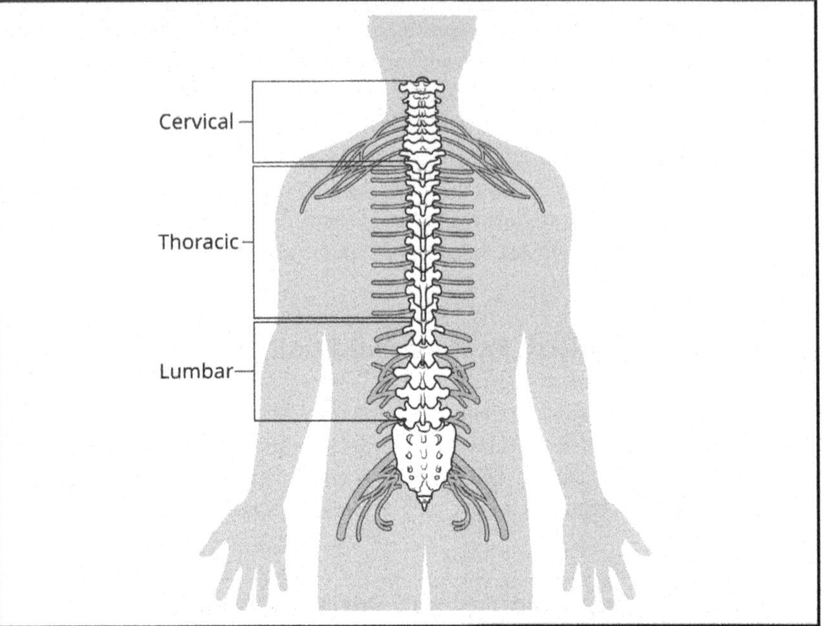

Note. From "Diagram of the Spinal Cord," by Cancer Research UK, 2014 (https://commons.wikimedia.org/wiki/File:Diagram_of_the_spinal_cord_CRUK_046.svg). Licensed under CC BY-SA 4.0 (https://creativecommons.org/licenses/by-sa/4.0/deed.en).

& Carrier, 2023). The nerve roots exit the spinal canal through their respective intervertebral foramina to supply the legs, bowel, bladder, and genitalia, and they serve as the anatomic connection between the central and peripheral nervous systems (Ko, 2022).

Location of Malignant Spinal Involvement

Several factors contribute to the likelihood of MSCC occurring in a specific region of the spine, including the propensity of a tumor to metastasize to vertebral bone, the volume of vertebral bone in the region, the width of the epidural space, and the patterns of venous blood flow to each region of the spine (Narang et al., 2020). The thoracic spine is the most common site of MSCC, accounting for 60%–80% of all cases (Narang et al., 2020). It has 12 vertebrae and contains the largest volume of bone and bone marrow, which supports the growth of tumor deposits; a narrow epidural space; and a poor blood supply. The lumbosacral spine (15%–30% of cases) and cervical spine (< 10%) follow with multiple level involvement in up to 50% of patients (Narang et al., 2020).

Based on a postmortem series, the incidence of MSCC was 70%–90% for patients with breast or prostate cancer, with the thoracic and lumbar spinal levels being the most often affected (Esperança-Martins et al., 2023).

Mechanisms Associated With Metastatic Spinal Cord Compression

Three pathologic mechanisms are associated with the development of MSCC. The most common occurs when a metastatic tumor within the vertebral body expands into the epidural space and compresses the spinal cord and the surrounding epidural venous plexus (Narang et al., 2020).

The second most common pathology involves the mechanical destruction of the cord that occurs when a metastatic tumor erodes and collapses the vertebral body, displacing bone fragments into the epidural space. The bone then compresses the spinal cord and the epidural venous plexus, causing spinal instability (Narang et al., 2020). Vertebral collapse is the most frequent mechanism associated with MSCC in patients with multiple myeloma (Zijlstra et al., 2020).

The third and least common mechanism of MSCC is direct extension of tumors into the epidural space without destruction of the bone. In instances of lung cancer, lymphoma, or retroperitoneal sarcoma, the cancer penetrates the epidural space through the intervertebral foramina (Narang et al., 2020). Direct tumor extension into vertebral structures and the epidural space may occur with Pancoast tumors of the lung apex and with cancers of the colon, kidney, prostate, head and neck, and esophagus.

MSCC damages the cord by direct compression, causing demyelination and injury to nerve axons. Destruction to the nerve axons in ascending nerve tracts, which carry sensory messages toward the brain, may result in pain and sensory changes. Acute compression of the anterior spinal cord obstructs the healthy flow of venous blood from the cord into the vertebral venous plexus, resulting in venous stasis and inflammation (Kaplow & Webster, 2022). Instituting corticosteroid therapy may reduce edema and inflammation and reverse this process (Narang et al., 2020).

Patient Assessment

History

For patients who present with spinal cord symptoms (e.g., back pain, motor or sensory changes, weakness of extremities, ataxia, changes in bowel and bladder habits), obtaining a health history is imperative. A detailed pain history augments decision-making and treatment planning. Localized pain is a frequent complaint in many patients at presentation (Laufer et al., 2024). Back pain is also a common occurrence, so it is important to ascertain the origin of this pain.

Nurses can assess cancer risk factors in patients without a known history of cancer by questioning them regarding family medical history; lifestyle choices (e.g., alcohol use, smoking history); environmental exposures (e.g., asbestos, radon gas); recent breast, prostate, or colorectal screening tests; suspicious skin lesions; unexplained weight loss; and changes in bladder and bowel habits. Patients with a known cancer who present with new-onset back pain and other symptoms should undergo a thorough assessment, with treatment decisions guided by the nature and severity of their symptoms.

Assessment should include having a high index of suspicion when seeing patients with a history of cancers that frequently metastasize to bone, such as breast, lung, prostate, non-Hodgkin lymphoma, renal, melanoma, seminoma, and myeloma. Patients with a history of ependymoma, astrocytoma, or gliomas can also develop metastatic disease in the spine. Inquiring if patients have a history of vertebral compression fractures assists in decision-making. It is not uncommon for patients with spinal cord compression symptoms to have metastatic disease at presentation (Laufer et al., 2024).

Physical Examination

A thorough, systematic examination is essential to determine the presence, location, and type of pain; assess motor function, coordination, gait, sensory status, and reflexes; identify signs of autonomic dysfunction; and determine functional impairments impacting activities of daily living (Bauder, 2024). A performance scoring system, such as the Karnofsky Performance Status Scale or the Eastern Cooperative Oncology Group Performance Status Scale, is used to assess patient functional status.

Pain Assessment

Back pain can be a common symptom described by patients. Pain usually precedes other symptoms of MSCC (Crommett, 2019). A thorough pain assessment should be conducted, including the location, description of pain, how long it has been occurring, and factors that exacerbate or relieve it. Pain is frequently described as dull or achy. Patients can point to the site of pain and rank its intensity using a visual analog scale. A complaint of neck or back pain in patients with cancer warrants evaluation (Bauder, 2024). Sudden onset pain in the neck or back may indicate a pathologic fracture, whereas pain with movement can indicate instability of the spine (Laufer et al., 2024).

Gentle palpation and percussion over the vertebrae can identify areas of tenderness over the level of compression (Bauder, 2024). Elicited pain may be bilateral or unilateral. The level of compression may be indicated if pain increases with movement, such as coughing, sneezing, or twisting, or when lying down or performing straight leg raises (Bauder, 2024). Epidural spinal cord compression occurs most often in the thoracic spine (Laufer et al., 2024). Compression in the thoracic cord region is frequently associated with bilateral pain and weakness and can be described like a band wrapping around the chest or abdomen (Laufer et al., 2024). Pain with movement only indicates spinal instability and requires imaging. Patients with spinal instability experiencing pain may not accurately indicate the level of compression. For example, patients with unstable thoracic metastases may have pain while lying down. Nocturnal pain is common. The description of pain can change over time (Laufer et al., 2024).

Musculoskeletal Assessment

Clinicians should observe patients for movement and arm swinging while walking and turning. Evaluation includes the ability to walk heel to toe in a straight line and stand on one leg at a time. Coordination is assessed by asking patients to touch the thumb of each hand with each finger in that hand in rapid succession and to alternately touch their nose and the examiner's finger as quickly as possible (Bickley et al., 2021). An ataxic gait, indicated by loss of balance, may be present even before apparent weakness and should be considered suspicious (Laufer et al., 2024).

Motor weakness begins in the proximal muscles of the leg and may be indicated by patient reports of leg stiffness or heaviness and difficulty rising from a seated position or climbing stairs. Clinicians can test leg strength by asking patients to do heel walking, toe walking, and deep knee bends or by having them perform active movements against the examiner's resistance, if capable (Bickley et al., 2021). Clinicians should evaluate each muscle group individually and compare the results from each side of the body for muscle strength and symmetry of movement (Bickley et al., 2021). The American Spinal Injury Association uses grading categories ranging from 0 (total paralysis) to 5 (active movement, full range of motion against gravity) to score muscle strength in the presence of spinal cord injury. It has created standardized forms that can be used at baseline and follow-up to classify existing motor and sensory function and impairment (Rupp et al., 2021).

Sensory Assessment

Sensory assessment is an essential part of a neurologic examination and includes evaluation of patients' ability to sense pain, temperature, light touch, vibration, and position (proprioception) (Bickley et al., 2021). This testing should take place when patients are as relaxed and comfortable as possible, as results may be unreliable when they are experiencing pain. Reduced sensation may be detected up to five segmental levels below or one to two segments above the level of neural damage (Laufer et al., 2024). Pinprick testing for pain localization involves alternately tapping a sharp and dull object against the skin along the lines of the dermatomes, applying equal pressure throughout. Patients' eyes should remain closed during this testing (Bickley et al., 2021). Their sensitivity to warm and cold temperatures can be evaluated using warmed and chilled metal tuning forks. The tuning fork is used over bony prominences to assess vibration sense. Sensitivity to light touch is evaluated by brushing a wisp of cotton or cotton-tipped applicator against the skin along a dermatome (Bickley et al., 2021). To assess proprioception, patients must stand with their feet together and eyes closed, known as the Romberg test. If they cannot maintain this posture and begin to sway or fall, this unsteadiness is considered a positive test and indicates involvement of the dorsal columns of the spinal cord (Bickley et al., 2021; Potter, 2025).

Loss of sensation for light touch, pain, or temperature, and diminished or absent sense of vibration or proprioception indicate progressive neurologic dysfunction (Potter, 2025). Patients with cauda equina syndrome, which develops when the level of compression is below the point where the spinal cord terminates at the first lumbar vertebra, may present with saddle sensory changes (Laufer et al., 2024).

Autonomic Function Assessment

Patient questioning focuses on changes in bladder and bowel habits as well as sexual dysfunction. Reports of frequent, small voids may indicate urinary retention, which can be detected by abdominal percussion (Laufer et al., 2024). To measure residual urine volume, patients should first urinate, after which the bladder is scanned or catheterized to determine the postvoid volume. The presence of urinary tract infection or distended bladder or bowel can result in extreme hypertension and headache.

Reflex Assessment

Deep tendon reflexes are an important indicator of neurologic status. Normal reflex response is brisk. Changes in reaction time and intensity may indicate the severity of neural damage. Deep tendon reflexes decrease at the level of compression and become hyperactive (Morimoto et al., 2024).

Hyperactive deep tendon reflexes in the lower extremities and extensor plantar responses indicate cord compression in the thoracic region. A positive Babinski sign is always an abnormal finding in adults and is a sensitive and specific sign of corticospinal tract dysfunction (Bickley et al., 2021). To elicit the Babinski sign, clinicians stroke a tool across the sole, from the heel to the small toe, then draw an arc across to under the big toe. Dorsiflexion of the great toe with fanning of the other toes indicates a positive response (Bickley et al., 2021).

To induce the Beevor sign, the examiner flexes a supine patient's head forward against resistance while observing the movement of the umbilicus. Movement in a caudal direction (toward the foot) indicates that nerve root involvement is above T10. Cephalad movement (toward the head) indicates the dysfunction is below T10 (Althagafi & Nadi, 2025).

In contrast to the hyperreflexia seen with higher lesions, compression at the level of the cauda equina produces hyporeflexia or areflexia in the legs (Bickley et al., 2021; Rider & Marra, 2023). Weakness of the hip flexor muscles and loss of the knee jerk reflexes indicate nerve root involvement of the upper lumbar plexus. Foot drop and a diminished ankle jerk reflex indicate lesions of the nerve roots of the lower lumbar plexus (Morimoto et al., 2024). Lesions of the conus medullaris present a mixed picture. The knee jerk, bulbocavernosus, and anal reflexes may be preserved, whereas the ankle and plantar reflexes are decreased to absent (Bickley et al., 2021).

Advanced Practice Considerations

Early recognition, prompt diagnosis, and appropriate treatment of spinal cord compression are crucial to limiting functional impairments and maintaining the quality of remaining life. Advanced practice nurses must be able to recognize which patients are at increased risk for MSCC and raise their level of suspicion at the appearance of the subtle and nonspecific signs and symptoms of this condition.

Imaging Studies

A magnetic resonance imaging scan is considered the imaging procedure of choice for evaluating MSCC (Laufer et al., 2024; Lawton et al., 2019). With and without contrast, a scan of the entire spine should be performed promptly on anyone suspected of having MSCC due to the possibility of having a synchronous multifocal MSCC (Narang et al., 2020). A magnetic resonance imaging scan has excellent soft tissue contrast resolution and allows for precise detection of marrow infiltration, tumor extension, paraspinal soft tissue involvement, and degree of spinal cord compression (Bai et al., 2022).

Laboratory Studies

No laboratory study can diagnose MSCC. For patients without a previous history of cancer, initial laboratory tests should include a complete blood count, erythrocyte sedimentation rate (inflammation marker), electrolytes, renal and liver function tests, and clotting parameters (Kaplow & Webster, 2022). Serum albumin levels should be reviewed in conjunction with ionized calcium because patients with bone metastases may be hypercalcemic (Kaplan, 2018).

Treatment Modalities

Treatment Goals

Optimizing patient quality of life with MSCC involves relieving pain, palliating symptoms, preventing irreversible disability, preserving or recovering motor and sphincter function, providing spinal stability and local tumor control, and extending the active portion of remaining life (Laufer et al., 2025; Van den Brande et al., 2022). An interprofessional team approach is essential for the optimal management of this oncologic emergency. In cases of previously undiagnosed cancer, emergency physicians are often the first to identify MSCC and initiate referral to appropriate specialists (Borke, 2023). However, misdiagnosis of MSCC in nontrauma patients is common in emergency departments, even when neurologic deficits are clearly present at the time of presentation. This can lead to significant delays in accurate diagnosis and timely interventions (Newman-Toker et al., 2022).

Supportive care with corticosteroids and pain management should be followed by therapy to decompress the spine using radiation therapy and surgery, either alone or in combination (Laufer et al., 2025). Administration of systemic therapy may be helpful to shrink tumors from the spinal cord in patients with cancers known to be chemosensitive (Bauder, 2024). Rehabilitation goals are considered on an individual basis depending on overall prognosis and goals for life. Multifaceted discharge planning facilitates rehabilitation placement or home health care, encourages quality-of-life discussions, and outlines options for supportive or palliative care (Lawton et al., 2019; Van den Brande et al., 2022). Nurses should provide counseling, education, and emotional support to patients and caregivers from the time of MSCC diagnosis.

Pain relief remains a priority regardless of prognosis (Lawton et al., 2019). Effective pain assessment, management, and evaluation of relief measures are essential nursing responsibilities and should begin at diagnosis. Corticosteroids may provide initial relief because of their anti-inflammatory properties. However, as pain intensifies over time, additional therapies—particularly around-the-clock opioid dosing—are often required (Lawton et al., 2019). Pain management interventions should be tailored to prognosis and life expectancy, which is typically three months.

Corticosteroids

Initial supportive therapy for patients who are symptomatic with MSCC is corticosteroids. These medications require urgent initiation, even before radiographic confirmation, in patients suspected of having MSCC (Singleton & Hefner, 2023). Steroids interrupt the inflammatory cascade, reduce vasogenic cord edema, and downregulate expression of vascular endothelial growth factor, resulting in improved neurologic symptoms and pain relief (Singleton & Hefner, 2023). Additionally, steroids have a direct oncolytic effect on some tumors, especially lymphomas and thymomas, and can complicate diagnosis because of tumor shrinkage. Thus, except in emergencies, corticosteroids should be held in patients suspected of lymphoma-associated MSCC. This precaution is especially important for young people without a prior history of cancer or a definitive diagnosis of MSCC. Corticosteroids should be avoided in these patients until diagnosis is confirmed (Laufer et al., 2025).

For patients with neurologic deficits and pain, initial corticosteroid therapy typically consists of 10 mg IV followed by 16 mg over 24 hours, then tapered (Laufer et al., 2025). Higher doses have been used but are associated with more side effects and have not demonstrated increased efficacy (Akanda & McKay, 2023).

Radiation Therapy

Conventional external beam radiation therapy alone has been the standard palliative treatment for MSCC for decades. It is effective in controlling pain, neurologic symptoms, and organ-specific obstructive symptoms (Alcorn et al., 2024). Conventional external beam radiation therapy is also the primary treatment option for most epidural metastases and spinal cord compression when there is no evidence of spinal instability.

Radiation dose and schedules are dependent on patient prognosis, symptom type, and whether radiation therapy is used in conjunction with surgery. Patients with a poor prognosis or mobility impairment may receive a single, large, fractionated dose of radiation (8 Gy). Patients with better prognosis and less overall compromise often receive 30 Gy divided into smaller doses over 10 days of therapy (Zaki et al., 2023). When radiation therapy follows decompressive surgery, it is typically delayed by one week to allow for postoperative healing. The desired outcomes of palliative radiation therapy for bone metastases include improved patient-reported pain and neurologic symptoms, as well as enhanced overall quality of life (Alcorn et al., 2024).

Assessment of patients with radiologic findings may indicate the need for surgery, such as impending cord compression, spinal instability, and bony retropulsion, along with reports of neurologic changes or pain requiring tissue diagnosis (Loblaw et al., 2020). Newer, minimally invasive surgical techniques have improved patient tolerance. For example, separation surgery was designed to decompress the thecal sac instead of completely removing the tumor so that space is available in the radiation field for radioresistant epidural metastatic disease. By creating an open area around the cord, this procedure allows radiation to be delivered without harm to the cord by using stereotactic body radiation therapy (Zhang et al., 2024). This approach enables a more effective radiation treatment dose. Stereotactic radiosurgery or stereotactic body radiation therapy can be considered following separation surgery, provided treatment planning is completed and insurance coverage is approved.

Surgery

Therapeutic advances in the treatment of cancer, such as targeted agents and immunotherapy, have improved survival rates. With extended longevity, the incidence of metastases has increased (Newman et al., 2020). Controversy remains as to which modality (i.e., radiation therapy or surgery) should be the initial definitive treatment for MSCC. Estimating life expectancy is an important consideration in decision-making. A survival projection of three months or longer is considered appropriate for surgical intervention (Park et al., 2022). Selection of the appropriate surgical approach depends on several factors, including tumor location and extent, tumor histology, integrity of adjacent segments, type of spinal reconstruction or stabilization required, and the patient's general condition (Rothrock et al., 2020). Spinal stabilization is a surgical management (Lawton et al., 2019). Patients benefit from interprofessional decision-making regarding potential surgical options. Hussain et al. (2019) validated the Spine Instability Neoplastic Score, which ranges from 0–6 (stable), 7–12 (pending instability), and 13–18 (unstable). The score also includes patient-reported outcomes, such as pain, and the University of Texas MD Anderson Symptom Inventory, which includes components specific to spinal tumor-related symptoms.

Laminectomy

Laminectomy is performed with a posterior approach; however, it is not effective in debulking anterior or circumferential tumor masses compressing the cord, as it contributes to further loss of spinal stability and neurologic deterioration (Laufer et al., 2025). Indications for decompressive laminectomy include the presence of posterior radioresistant tumors, worsening neurologic status following radiation therapy, absence of vertebral involvement, or the need to obtain a tissue diagnosis (Laufer et al., 2025).

Advances in surgical techniques and spinal instrumentation have made it possible to decompress the spinal cord using anterior, posterior, or combined approaches and to immediately reconstruct and stabilize the spine. Percutaneous procedures, such as vertebroplasty or kyphoplasty, can be effective for pain relief from collapsed vertebrae in select patients who do not have neurologic deficits (Al Farii et al., 2023).

Anterior Vertebral Body Resection With Stabilization

In 85% of MSCC cases, the location of metastatic disease is anterior to the spinal cord; hence, the ability to perform corpectomy and vertebral body replacements with expandable cages was an important advance (Loblaw et al., 2020). Resecting the tumor anteriorly, however, has a higher rate of morbidity and therefore is usually reserved for patients with a good prognosis and minimal comorbidities (Loblaw et al., 2020).

Vertebral body resection results in a defect in the anterior spinal column that must be reconstructed using a stabilizing device. The bone cement filler, polymethyl methacrylate, is used in conjunction with internal fixation devices to reconstruct the spine and reestablish stability for the remainder of the patient's life. Metallic fixation devices (i.e., pins, rods, plates, or expandable titanium cages) are anchored to intact vertebral bodies above and below the metastatic site to achieve immediate spinal stability.

Renal cell carcinoma, thyroid malignancies, and hepatocellular metastases are highly vascular tumors resulting in blood loss during vertebral body resection, which can be life threatening. To minimize intraoperative blood loss, these tumors are usually embolized prior to surgery (Loblaw et al., 2020). In addition to blood loss, other examples of morbidity include deep vein thrombosis, pulmonary embolism, wound infection, stabilization failure, hematoma, pneumonia, and cardiac infarction (Laufer et al., 2025).

Patients with a life expectancy of less than six months who are poor surgical candidates but have pain without neurologic manifestations related to their MSCC may have improved quality of life with a less invasive vertebral augmentation technique, such as vertebroplasty or kyphoplasty (Loblaw et al., 2020). These procedures use a more focused surgical tumor resection that exposes the tumor bed for the use of stereotactic radiosurgery (Loblaw et al., 2020).

Vertebroplasty

Vertebroplasty is a minimally invasive, image-guided, percutaneous procedure that was initially developed for the treatment of painful compression fractures associated with osteoporosis. It is also used for restabilizing collapsed vertebrae from MSCC with the insertion of cement into the compromised vertebrae's collapsed bone (Loblaw et al., 2020). Vertebroplasty's primary goal is to increase the stability of the spine's anterior column (Loblaw et al., 2020). In vertebroplasty, the bone cement filler is injected directly into the vertebral body through a hollow-bore needle under fluoroscopic or computed tomography scan guidance with the patient under sedation or general anesthesia (Al Farii et al., 2023). Pain relief is usually immediate (within 72 hours) and lasting.

Kyphoplasty

Similar to vertebroplasty, percutaneous kyphoplasty is a minimally invasive procedure in which a balloon is inserted into the vertebral body under fluoroscopic guidance. The balloon is then expanded to help restore vertebral height. Upon removal, a cavity is created into which the cement bone filler is injected. The newly filled cavity restores stability of the fractured vertebral body, restores height, and reduces kyphosis and its associated pain (Loblaw et al., 2020). Pain relief is often dramatic, and complication rates are low (Al Farii et al., 2023). Indications for kyphoplasty include painful vertebral body metastases or spinal instability without associated neurologic deficits. Burst fractures, spinal instability, and symptomatic radiculopathy are considered relative contraindications to both vertebroplasty and kyphoplasty (Loblaw et al., 2020). Kyphoplasty may also be used in combination with conventional radiation therapy or stereotactic body radiation therapy (Al Farii et al., 2023).

Antineoplastic Therapy

Systemic drug therapy delivered in conjunction with radiation therapy may be an effective adjunct in treating MSCC associated with chemosensitive tumors (e.g., Hodgkin lymphoma, non-Hodgkin lymphoma, neuroblastoma, germ cell tumors, breast cancer). Hormone therapy with tamoxifen, aromatase inhibitors, or androgen blockade may be beneficial in metastatic breast and prostate cancers not previously exposed to hormones. Hence, molecular studies of the tumor need to be reviewed in these two patient populations (Newman et al., 2020). Patients often receive chemotherapy and hormone treatments in combination with more rapidly effective modalities, such as radiation therapy or surgery. Chemotherapy alone may be effective as the sole treatment for MSCC caused by non-Hodgkin lymphoma, which is highly chemosensitive (Laufer et al., 2025).

Bisphosphonates and Denosumab

Agents that prevent bone decomposition may be included in the treatment regimens of patients with MSCC. These include bisphosphonates, such as zoledronate and pamidronate, and denosumab, a synthetic fully human monoclonal antibody (Kaplan, 2018). Bisphosphonates are widely used to prevent bone destruction, including in patients with bone metastases from cancer. Denosumab is approved for the prevention of skeletal-related events in patients with bone metastases from solid tumors and for those with associated multiple myeloma (Hildebrand et al., 2024). Both types of agents inhibit tumor-induced bone resorption and reduce complications of vertebral metastases, such as pain, vertebral fractures, and hypercalcemia. However, bisphosphonates and denosumab are associated with adverse effects, namely osteonecrosis of the jaw and atypical femoral fractures (Kaplan, 2018).

Nursing Management

Comprehensive, individualized nursing care is a cornerstone of MSCC management. Nursing responsibilities evolve as patients progress along a continuum—from early detection and diagnosis to emergent and definitive treatments, followed by rehabilitation and supportive palliative care. Nurses are pivotal in recognizing the subtle signs and symptoms of spinal cord compression and initiating prompt diagnostic evaluation. Once MSCC is confirmed and treatment begins, nursing care should be tailored to patients' neurologic status and degree of spinal stability. Key nursing focuses should include pain relief; assessment and management of motor and sensory deficits, as well as bladder and bowel dysfunction; education about treatment and side effects; promotion of safety; maintenance of skin integrity; caregiver support; and reduction of psychosocial distress. Nurses need to incorporate rehabilitation principles into care planning to maximize and restore function, prevent injuries, coordinate care with the interprofessional team, and prepare patients for discharge to home or hospice. Patient and caregiver education is customized to address coping mechanisms and specific informational needs. Encouragement and emotional support are essential throughout the entire continuum of care. When functional compromise is significant, nurses should anticipate substantial caregiver burden and offer preparatory guidance to family members (Fallon et al., 2018). General nursing interventions in the care of patients with MSCC include the following (Lawton et al., 2019; Potter et al., 2025):

- Institute pain relief measures and evaluate their effectiveness.
- Conduct ongoing assessment of sensory and motor functions.
- Measure vital signs with attention to respiration and fluid intake and output.
- Provide education and reassurance related to treatment modalities.
- Evaluate objective and subjective responses to therapy.
- Institute safety measures to prevent injury and further neurologic damage.
- Mobilize patients and assist them with weight-bearing activities and proper body mechanics as appropriate.
- Manage a preventive skin care regimen.
- Monitor nutrition and fluid status.
- Assess bladder distension and need for urinary catheter.
- Assess bowel function and establish an elimination program.
- Coordinate activity regimen and rehabilitation program.
- Assess coping mechanisms related to cancer diagnosis, altered body image, and changes in sexual function.
- Facilitate adaptation to neurologic deficits and advancing disease.
- Support patients and caregivers in accepting functional limitations.
- Provide emotional support to patients and caregivers as they deal with end-of-life issues.

Pain Management

Management of pain is of high priority in patients with MSCC. Pain should be assessed by patient self-report. A baseline pain assessment is essential, noting the pain quality and intensity, location, pattern (local or radiating), actions that increase pain or provide relief, and past treatments that have been effective (Laufer et al., 2025). The analgesic regimen correlates with the presentation of MSCC. Administration of corticosteroids immediately after diagnosis provides initial pain relief, but additional pain therapy is usually needed (Lawton et al., 2019). Inadequate pain relief has a significant negative effect on functional capacity and quality of life; thus, ongoing pain assessment is necessary throughout treatment.

Nurses should be familiar with the pharmacologic principles of analgesia and equianalgesic dose, including the risks, benefits, and costs of different drug regimens. Nonpharmacologic behavioral approaches to manage pain should also be considered, such as relaxation techniques, acupressure, and guided imagery (Stie et al., 2022). Often, adjuvant drugs (e.g., anticonvulsants, antidepressants, anxiolytics) are added to enhance the management of moderate and severe pain (Lawton et al., 2019).

Patients should be questioned about their pain levels and response to analgesics over time so that doses can be modified or adjuvant drugs added if necessary. Chronic opioid therapy is often required for persistent pain and should be prescribed on an around-the-clock or fixed schedule (Lawton et al., 2019). Opioids have constipating effects; therefore, a combination of stimulant laxatives and stool softeners is needed to increase bowel motility and should begin concurrently with opioid therapy initiation. Patients on opioids should be evaluated and treated prophylactically for constipation (Lawton et al., 2019).

Adjuvant analgesics, commonly called coanalgesics, may be used to provide pain relief. Coanalgesics are classified as drugs that relieve pain through complementary pharmacologic pathways. Antiepileptic drugs, antidepressants, and corticosteroids are coanalgesics recommended for treating neuropathic cancer pain (Lawton et al., 2019). When refractory pain evolves, a neuroablative procedure may be necessary to provide pain relief. Nerve blocks are used for the head, neck, and upper extremities, and lumbar sympathetic blocks are used to ablate pain in the lower extremities (Fallon et al., 2018).

Mobility and Safety Issues

Although the care of patients with MSCC is highly individualized, patient comfort and safety remain of utmost importance. Patients with tenderness or symptoms associated with suspected involvement of the cervical spine should be immobilized and have a cervical collar placed to stabilize the area until results of the diagnostic evaluation are known (Laufer et al., 2025). Patients with spinal instability demonstrated on magnetic resonance imaging scans are often confined to total bed rest and are moved with great caution (Laufer et al., 2025). These patients are at risk for pressure injuries, thrombotic events, and respiratory infections, so prevention and early detection are critical. Strategies to prevent deep vein thrombosis include prophylactic administration of low-molecular-weight heparin. Elastic compression stockings and intermittent pneumatic compression devices are typically applied in order to avoid deep vein thrombosis (Laufer et al., 2025). If vertebral fractures are present, patients may be fitted with a brace to provide external immobilization until surgery can be performed. Following surgical intervention, the principles of postoperative nursing care include serial neurologic assessment, pain management, wound care, body alignment, and maintenance of spinal stability.

Patients who have lesions of the cervical or upper thoracic spine are at risk for acute respiratory insufficiency and autonomic dysreflexia. Nurses should institute pulmonary hygiene measures as ordered to prevent hypoventilation, atelectasis, and pneumonia, and consider the possibility of mechanical ventilation necessity. Signs indicative of autonomic dysreflexia (i.e., elevated blood pressure, bradycardia, pounding headache, chest pain, vasodilation, flushing, and profuse sweating above the level of the spinal block) require immediate attention.

Skin Care

Patients with MSCC are frequently malnourished and less mobile, elevating their risk for skin breakdown. Those with major sensory deficits due to MSCC or who are sedentary are at risk for pressure injuries and contractures. Nursing measures should be considered, such as meticulous skin inspection and preventive interventions (e.g., position changes every two hours, safe transfer techniques, the use of heel protectors, decreasing vulnerable pressure areas, specialty mattresses). Physical therapy support and range-of-motion exercises are also important interventions to consider (Lawton et al., 2019). Skin alterations related to reduced mobility may be exacerbated by radiation-related dermatologic changes. Nurses should monitor patients' skin for redness in the radiated treatment field and provide skin care instructions.

Bowel and Bladder Function

MSCC-related bladder dysfunction is often evidenced by the inability to fully empty the bladder, which results in urinary retention, bladder distension, and chronic urinary tract infections (UTIs). Monitoring fluid intake and output and assessing for bladder distension are required. The presence of residual urine after voiding is evaluated by means of a bladder scan or catheterization (Carter, 2024). If retained urine is present, a schedule of intermittent catheterization may be instituted during the acute phase of MSCC to reduce the risk of UTIs and renal damage. Patients with involvement below the level of C7 can usually manage self-catheterization. Otherwise, a permanent indwelling urinary catheter may be placed (Carter, 2024). Nursing measures to reduce the risk of UTIs from an indwelling urinary catheter include maintaining fluid intake greater than 2 L/day, daily catheter care and perineal hygiene, and regular catheter changes. Nurses should report signs and symptoms of UTIs, monitor the results of urinalysis and cultures, and assess the effectiveness of antibiotic therapy sensitive to the identified infectious organisms (Potter et al., 2025). Patients with lower motor neuron lesions experience flaccidity of the sphincter and incontinence. These patients may benefit from timed voiding and bladder training (Lawton et al., 2019). Nurses should instruct patients and their caregivers on intermittent self-catheterization and recognizing the signs of UTI.

Autonomic dysfunction in patients with MSCC also results in constipation caused by the loss of voluntary and reflex constriction of the anal sphincter and loss of perineal sensation (Laufer et al., 2025). Constipation can progress to fecal impaction and loss of sphincter control to stool incontinence. It is also a common side effect of older age, inadequate fluid intake, inactivity, and immobility (Lawton et al., 2019). For patients with sphincter control, a bowel maintenance program incorporating the use of a stool softener, a stimulant, and an osmotic laxative is recommended to promote bowel evacuation at least every one to two days. Nurses should inspect, auscultate, palpate, and percuss the abdomen for signs of distension and presence or absence of bowel sounds and check for stool impaction daily, documenting and reporting abnormalities (Bauder, 2024). Patients should be encouraged to increase their daily fluid intake as well as consume a high-fiber diet. Psyllium for bulking can be added (Lawton et al., 2019).

Psychosocial Support and Palliative Care

Changes in self-image, loss of independence and ability to work, and role deterioration within the family and community contribute to emotional distress in patients with MSCC. Nurses can assist patients and caregivers in coping with increasing dependence by encouraging them to express their feelings, fears, and concerns, referring them to team members as appropriate, and supporting them in establishing realistic rehabilitation goals. For patients with limited life expectancy, usually less than six months, supportive or palliative care goals shift toward caregiver involvement and dependent care. These goals emphasize pain relief, comfort measures, prevention of further injury, and management of bladder and bowel elimination (Lawton et al., 2019).

Evidence of MSCC characterizes cancer progression and approaching mortality. Because nurses have established a unique bond with patients and caregivers over time, they are the ideal healthcare providers to offer emotional support and make referrals for professional assistance as needed. Patients with irreversible or progressive neurologic decline or those with end-stage disease may require more intensive nursing care and referral to hospice or comprehensive palliative homecare services to maintain their quality of life. This specialized interprofessional team supports patients and their caregivers coping with the disabling sequelae of MSCC by intervening with psychological and spiritual support.

Rehabilitation and Palliative Care

General rehabilitation goals are to improve ambulation, achieve weight-bearing and transfer ability, restore bladder and bowel function when possible, and protect the skin (Lawton et al., 2019). Loss of bladder and bowel control, pain, and alterations in body image can diminish libido. A nurse-led interprofessional approach is optimal for addressing these complex needs. Physical and occupational therapy, social services, and home health professionals contribute expertise tailored to patient and caregiver needs. Nurses can also facilitate communication between patients and their partners, promoting alternative forms of physical intimacy, such as holding hands, cuddling, or gentle massages, to help maintain emotional connection and reduce distress (Poullard & Charles, 2024).

Discharge Planning

Ongoing assessment of pain, functional status, and signs of disease progression is essential. During these visits, providers instruct patients and caregivers regarding pain management, techniques for transfers and ambulation, safety measures and fall prevention, and regulation of bladder and bowel elimination. Physical and occupational therapists evaluate patients' functional abilities and need for assistive devices and medical equipment, such as specialized hospital beds, wheelchairs, or home ramps. They also provide instruction in range-of-motion exercises, safe transfer methods, and the use of assistive devices (Lawton et al., 2019).

Patient and Caregiver Education

Patients at high risk for spinal cord compression, particularly those with known bone metastases from lymphoma, myeloma, and cancers of the lung, breast, or prostate, should be taught the importance of promptly reporting all back pain, whether a new onset or a change in existing pain. These individuals should also be instructed to call their healthcare provider within 24 hours of new or worsening back pain or immediately if they develop neurologic symptoms in the lower extremities.

Pressure injury prevention measures, such as regular skin inspection, proper positioning, turning, and safe transfer methods, as well as the use of skin-protecting products and pressure-reducing support surfaces, are taught as indicated (Potter et al., 2025). Patients and caregivers also receive instructions on medication management and the importance of scheduled follow-up visits.

Summary

MSCC is a structural oncologic emergency that, if left untreated, evolves into a relentless trajectory of significant pain, progressive neurologic decline, increased disability, dependence, and death. Most patients with MSCC have a life expectancy of months, but up to one-third will survive beyond one year. Delays in early diagnosis and treatment can result in rapid, irreversible loss of function. Nursing patients with known bone metastases requires a high index of suspicion for this complication. Prompt recognition, diagnosis, and treatment may mean the difference between patients maintaining their functional independence and a reasonable quality of life or spending the remainder of their lives incapacitated and dependent on others.

The authors would like to acknowledge Marcelle Kaplan, MS, RN, CNS, for her contribution to this chapter that remains unchanged from the previous edition of this book.

References

Akanda, Z.Z., & McKay, M.J. (2023). Narrative review—diagnosing and managing malignant epidural spinal cord compression: An evidence-based approach. *Annals of Translational Medicine, 11*(11), 386. https://doi.org/10.21037/atm-22-3076

Al Farii, H., Aoude, A., Al Shammasi, A., Reynolds, J., & Weber, M. (2023). Surgical management of the metastatic spine disease: A review of the literature and proposed algorithm. *Global Spine Journal, 13*(2), 486–498. https://doi.org/10.1177/21925682221146741

Alcorn, S., Cortés, Á.A., Bradfield, L., Brennan, M., Dennis, K., Diaz, D.A., ... Balboni, T. (2024). External beam radiation therapy for palliation of symptomatic bone metastases: An ASTRO Clinical Practice Guideline. *Practical Radiation Oncology, 14*(5), 377–397. https://doi.org/10.1016/j.prro.2024.04.018

Althagafi, A., & Nadi, M. (2025). Beevor sign. In *StatPearls*. StatPearls Publishing. https://www.ncbi.nlm.nih.gov/books/NBK545262

Bai, J., Grant, K., Hussien, A., & Kawakyu-O'Connor, D. (2022). Imaging of metastatic epidural spinal cord compression. *Frontiers in Radiology, 2*, 962797. https://doi.org/10.3389/fradi.2022.962797

Bauder, N. (2024). Spinal cord compression. In J.M. Brant, D.G. Cope, & M.G. Saría (Eds.), *Core curriculum for oncology nursing* (7th ed., pp. 484–486). Elsevier.

Berg, E.J., & Ashurst, J.V. (2023). Anatomy, back, cauda equina. In *StatPearls*. StatPearls Publishing. https://www.ncbi.nlm.nih.gov/books/NBK513251

Bickley, L.S., Szilagyi, P.G., Hoffman, R.M., & Soriano, R.P. (2021). *Bates' guide to physical examination and history taking* (13th ed.). Wolters Kluwer.

Borke, J. (2023, May 15). Spinal cord neoplasms. *Medscape.* https://emedicine.medscape.com/article/779872-overview

Carter, G.T. (2024 , December 23). Bladder dysfunction. *Medscape.* https://emedicine.medscape.com/article/321273-overview

Coon, E. (2025). Horner syndrome. In M.C. Levin (Ed.), *Merck manual professional version: Neurologic disorders: Autonomic nervous system.* Merck. https://www.merckmanuals.com/professional/neurologic-disorders/autonomic-nervous-system/horner-syndrome

Crommett, J.W. (2019). Metastatic spinal cord compression. In J. Nates & K. Price (Eds.), *Oncologic critical care.* Springer. https://doi.org/10.1007/978-3-319-74698-2_41-1

Dzhafarov, V., Rzaev, J., Moysak, G., & Voronina, E. (2020). Facial pain as an initial manifestation of intramedullary cervical spinal cord tumor: A case report and literature review. *Surgical Neurology International, 11,* 173. https://doi.org/10.25259/SNI_546_2019

Esperança-Martins, M., Roque, D., Barroso, T., Abrunhosa-Branquinho, A., Belo, D., Simas, N., & Costa, L. (2023). Multidisciplinary approach to spinal metastases and metastatic spinal cord compression—A new integrative flowchart for patient management. *Cancers, 15*(6), 1796. https://doi.org/10.3390/cancers15061796

Fallon, M., Giusti, R., Aielli, F., Hoskin, P., Rolke, R., Sharma, M., & Ripamonti, C.I. (2018). Management of cancer pain in adult patients: ESMO Clinical Practice Guidelines. *Annals of Oncology, 29*(4, Suppl.), iv166–iv191. https://doi.org/10.1093/annonc/mdy152

Fridley, J.S., Syed, S., Niu, T., Leary, O.P., & Gokaslan, Z.L. (2020). Presentation of spinal cord and column tumors. *Neuro-Oncology Practice, 7*(1, Suppl.), i18–i24. https://doi.org/10.1093/nop/npaa051

Hawkins, J.E., Dworzynski, K., & Haden, N. (2023). Spinal metastases and metastatic spinal cord compression: Summary of updated NICE guidance. *BMJ, 383,* 1973. https://doi.org/10.1136/bmj.p1973

Hildebrand, G.K., Patel, P., & Kasi, A. (2024). Denosumab. In *StatPearls.* StatPearls Publishing. https://https://www.ncbi.nlm.nih.gov/books/NBK535388

Hussain, I., Barzilai, O., Reiner, A.S., McLaughlin, L., DiStefano, N.M., Ogilvie, S., ... Laufer, I. (2019). Spinal instability neoplastic score component validation using patient-reported outcomes. *Journal of Neurosurgery: Spine SPI, 30*(4), 432–438. https://doi.org/10.3171/2018.9.spine18147

Kaplan, M. (2018). Hypercalcemia of malignancy. In C.H. Yarbro, D. Wujcik, & B.H. Gobel (Eds.), *Cancer nursing: Principles and practice* (8th ed., pp. 1107–1134). Jones and Bartlett Learning.

Kaplow, R., & Webster, J. (2022). Malignant spinal cord compression. *Journal of Radiology Nursing, 41*(3), 207–213. https://doi.org/10.1016/j.jradnu.2022.05.009

Ko, H.-Y. (2022). *Management and rehabilitation of spinal cord injuries* (2nd ed.). Springer. https://doi.org/10.1007/978-981-19-0228-4_11

Laufer, I., Bilsky, M., Schiff, D., & Brown, P. (2025). Treatment and prognosis of neoplastic epidural spinal cord compression. In A.F. Eichler & S.R. Vora (Eds.), *UpToDate.* Retrieved October 3, 2025, from https://www.uptodate.com/contents/treatment-and-prognosis-of-neoplastic-epidural-spinal-cord-compression

Laufer, I., Schiff, D., Kelly, H.R., & Bilsky, M. (2024). Clinical features and diagnosis of neoplastic epidural spinal cord compression. In A.F. Eichler (Ed.), *UpToDate.* Retrieved October 3, 2025, from https://www.uptodate.com/contents/clinical-features-and-diagnosis-of-neoplastic-epidural-spinal-cord-compression

Lavignolle, B. (2020). Spinal nerves (Innervation of the spine). In J. Vital & D. Cawley (Eds.), *Spinal anatomy* (pp. 391–401). Springer. https://doi.org/10.1007/978-3-030-20925-4_25

Lawton, A.J., Lee, K.A., Cheville, A.L., Ferrone, M.L., Rades, D., Balboni, T.A., & Abrahm, J.L. (2019). Assessment and management of patients with metastatic spinal cord compression: A multidisciplinary review. *Journal of Clinical Oncology, 37*(1), 61–71. https://doi.org/10.1200/JCO.2018.78.1211

Lin, A.L., & Avila, E.K. (2017). Neurologic emergencies in the patients with cancer: Diagnosis and management. *Journal of Intensive Care Medicine, 32*(2), 99–115. https://doi.org/10.1177/0885066615619582

Loblaw, A., George, K.J., & Misra, V. (2020). Surgical and radiotherapeutic management of malignant extradural spinal cord compression. *Clinical Oncology, 32*(11), 745–752. https://doi.org/10.1016/j.clon.2020.07.022

Marino, H., & Kaplow, R. (2025). Malignant spinal cord compression. *Journal of Radiology Nursing, 44*(2), 179–183. https://doi.org/10.1016/j.jradnu.2024.12.009

Morimoto, T., Hirata, H., Watanabe, K., Kato, K., Otani, K., Mawatari, M., & Nikaido, T. (2024). The usefulness of deep tendon reflexes in the diagnosis of lumbar spine diseases: A narrative review. *Cureus, 16*(3), e55772. https://doi.org/10.7759/cureus.55772

Narang, M., Mohindra, P., Mishra, M., Regine, W., & Kwok, Y. (2020). Radiation oncology emergencies. *Hematology/Oncology Clinics of North America, 34*(1), 279–292. https://doi.org/10.1016/j.hoc.2019.09.004

Newman, W.C., Laufer, I., & Bilsky, M.H. (2020). Neurologic, oncologic, mechanical, and systemic and other decision frameworks for spinal disease. *Neurosurgery Clinics of North America, 31*(2), 151–166. https://doi.org/10.1016/j.nec.2019.11.005

Newman-Toker, D.E., Peterson, S.M., Badihian, S., Hassoon, A., Nassery, N., Parizadeh, D., ... Robinson, K.A. (2022). *Diagnostic errors in the emergency department: A systematic review.* Agency for Healthcare Research and Quality. https://www.ncbi.nlm.nih.gov/books/NBK588118

Park, S.-J., Ma, C.-H., Lee, C.-S., Jeon, C.-Y., Shin, T.-S., & Park, J.-S. (2022). Survival and functional outcomes after surgical treatment for spinal metastasis in patients with a short life expectancy. *Journal of Clinical Medicine, 12*(1), 46. https://doi.org/10.3390/jcm12010046

Phillips, K., & Schiff, D. (2022). Epidural metastasis and spinal cord compression. In H.B. Newton & M.G. Malkin (Eds.), *Neurological complications of systemic cancer and antineoplastic therapy* (2nd ed., pp. 115–131). https://doi.org/10.1016/B978-0-12-821976-8.00011-6

Potter, P. (2025). Chapter 6: Health assessment. In A.G. Perry, P.A. Potter, W.R. Ostendorf, & N. Laplante (Eds.), *Clinical nursing skills and techniques* (11th ed., pp. 110–176). Mosby.

Potter, P., Perry, A., Stockert, P., Hall, A., & Ostendorf, W. (2025). *Fundamentals of nursing* (12th ed.). Elsevier.

Poullard, A., & Charles, S. (2024). Advanced practice providers' role in intimacy in advanced cancer patients. *Journal of the Advanced Practitioner in Oncology, 15*(1), 56–58. https://doi.org/10.6004/jadpro.2024.15.1.6

Rades, D., Janssen, S., Conde-Moreno, A.J., Cacicedo, J., Metz, M., Veninga, T., ... Schild, S.E. (2017). Role of the overall treatment time of radiotherapy with 10 × 3 Gy for outcomes in patients with metastatic spinal cord compression. *Journal of Medical Imaging and Radiation Oncology, 61*(3), 388–393. https://doi.org/10.1111/1754–9485.12553

Rider, L.S., & Marra, E.M. (2023). Cauda equina and conus medullaris syndromes. In *StatPearls.* StatPearls Publishing. https://www.ncbi.nlm.nih.gov/books/NBK537200

Rothrock, R., Pennington, Z., Ehresman, J., Bilsky, M.H., Barzilai, O., Szerlip, N.J., & Sciubba, D.M. (2020). Hybrid therapy for spinal metastases. *Neurosurgery Clinics of North America, 31*(2), 191–200. https://doi.org/10.1016/j.nec.2019.11.001

Rupp, R., Biering-Sørensen, F., Burns, S.P., Graves, D.E., Guest, J., Jones, L., ... Kirshblum, S. (2021). International standards for neurological classification of spinal cord injury: Revised 2019. *Topics in Spinal Cord Injury Rehabilitation, 27*(2), 1–22. https://doi.org/10.46292/sci2702-1

Sassack, B., & Carrier, J.D. (2023). Anatomy, back, lumbar spine. In *StatPearls.* StatPearls Publishing. https://www.ncbi.nlm.nih.gov/books/NBK557616

Shah, S., Kutka, M., Lees, K., Abson, C., Hadaki, M., Cooke, D., ... Boussios, S. (2021). Management of metastatic spinal cord compression in secondary care: A practice reflection from Medway Maritime Hospital, Kent, UK. *Journal of Personalized Medicine, 11*(2), 110. https://doi.org/10.3390/jpm11020110

Singleton, J.M., & Hefner, M. (2023). Spinal cord compression. In *StatPearls.* StatPearls Publishing. https://www.ncbi.nlm.nih.gov/books/NBK557604

Stephenson, R., & Berliner, J. (2024, March 19). Autonomic dysreflexia in spinal cord injury. *Medscape.* https://emedicine.medscape.com/article/322809-overview

Stie, M., Delmar, C., Nørgaard, B., & Jensen, L.H. (2022). Impact of open dialogue about complementary alternative medicine—A phase II randomized controlled trial. *Cancers, 14*(4), 952. https://doi.org/10.3390/cancers14040952

Van den Brande, R., Cornips, E.M.J., Peeters, M., Ost, P., Billiet, C., & Van de Kelft, E. (2022). Epidemiology of spinal metastases, metastatic epidural spinal cord compression and pathologic vertebral compression fractures in patients with solid tumors: A systematic review. *Journal of Bone Oncology, 35,* 100446. https://doi.org/10.1016/j.jbo.2022.100446

Vassiliou, A., Osunronbi, T., Enyioma, S., Rago, G., Karathanasi, A., Ghose, A., ... Boussios, S. (2023). Prognostic factors in patients with metastatic spinal cord compression secondary to lung cancer—A retrospective UK single-centre study. *Cancers, 15*(18), 4432. https://doi.org/10.3390/cancers15184432

Vavourakis, M., Sakellariou, E., Galanis, A., Karampinas, P., Zachariou, D., Tsalimas, G., ... Pneumatikos, S.G. (2024). Comprehensive insights into metastasis-associated spinal cord compression: Pathophysiology, diagnosis, treatment, and prognosis: A state-of-the-art systematic review. *Journal of Clinical Medicine, 13*(12), 3590. https://doi.org/10.3390/jcm13123590

Weber-Levine, C., Jiang, K., Al-Mistarehi, A., Welland, J., Hersh, A., Horowitz, M., ... Lubelski, D. (2025). The role of combination surgery and radiotherapy in patients with metastatic spinal cord compression: What are the remaining grey areas? A systematic review. *Clinical Neurology and Neurosurgery, 248,* 108632. https://doi.org/10.1016/j.clineuro.2024.108632

Zaki, P., Barbour, A., Zaki, M., Tseng, Y., Amin, A., Venur, V., ... Schaub, S. (2023). Emergent radiotherapy for spinal cord compression/impingement–A narrative review. *Annals of Palliative Medicine, 12*(6), 1447–1462. https://doi.org/10.21037/apm-23-342

Zhang, X., Giantini Larsen, A., Kharas, N., Bilsky, M.H., & Newman, W.C. (2024). Separation surgery for metastatic spine tumors: How less became more. *Neuro-Oncology Advances, 6*(3, Suppl.), iii94–iii100. https://doi.org/10.1093/noajnl/vdae017

Zijlstra, H., Wolterbeek, N., Drost, R.W., Koene, H.R., van der Woude, H.J., Terpstra, W.E., ... Kempen, D.H.R. (2020). Identifying predictive factors for vertebral collapse fractures in multiple myeloma patients. *Spine Journal, 20*(11), 1832–1839. https://doi.org/10.1016/j.spinee.2020.07.004

Linda Bloom, MPA, RN, OCN®,
and Joaquin Buitrago, PhD, RN, OCN®

CHAPTER 7

Increased Intracranial Pressure

FAST FACTS

- **Description:** The cranium encloses brain tissue, blood, and cerebrospinal fluid in a delicate balance. Alteration of these elements or the presence of additional components (e.g., brain tumor) causes compression within the brain and pressure-induced dysfunction of healthy brain functions.
- **Incidence:** The most common causes of oncology-related increased intracranial pressure are primary and metastatic brain tumors, especially lung, breast, and renal cancers, as well as melanoma. Other etiologies include poor cerebrospinal fluid circulation, infectious invasion of the brain or meninges, and intracranial bleeding.
- **Clinical Manifestations:** Symptoms of increased intracranial pressure can vary, ranging from mild neurologic changes to severe, life-threatening neurologic deterioration. The most sensitive indicator of increased intracranial pressure is altered mental status. Nausea, headache, hypertension, and bradycardia may also occur. Focal neurologic deficits (e.g., behavior changes, sensory changes, motor deficits, plegias) may reflect the specific area of brain compression.
- **Risk Factors and Etiology:** Patients with cancer have an increased risk of developing high intracranial pressure related to a space-occupying primary brain lesion, leptomeningeal metastases, interruption in the cerebrospinal fluid, cerebral hemorrhage, and any cerebral vasogenic edema which may occur with these pathologies.
- **Pathophysiology and Patient Evaluation:** Any pressure increase can cause elevated intracranial pressure. This can result in an intracranial herniation, a fatal condition that can lead to brain death. Rapid evaluation and expeditious clinical intervention is critical to preserving neurologic function and patient outcomes.
- **Advanced Practice Considerations:** The initial diagnostic test for increased intracranial pressure is a head computed tomography scan without contrast to detect major structural changes or bleeding. Brain magnetic resonance imaging may follow. Lumbar puncture is performed for suspected meningitis, but only after a computed tomography scan rules out hemorrhage.
- **Treatment Modalities:** Initial treatment focuses on reducing fluid volume in the brain and may include an osmotic diuretic (e.g., mannitol), corticosteroids to reduce edema, and hyperventilation to cause cerebral vasoconstriction. Other therapies, if indicated, include surgery to debulk the tumor, radiation therapy, or direct intrathecal injection of medications if increased intracranial pressure is not exacerbated.
- **Nursing Management:** Nurses should perform frequent neurologic assessments to evaluate the progression of pressure-related injury or response to interventions. Mea-

sures to minimize pressure and resultant clinical effects include elevating the head of the bed, maintaining airway protection, controlling cerebral blood flow, and directly supporting neurologic deficits. Evaluation tools, such as the Glasgow Coma Scale, are available to assess motor response, visual acuity, speech, memory, and the ability to follow commands.

- **Outcomes:** Prompt recognition of manifestations of increased intracranial pressure and potential etiologies permits rapid assessment and diagnosis. Interventions and outcomes vary based on the specific etiology. A successful surgical resection of a brain lesion is the best predictor of a positive clinical outcome.

Introduction

Increased intracranial pressure (ICP) is a potentially fatal neuro-oncology emergency characterized by elevated pressure within the cranial vault. It is often caused by disruptions in cerebrospinal fluid (CSF)—the protective fluid for the brain and spinal cord—as well as impaired circulation, cerebral swelling, or bleeding in the brain (Saria & Kesari, 2021). Uncontrolled, high-pressure states within the solid, nonexpansile skull can lead to catastrophic permanent neurologic deficits or death. Usually, the CSF serves as a filter to remove metabolic waste and deliver nutrients to the central nervous system (CNS). It acts as a cushion to protect the brain and spinal cord (Javed et al., 2023). Under normal circumstances, CSF circulates in the brain, cerebral ventricular system, and spinal cord, and ICP is maintained within a narrow range of 5–15 mm Hg (Kareemi et al., 2023). However, a variety of factors can increase this pressure, including the presence of primary or metastatic brain tumors and the vasogenic edema which frequently accompanies them; blockage of CSF flow; cerebral bleeding or hemorrhages; ischemia; trauma; leptomeningeal disease; and infection of the brain or meninges (Faraj et al., 2022; Pandhi et al., 2020; Saria & Kesari, 2021). Neurologic manifestations of increased ICP range from subtle behavior changes to obvious expressive or receptive aphasia with motor deficits. The onset may be gradual or sudden, and the severity may range from insignificant to severely disabling. Specific, localized symptoms depend on the intracranial location affected by the pressure injury and may be more devastating than the presence of a malignancy.

Early recognition of increased ICP can preserve patients' cognitive and physical functioning. If left untreated, rising ICP can cause brain stem herniation, cessation of vital functions, and death. Oncology nurses are in an ideal position to recognize the subtle alterations in physical and cognitive functioning that are the earliest detectable indicators of increased ICP. Prompt recognition and intervention in this oncologic emergency are paramount for improving survival and minimizing its consequences (Liebman & Makic, 2022).

In patients with a primary or metastatic brain malignancy, a significant increase in brain tissue volume due to the tumor's growth causes crowding in the cranium and the development of cerebral edema. Primary or metastatic lesions may be accompanied by vasogenic edema, obstruction of the CSF flow, cerebral bleeding or ischemia, trauma, and infection of the brain or meninges (Pandhi et al., 2020; Saria & Kesari, 2021). Any tumor or leptomeningeal lesion may hemorrhage within (intraparenchymal or intraventricular hemorrhage) or outside of the brain (subarachnoid, subdural, or epidural hematoma), adding to existing increased ICP. If a tumor or a clot blocks the CSF, a compensatory correction of increased ICP occurs by shunting CSF out of the cranial vault through the ventricles.

Although this process can decrease ICP to a small degree, it produces only a limited benefit. Once this compensation is exhausted, any additional increases in intracranial volume can result in a significant rise in ICP, which may lead to intracranial hypertension (IH), a condition characterized by increased pressure within the skull, affecting the brain and normal homeostatic mechanisms that regulate CSF, requiring immediate medical or surgical interventions (Saha & Tapuria, 2024).

Incidence

The incidence of increased ICP or IH among patients with cancer is ill-defined (Pinto & Adeyinka, 2025). The literature suggests that approximately 10% of patients with cancer develop brain metastases annually. These patients represent 17.9% of individuals with cancer who present to emergency departments of academic medical centers with neurologic symptoms (Lamba et al., 2021). However, cancer and its related consequences remain a leading cause of morbidity and mortality, accounting for 14%–22% of all intensive care unit admissions (Saria & Kesari, 2021).

Although brain cancer comprises 1.3% of all cancers, it was responsible for 3.1% of all cancer-related deaths in 2024, underscoring its disproportionately high mortality rate (National Cancer Institute Surveillance, Epidemiology, and End Results Program, 2025). With advances in treatment, the five-year relative survival rate for malignant primary brain and CNS cancers has increased to 58%. Factors such as tumor location, surgical resection, and age all play a part in patient outcomes (National Cancer Institute Surveillance, Epidemiology, and End Results Program, 2025). Table 7-1 lists the common types and characteristics of primary malignant and metastatic brain tumors.

Leptomeningeal disease, also referred to as leptomeningeal metastases or carcinomatosis, occurs in approximately 20%–40% of patients with cancer (Lamba et al., 2021). Patients with lung and breast cancer, in addition to melanoma, are at most significant risk for developing brain metastases. However, leptomeningeal disease is also seen in patients with advanced renal cell and colorectal cancers (Lamba et al., 2021). Leptomeningeal disease develops most commonly in patients with primary brain tumors (10%–20%), hematologic malignancies (5%–15%), and solid tumors (1%– 8%) (T. Nguyen et al., 2022).

The diffuse nature of leptomeningeal disease defies easy diagnosis (the true incidence is likely underdiagnosed) and may account for 1%–8% of patients with cancer, with 110,000 cases reported annually in the United States (T. Nguyen et al., 2022). Among patients with cancer, autopsy studies indicate that leptomeningeal disease from systemic malignancies comprises approximately 5%–20% (Wilcox et al., 2022).

TABLE 7-1
Common Types of Primary and Metastatic Brain Tumors

Type of Tumor	Description	Location	Treatment	Prognosis
Anaplastic astrocytoma (grade 3)	Cellular anaplasia	Cerebral hemispheres	Gross total resection Radiation therapy Chemotherapy	2–5 years median survival
Astrocytoma (grade 1–2)	Grade 1: well-defined cells Grade 2: less cell differentiation	Cerebral hemispheres	Gross total resection recommended Radiation is controversial; not usually for grade 1	5–7 years median survival
Ependymoma	Slow growing from ependymal cells (lining of the ventricular system)	Ventricular system	Surgery, if accessible Chemotherapy not helpful Radiation controversial; may use craniospinal radiation	5–10 years survival; depends on location
Glioblastoma multiforme (grade 4)	Highly infiltrative Most common, fast-growing Area of necrosis within the tumor	Cerebral hemispheres	Gross total resection Radiation therapy Chemotherapy	12–18 months median survival
Meningioma	Slow growing From meningeal cells Well circumscribed Usually benign	Parasagittal sinus, sphenoid ridge	Usually, gross total resection Observation, depending on size and location	Cure with total removal
Metastatic brain tumors	Spherical, contrast-enhancing with a necrotic center Peritumoral edema Occurs in the gray matter near major arteries	Common primary sites: • Lung: 50% • Breast: 15%–20% • Melanoma: 10% • Unknown primary: 10% • Gastrointestinal tract: 5%	Surgery common with a single lesion Radiation therapy: often radiosensitive lesions	Depends on the presence or absence of systemic disease

(Continued on next page)

TABLE 7-1
Common Types of Primary and Metastatic Brain Tumors *(Continued)*

Type of Tumor	Description	Location	Treatment	Prognosis
Oligodendroglioma (grade 2–3)	May be calcified Usually slow growing	Cerebral hemispheres Occurs in children and adults	Gross total resection Radiation therapy Chemotherapy	5–10 years median survival; depends on grade and loss of heterozygosity on chromosomes 1p/19q

Note. Based on information from Dorsey et al., 2020; Kaidar-Person et al., 2020; Louis et al., 2021; Neiderhuber et al., 2020; Rezaei & Hanaei, 2023; Seano, 2021; Zaky et al., 2024; Zoghbi et al., 2024.

Malignant cells in the CSF have been detected in 50% of melanomas, 48% of metastatic breast cancers, and 28% of lung cancers (Jeffus et al., 2024). Acute leukemia and non-Hodgkin lymphoma historically had a reported incidence of leptomeningeal disease as high as 30% (A. Nguyen et al., 2023). However, with routine CNS prophylaxis, this number has been reduced to less than 10% (Ozcan et al., 2023). The incidence of leptomeningeal disease in breast and lung cancers and melanoma is increasing, possibly related to chemotherapies that better control systemic disease but have suboptimal CNS penetration, potentially leading to poor disease control in the CNS (Gwak, 2023). These metastatic tumors are difficult to treat medically and are a poor prognostic indicator. Unfortunately, because of the mass effect of leptomeningeal metastases, neurologic sequelae and increased ICP may be the presenting sign of a late cancer diagnosis (Achrol et al., 2019).

Clinical Manifestations

Clinical signs of increased ICP vary based on the source, rate, and severity of pressure. The hallmark symptom is altered mental status (Pandhi et al., 2020; Saria & Kesari, 2021). Early signs include headache, nausea, vomiting, visual disturbances, pupillary or behavioral changes, confusion, and vital sign shifts (e.g., bradycardia, hypotension). Late signs, such as the Cushing triad, stupor, coma, and abnormal posturing, often signal impending herniation (Hinkle et al., 2021; Pinto & Adeyinka, 2025).

Headaches are common and may worsen over time or after activities. They often resist standard pain relievers but may improve briefly after vomiting (Burleson et al., 2023). Vomiting, particularly projectile and unaccompanied by nausea, suggests infratentorial lesions. In leptomeningeal disease, headaches—often bifrontal or at the skull base—are frequent and may be accompanied by nausea and vomiting (Wilcox et al., 2023). Posterior reversible encephalopathy syndrome (PRES) is caused by brain swelling and is usually diagnosed with imaging (e.g., magnetic resonance imaging [MRI]) (Zelaya & Al-Khoury, 2024). It can also present with a headache, which is typically occipital and dull. As ICP increases, altered consciousness, hemiplegia, and posturing may develop, possibly progressing to death (Niederhuber et al., 2020). Nurses must recognize that neurologic deficits do not always correlate with ICP levels and should perform regular, detailed neurologic assessments, including cognition, memory, orientation, speech, and motor/sensory function, to detect subtle changes (Morrison et al., 2022).

Increased Focal Pressure

Focal pressure changes within the brain develop as a result of a localized tumor, vasogenic edema, obstruction, or injury to a specific area, causing alterations of site-specific neurologic functions. Symptoms can include changes in handwriting, memory, counting, speaking (e.g., slurring, word substitution), limb usage, gait, and vision (e.g., blurring, diplopia, field cut). Hemiplegia and receptive and expressive aphasia are also common features of elevated focal pressure (Ghandour et al., 2021). Motor weakness may develop in the leg and arm on the side of the body opposite to the intracranial mass because of the pressure on the pyramidal tracts (Buitrago et al., 2019; Rees, 2022). Additionally, changes in visual acuity and blurring of vision can occur because of early swelling in the cerebral hemisphere. Also, diplopia results from weakness of one or more of the extraocular muscles. Assessment of extraocular movements may determine which cranial nerves are affected by the increasing pressure and provide information about brain stem functioning. Cranial nerves III, IV, and VI participate in extraocular movements (Buitrago et al., 2019; Rees, 2022).

Effects on Vital Signs

Vital signs can indicate increased ICP. Temperature remains normal unless hypothalamic damage occurs, causing elevated temperature, typically in the decompensatory phase (Hinkle et al., 2021; Morrison et al., 2022; Pinto & Adeyinka, 2025). Blood pressure initially rises as a compensatory response, leading to widened pulse pressure. When PRES occurs, it may be caused by intracerebral hemorrhage, and high blood pressure may be more common. As ICP rises further, blood pressure decreases in the decompensatory phase. Pulse remains stable until brain stem herniation occurs, causing bradycardia, and later, irregular, rapid, and thready pulses leading to cardiac arrest (Hickey & Strayer, 2019; Pandhi et al., 2020). Respiratory patterns change as ICP increases, starting with Cheyne-Stokes respirations, progressing to ataxic or agonal breathing, and finally apnea with brain stem herniation (Hinkle et al., 2021; Morrison et al., 2022; Pinto & Adeyinka, 2025). Late signs include the Cushing triad (hypertension with widening pulse pressure, bradycardia, and abnormal respirations), signaling brain stem dysfunction and low brain compliance, often with comatose states and cerebral herniation (Hickey & Strayer, 2019; Pandhi et al., 2020).

Infections and Inflammation

Brain infections lead to vasogenic edema, abscess, or diffuse infiltration with white blood cells—all of which shift the normal structures within the brain and lead to increased ICP. Symptoms of brain abscess include headache (most common) and focal deficits based on location, but fever is not usual. Urgent signs and symptoms include a headache that suddenly becomes severe and is associated with neck stiffness or photophobia (T. Nguyen et al., 2022; Nolan et al., 2021). These manifestations usually indicate that the abscess has reached a ventricle, raising the risk of death to as high as 80% (Pinto & Adeyinka, 2025).

Brain inflammation may involve the meninges (meningitis) or the cerebral tissue. Common signs of meningitis are fever, chills, nausea, vomiting, photophobia, nuchal rigidity (stiff neck), cognitive impairment, agitation, somnolence, and an associated rash or seizure. Encephalitis is characterized by somnolence, confusion, location-specific focal deficits, and seizures. PRES is rare and typically presents in the posterior cerebrum. Clinical symptoms related to PRES usually include headache, encephalopathy, visual disturbances, altered mental status, and seizures (Guevara et al., 2022; Zelaya & Al-Khoury, 2024).

Radiation Necrosis

Radiation necrosis is a late complication of radiation therapy (RT) to the brain that can cause an inflammatory process that typically affects the white matter. The incidence of this complication may be as high as 25% (Mayo et al., 2023). Radiation necrosis can develop in any region of the brain where a tumor has been irradiated and is almost indistinguishable from tumor progression. Local necrosis and edema may result (Mayo et al., 2023; Zoghbi et al., 2024). Depending on the location, extent, and the amount of edema it causes, signs and symptoms of necrosis can range from focal neurologic deficits to the most advanced presentation of increased ICP and IH (Mayo et al., 2023; Rashidi et al., 2025). Factors associated with an increased risk of radiation necrosis include the volume of tissue irradiated, dose fractionation schedule, prior treatment with RT, and radiation-sensitizing chemotherapy (Mayo et al., 2023). Patients with necrosis of the temporal lobe will have cognitive impairment affecting memory, language, and executive function (Dixit & Kumthekar, 2020). This delayed complication may develop within months or years after radiation exposure (Zoghbi et al., 2024). Although no standardized treatment exists for radiation necrosis, some patients have benefited from high-dose corticosteroids, hyperbaric oxygen, or administration of a vascular endothelial growth factor inhibitor (e.g., bevacizumab), which helps reduce vascular permeability of the blood–brain barrier (BBB) (Mayo et al., 2023; Niederhuber et al., 2020).

Risk Factors and Etiology

Increased ICP is a common neurologic complication in patients with cancer and occurs most frequently in the presence of primary brain tumors, metastatic brain lesions, meningeal malignancies, intracranial hemorrhage (ICH), and central nervous system infections. Primary or metastatic tumors increase intracranial volume through direct mass effect and by promoting vasogenic edema, thereby contributing to elevated ICP (Pandhi et al., 2020).

Additional factors include tumor-related hemorrhage, obstruction of cerebral blood flow, and both direct and indirect brain injury (Jeffus et al., 2024). Obstruction of cerebrospinal fluid flow caused by tumors or clots, cerebral bleeding, ischemia, trauma, leptomeningeal disease, and infections of the brain or meninges can lead to intracranial overcrowding and progressive increases in ICP (Pandhi et al., 2020; Saria & Kesari, 2021). Tumors or metastatic lesions may also result in obstructive hydrocephalus or hemorrhage within the brain parenchyma or ventricles, or in extra-axial spaces such as subarachnoid, subdural, or epidural compartments (Saha & Tapuria, 2024).

Certain treatment modalities, such as immunotherapies (e.g., chimeric antigen receptor [CAR] T-cell therapy), chemotherapy, or RT, may also lead to cerebral edema, a volume shift inside the cranium, or an infection (Ahmed et al., 2021; Patel et al., 2023).

Once ICP elevation rises to life-threatening levels (> 20 mm Hg), IH can occur (Hinkle et al., 2021; Pandhi et al., 2020; Patel et al., 2023; Saria & Kesari, 2021). If left untreated, IH leads to decreased brain perfusion, cessation of vital functions, and death (Pinto & Adeyinka, 2025). Prompt intervention is needed and can interrupt this destructive cycle and preserve cognitive and physical functioning (Morrison et al., 2022). Learning to quickly recognize the subtle alterations in the physical and cognitive functioning of rising ICP can prevent brain herniation (see Table 7-2).

TABLE 7-2
Conditions Associated With the Development of Increased Intracranial Pressure

Factor	Explanation
Astrocytoma (grade 1–2)	Benign or well differentiated Occurs primarily in the cerebral cortex
Anaplastic astrocytoma (grade 3)	Malignant Occurs primarily in the cerebral cortex, can occur in the cerebellum and spine
Glioblastoma multiforme (grade 4)	Rapidly growing; malignant Usually occurs in the cerebral cortex, but can occur in the cerebellum and spine Accounts for 55% of all gliomas
Ependymoma	Occurs in the lining of the ventricles; responds best to surgery and radiation

(Continued on next page)

TABLE 7-2.
Conditions Associated With the Development of Increased Intracranial Pressure *(Continued)*

Factor	Explanation
Oligodendroglioma	May be well differentiated, low grade Occurs in the cerebral cortex; calcification within the tumor common Improved survival in subtypes with deletions on chromosomes 1p and 19q
Metastatic brain tumor	Occurs in 20%–40% of patients with cancer; most frequently associated with cancers of the lung, breast, colon, and rectum
Diffuse cerebral edema with leukemia	Attributable to leukostasis—blast counts > 400,000 cells/mcl
Encephalopathy syndromes	Causes vasogenic edema due to infection or inflammation of the brain; may be a direct toxic effect or from endothelial injury
Disseminated intravascular coagulation	Causes diffuse cerebral hemorrhages
Herpes simplex encephalitis	Causes extensive vasogenic edema
Leptomeningeal metastasis	Often obstructs the flow of cerebrospinal fluid
Opportunistic infection	Often present with signs of increased intracranial pressure (e.g., cerebral toxoplasmosis, aspergillosis, candidiasis)
Radiation necrosis	Increased intracranial pressure from vascular damage postradiation therapy
Syndrome of inappropriate antidiuretic hormone secretion	Causes increased intracellular water and sodium content in brain cells, resulting in cerebral edema
Cranial irradiation, acute reaction	Vasogenic edema caused by tissue damage from radiation

Note. Based on information from Achrol et al., 2019; Delawan et al., 2024; Faraj et al., 2022; Niederhuber et al., 2020; Odom-Forren, 2024; Sobti et al., 2024; Yust-Katz et al., 2020.

Direct Tumor Effects

Malignant tumors within the brain can increase ICP through a variety of mechanisms, ranging from direct tumor compression of brain tissue or vasculature to infiltration of the meninges. The presence of brain tumors enhances the release of tissue thromboplastin from glial cells, creating a hypercoagulability state and increasing the risk for ischemic stroke, meningitis, and encephalitis. Cerebral venous sinus thrombosis, a rare form of ischemic brain injury, may be directly caused by vascular injury from a tumor or indirectly caused by hypercoagulability. It is commonly seen with dehydration, intracranial infections, and acute lymphoblastic leukemia (Khaddam et al., 2024; T. Nguyen et al., 2022).

Ommaya Reservoir Complications

The Ommaya reservoir, implanted into the cerebral ventricles, is a ventricular access device that provides access to the intrathecal space. It is a highly effective implant that allows for long-term access to the CSF and can be used for the administration of antineoplastic, antimicrobial, and analgesic medications directly into the brain (Hall & De Jesus, 2025). It is important to remember that when chemotherapy agents are delivered through the shunt into the CSF for a malignancy that involves the meninges, there is a risk of increasing ICP. The most frequent complications of ventricular reservoir placement are infection, suboptimal position, subdural hematoma, mechanical device failure, and leukoencephalopathy.

Obstruction of Cerebrospinal Fluid Flow

Increased ICP can result from tumor cells obstructing the flow of CSF, an occluded Ommaya reservoir, the presence of leptomeningeal disease, or blood products that may impede the CSF reabsorption process, which can lead to a multitude of symptoms attributed to cerebral edema, cranial and spinal dysfunction, and hydrocephalus (Khosla et al., 2023). A tumor can obstruct CSF flow, primarily when it is located at a bottleneck in the CSF pathway, such as the foramen of Monro or the aqueduct of Sylvius (see Figure 7-1).

Infection

Patients who are immunocompromised with primary CNS tumors or leptomeningeal metastases are at heightened risk for intracranial infections, including abscesses, meningitis, and encephalitis caused by bacterial, viral, or fungal pathogens (Al-asady et al., 2024; Freifield & Kaul, 2020; Zinserling, 2022). These infections may result from CNS surgery, traumatic injury, hematogenous spread, or devices such as Ommaya reservoirs and shunts (Farkas, 2022; Hall & De Jesus, 2022). Effective assessment and thorough monitoring of implanted devices, such as Ommaya reservoirs and central vascular catheters, are essential to identify and prevent infections, including those of the CNS. Common pathogens include *Streptococcus pneumoniae*, *Neisseria meningitidis*, *Haemophilus influenzae*, *Toxoplasma gondii*, *Taenia solium*, *Aspergillus*, and *Nocardia* (Arjarquah et al., 2022; Tawfik et al., 2022; Yanagida et al., 2024). Opportunistic infections are especially prevalent in patients with HIV, hematologic malignancies, or those undergoing transplantation (Owusu & Abebrese, 2023). Viral encephalitis may be caused by herpes

FIGURE 7-1. Brain Herniation Syndromes

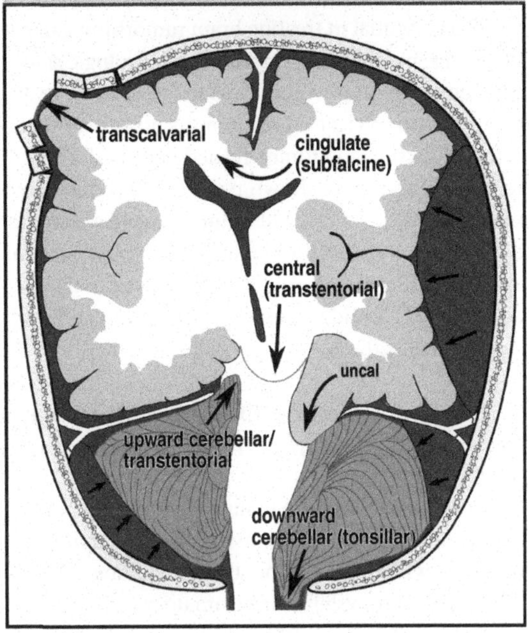

Note. Image courtesy of RupertMillard (https://commons.wikimedia.org/wiki/File:Brain_herniation_types-2.svg). Licensed under CC BY-SA 3.0 (https://creativecommons.org/licenses/by-sa/3.0/deed.en).

simplex virus, varicella zoster virus, Epstein-Barr virus, or human polyomavirus 2, commonly referred to as the John Cunningham virus. Along with rituximab, John Cunningham virus has been linked to progressive multifocal leukoencephalopathy (Farkas, 2022; Tcyganov et al., 2021). Fungal mycotic aneurysms and generalized CSF infections, occurring in 10%–25% of recipients of intraventricular chemotherapy, are also relevant concerns (Tawfik et al., 2022; Yanagida et al., 2024).

ICH, the most fatal form of stroke, can occur in intracerebral, subarachnoid, subdural, or epidural spaces and is particularly common in patients with cancer because of coagulopathies, thrombocytopenia, infection, or tumor-related bleeding (Khorchid & Malkoff, 2020; Qdaisat et al., 2022). Intraparenchymal hemorrhage is most frequent, followed by other compartments. Highly vascular tumors, including metastases from melanoma, lung and breast cancers, glioblastoma, and hematologic malignancies, significantly increase ICH risk. Antiangiogenic agents, such as bevacizumab, have also been associated with ICH (Wang et al., 2024). Among patients with leukemia, especially those with acute promyelocytic leukemia, ICH is linked to disseminated intravascular coagulation, leukemic infiltration, and fungal infections, representing a significant cause of mortality (Kannan et al., 2023). It leads to hospitalizations in up to 15% of cases and has a mortality rate of 25.6% among patients with cancer (Qdaisat et al., 2022).

Cerebral Edema

Local vasogenic edema that develops around any brain tumor contributes to a global increase in ICP. Common imaging findings in patients with cancer show brain edema at 47% and midline shifts at 34% (Qdaisat et al., 2022). Cranial irradiation, used to treat benign and malignant low- or high-grade brain tumors, frequently causes local swelling and an increase in ICP (Qdaisat et al., 2022).

Radiation Therapy Complications

RT is essential in treating brain tumors but can cause both acute and delayed complications, including increased ICP. Neurologic side effects depend on dose, treatment fractions, and brain volume irradiated (Khosla et al., 2023). Acute reactions typically occur within weeks to three months post-treatment and may involve worsening neurologic function and tumor-related deficits. Techniques sparing the hippocampus and temporal lobes have shown potential in reducing cognitive decline in patients with brain metastases. A rare but serious delayed effect, radiation necrosis, arises six months to three years after RT and may lead to irreversible neurologic decline and stroke-like symptoms (Zoghbi et al., 2024). RT-related ischemic strokes may result from vascular damage and carotid stenosis following head and neck irradiation (Khosla et al., 2023; Zoghbi et al., 2024).

Immune Effector Cell Therapy–Associated Increased Intracranial Pressure

CAR T-cell therapy has shown promising outcomes in treating a variety of B-cell malignancies. However, it is associated with unique and severe toxicities not commonly observed with other cell therapies, including cytokine release syndrome, a potentially life-threatening systemic inflammatory response. Cytokine release syndrome is often characterized by high fever, flu-like symptoms, and potential progression to severe complications, including hypotension, hypoxia, and multiorgan dysfunction (Bangolo et al., 2025). In addition to CAR T cells, bispecific T-cell engagers and bispecific antibodies are targeted therapies that may have similar toxicity profiles.

Immune effector cell–associated neurotoxicity syndrome (ICANS) is another well-recognized potential side effect of CAR T-cell therapy and is usually reversible with the use of steroids. It is generally expressed by confusion, word-finding difficulties, impaired fine motor skills, headache, lethargy, agitation, hallucinations, tremors, memory loss, and personality changes ranging from mild to severe. Worse cases present with seizures, coma, cerebral edema, and brain hemorrhage (Rees, 2022).

Additional Factors

Various activities (e.g., coughing, vomiting, Valsalva maneuver) can transiently raise ICP, whereas sustained increases may result from hypertension, seizures, hyperthermia, and hepatic encephalopathy linked to ammonia accumulation (Davidson & Kumar, 2024; Mendoza Vasquez et al., 2023; Yiangou et al., 2024). Neurotoxic effects from treatments, including as intrathecal methotrexate, L-asparaginase, and intra-arterial chemotherapy, have also been implicated (Jung et al., 2024). Paraneoplastic limbic encephalopathy, often seen in late-stage cancers such as small cell lung or testicular, can cause seizures, memory loss, and increased ICP (Altabakhi et al., 2024; T. Nguyen et al., 2022). Chemotherapy-induced neurologic deficits may include encephalopathy, ataxia, and polyneuropathy. Ifosfamide-related limbic encephalopathy can also present with symptoms of elevated ICP. Additionally, PRES, linked to multiple cancer therapies, involves vasogenic edema and symptoms such as headaches, vision changes, seizures, and altered mental status (T. Nguyen et al., 2022).

Neurotoxicity in the context of CAR T-cell therapy is typically characterized by encephalopathy, which presents with symptoms such as confusion, delirium, cognitive impairment, and language disturbances, often leading to compromised handwriting and motor weakness. Expressive aphasia is a hallmark of severe neurotoxicity. Although rare, cerebral edema can develop rapidly, leading to brain death within 24 hours. Seizures are also observed, especially in patients with specific CAR T-cell constructs, such as axicabtagene ciloleucel or idecabtagene vicleucel (Santomasso et al., 2023; Velasco et al., 2023). Neurologic toxicities, including ICP, myoclonic seizures, and transient ischemic attacks, may occur for weeks post-infusion of CAR T cells. These can manifest as headaches, neuropsychiatric disorders (e.g., depression, suicidal attempts), coordination problems, weakness, confusion, and aphasia (Buitrago et al., 2019).

Pathophysiology and Patient Evaluation

Understanding Pathophysiologic Processes

Healthy Brain Physiology

Intracranial volume can be divided into three components: brain tissue (80%), blood (10%), and CSF (10%). In a healthy adult with an intact skull, the three components of the brain remain in a constant relationship (Davidson & Kumar, 2024) (see Table 7-3 for formulas and definitions related to intracranial volume). The Monro-Kellie doctrine (Monro, 1783) states that to maintain a normal ICP in the fixed space of the cranium, the brain parenchyma, blood, and CSF should remain at a steady volume of 1,400–1,700 ml. If the volume of any one of these components increases, another must decrease to maintain this dynamic equilibrium. Without this reciprocal relationship, ICP could increase above the normal acceptable range of 5–15 mm Hg (Kareemi et al., 2023). If ICP should rise above 5–15 mm Hg, the assessment and management of the increase is critical to ensure the best outcomes for patients (Kareemi et al., 2023; Liebman & Makic, 2022).

Cerebral Hemodynamics

Cerebral perfusion pressure (CPP), ideally between 70–100 mm Hg, is a function of both the mean arterial pressure (MAP) and ICP. An increase in ICP or a decrease in MAP can lower CPP, raising the risk for ischemia and infarction. Compensatory mechanisms, such as CSF displacement, help to manage minor pressure changes, but larger shifts can be dangerous (Liebman & Makic, 2022; Saha & Tapuria, 2024).

Normal cerebral blood flow is 50 ml/100 g/minute, with gray matter receiving significantly more than white matter. The CSF, primarily produced in the choroid plexus, circulates through the brain ventricles and subarachnoid space via the foramina of Luschka and Magendie. To reduce ICP, CSF can be drained, or cerebral blood volume reduced through vasoconstriction. Because the brain relies on glucose for energy and cannot store it, adequate blood flow is critical (Pinto & Adeyinka, 2025; Saha & Tapuria, 2024).

TABLE 7-3
Terminology Related to Intracranial Volume

Term	Definitions and Formulas
Intracranial pressure (ICP)	The pressure normally exerted by the cerebrospinal fluid, which circulates around the brain and spinal cord Normal range ICP: 0–10 mm Hg (15 = high normal)
Intracranial compliance	Adaptability of the brain to maintain volume and pressure equilibrium Compliance (C): the ratio of change in cerebral volume to the resulting change in pressure (C = dV/dP [change in volume/change in pressure])
Intracranial elastance	Inverse of compliance; refers to pressure changes for a given change in volume
Mean arterial pressure (MAP)	MAP = [(2 × diastolic blood pressure) + systolic blood pressure] / 3 MAP < 70 mm Hg: possible reduction in cerebral blood flow, but also reduces cerebral perfusion pressure Normal MAP > 65 mm Hg
Central venous pressure (CVP)	Right atrial pressure
Cerebral blood flow (CBF)	CBF = CPP/CVR (cerebrovascular resistance)
Cerebral perfusion pressure (CPP)	Blood pressure gradient of the brain: CPP = MAP – CVP Normal range: 70–100 mm Hg

Note. Based on information from Faraj et al., 2022; Liebman & Makic, 2022; Odom-Forren, 2024; Pandhi et al., 2020.

Intracranial Pressure Concepts and Changes

ICP is the pressure exerted by the CSF around the brain and spinal cord, regulated by the brain's elastance and compliance. In this instance, compliance refers to the brain's adaptability, whereas elastance refers to its stiffness—both influence pressure–volume dynamics. When the brain's compensatory mechanisms (e.g., CSF, blood displacement) are exceeded, ICP increases (Liebman & Makic, 2022; Saha & Tapuria, 2024).

The BBB protects the CNS by restricting harmful substances from entering the brain. Formed by tightly joined capillary cells, the BBB allows fat-soluble molecules to pass but blocks water-soluble substances. Although it protects the brain from toxins and pathogens, it also prevents most chemotherapy agents from entering it. High-dose chemotherapy can partially overcome this; however, the necessary doses can be too toxic for safe use, potentially allowing unchecked tumor growth (Davidson & Kumar, 2024).

The skull cannot accommodate expanding masses, vasogenic edema, increased CSF, or excess intracerebral volume caused by treatments such as RT, chemotherapy, or immunotherapy (Asioli et al., 2024). Vasogenic edema, resulting from increased capillary permeability at the BBB, leads to extracellular fluid leakage from brain lesions, trauma, or abscesses. Cytotoxic edema, caused by oncologic treatments, results in fluid accumulation in brain cells due to sodium–potassium pump failure, resulting in diffuse brain swelling. This can also occur in conditions such as syndrome of inappropriate antidiuretic hormone (Hladky & Barrand, 2024).

As ICP increases and compensatory mechanisms fail, mass effect and cerebral tissue shifts may lead to herniation, a potentially fatal downward displacement of brain tissue (Faraj et al., 2022). Common types include central and uncal herniation. Central herniation compresses the brain stem and causes rapid neurologic decline, whereas uncal herniation can cause pupillary dilation due to pressure on the oculomotor nerve (Hladky & Barrand, 2024). When ICP equals MAP, blood flow stops, leading to permanent damage. Early diagnosis and treatment are imperative to prevent irreversible damage, coma, or death (Bhalla et al., 2024; Faraj et al., 2022).

Brain Tumors

Brain tumors, both primary and metastatic, can increase ICP by expanding intracranial tissue, blocking CSF flow, and causing vasogenic edema (Saria & Kesari, 2021). Cancer-related inflammation of the meninges, known as carcinomatous meningitis, occurs when tumor cells infiltrate the leptomeninges and spread through the CSF, often collecting along nerve routes (Javed et al., 2023; Saria & Kesari, 2021).

Treatment options for brain tumors, including RT, surgery, chemotherapy, and antiangiogenesis agents, have greatly improved survival rates (Dixit & Kumthekar, 2020). Multimodal strategies may include chemotherapy wafers and radiosensitizing agents (Bouché et al., 2021). RT, used for both benign and malignant tumors, can lead to radiation necrosis, a complication that increases ICP due to brain vascular injury and edema, particularly in patients receiving whole-brain radiation or stereotactic radiosurgery (Rashidi et al., 2025). Radiation necrosis affects 5%–24% of patients receiving whole-brain radiation and 2%–10% of those undergoing stereotactic radiosurgery. Risk factors include high radiation doses, chemotherapy, and comorbidities such as hypertension and diabetes (Rashidi et al., 2025).

Brain Infections and Inflammatory Disorders

Brain infections are uncommon due to the protective cranium, increased vaccination rates, and the actions of the BBB; however, when brain infections occur, they can cause increased ICP due to inflammatory edema associated with mass-occupying lesions such as an abscess (Guevara et al., 2022). An abscess is a collection of microorganisms and infected tissue that has accumulated in one particular region of the brain. *Encephalitis*, *meningitis*, and *encephalomyelitis* are terms for the diffuse inflammation within the brain, meninges, or spinal cord. CNS infections most often result from a microorganism that was introduced during surgery or a penetrating wound, which can lead to a local abscess. Microorganisms, such as *Neisseria meningitidis* and *Haemophilus influenzae type b*, can also infiltrate the BBB via the sinuses or paranasal structures. Those that travel to the CNS from another part of the body are more likely to result in meningitis or encephalitis and can occur with infections from dental procedures, heart vegetation, primary syphilis, viral diseases, or spread from an infected carrier of meningitis (Al-asady et al., 2024; Guevara et al., 2022).

Paraneoplastic and drug-induced limbic encephalitis leads to focal vasogenic edema and inflammatory vascular permeability. This inflammation may be generalized throughout the body (from paraneoplastic methotrexate or ifosfamide-induced toxicity) or focal (located in the brain within the posterior and occipital cortical and subcortical white matter) (Guevara et al., 2022).

Patient Assessment

History

Patient assessment is necessary for identifying neurologic changes related to increasing ICP, with localized symptoms varying depending on the intracranial location of pressure (Rai et al., 2021). Nurses should consider patients' personal and family medical history, including non-oncologic risks, such as cardiovascular disease, cerebral arteriovenous malformation, diabetes, and hypertension, as well as oncologic risks, such as cancers prone to brain metastases (Knox et al., 2024; Pinto & Adeyinka, 2025; Talleur et al., 2024). RT for brain tumors can cause temporary edema, raising ICP. Specific chemotherapy agents may also induce hyponatremia or syndrome of inappropriate antidiuretic hormone, which can also increase ICP. Prolonged neutropenia elevates the risk of brain infections, which should be suspected in patients with persistent fever or new neurologic symptoms (Nolan et al., 2021; Shalabi et al., 2022). Additional risk factors include coagulopathy, hepatic disease, and renal dysfunction.

Physical Examination

Early recognition of increased ICP is critical, as timely intervention can reverse damage before brain stem involvement causes permanent deficits. Nurses are integral in identifying early signs, such as mental status changes, headache, vomiting, and vision disturbances, through regular, structured neurologic assessments (Liebman & Makic, 2022). Vital sign monitoring is key for detecting Cushing triad, which signals possible impending herniation (Pinto & Adeyinka, 2025). In addition, during physical examination, identification of potential meningitis related to implanted devices or surgical site infections, which usually occur during the immediate postoperative period (e.g., redness, swelling, wound dehiscence), can help to prevent meningitis and its related increase in ICP.

Cranial nerve assessments help identify brain stem involvement. For example, cranial nerve I is linked to olfaction (smell) but can be difficult to test; compression of cranial nerve II leads to vision loss; and cranial nerve III dysfunction presents as pupil dilation (see Table 7-4). Pupils should be assessed for size, shape, symmetry, and light response—sluggish or unequal pupils can indicate early or advanced increased ICP (Godase et al., 2024). Ocular movement abnormalities involving cranial nerves III, IV, and VI are associated with eye movement. If any of these nerves are affected, nystagmus or dysconjugate gaze may occur, which is also suggestive of increased ICP (Balasubaramaniam et al., 2023). Motor function is commonly assessed using the

Glasgow Coma Scale (GCS) (see Table 7-5), which helps quantify ocular, verbal, and motor responses. Motor symptoms can range from weakness to hemiplegia (Patel et al., 2023). Transient increases in ICP may result from coughing, vomiting, or the Valsalva maneuver, leading to short-term symptoms such as headache, speech issues, visual changes, or motor dysfunction, making vigilance during patient care a priority (Saha & Tapuria, 2024).

TABLE 7-4
Cranial Nerve Assessment

Function	Cranial Nerve (CN)	Assessment
Olfaction (smell)	CN I	Difficult to test; identify if scent is unfamiliar or loss of smell is present.
Vision	CN II: visual fields CN II, III: pupillary light reflex CN III, IV, VI: eye movements	Assess eye movement by asking patient to follow fingers (8 cardinal points). Monitor pupil constriction.
Facial sensation	CN V	Lightly touch right side of patient's face and repeat on other side. Note deviations in sensation.
Facial strength	CN V: mastication CN VII: facial expression	Have patient smile, look up, and wrinkle forehead. Monitor for deviations from side to side.
Hearing	CN VIII	Hold fingers inches away from patient's ear and rub together softly, testing each ear separately.
Vestibular function	CN VIII	Assess patient's gait and balance.
Palate movement	CN IX CN X	Ask patient to say "ahhhh" or to yawn, and look for symmetrical movement of the palate.
Dysarthria—impairments of speech	CN IX CN X CN XII	Assess gag reflex and abnormalities in swallowing. Monitor for abnormal voice quality, irregular rhythm with speech, and errors in articulation.
Head rotation/ shoulder elevation	CN XI	Have patient turn head against resistance and shrug shoulders.
Tongue movement	CN XII	Ask patient to stick out and wiggle tongue.

Note. Reprinted with permission from the American Society of PeriAnesthesia Nurses (ASPAN). *2024 Redi-Ref for Perianesthesia Practices*. ASPAN: 2024.

TABLE 7-5
Glasgow Coma Scale

Category	Response	Score
Eye opening	Spontaneously	4
	To speech	3
	To pain	2
	None	1
Best verbal response	Oriented to person, place, and time	5
	Confused (unable to state name, location, or date)	4
	Inappropriate words	3
	Incomprehensible sounds	2
	None	1
Best motor response	Obeys commands	6
	Localizes pain (attempts to remove stimuli)	5
	Withdraws from pain (pulls away from stimuli)	4
	Abnormal flexion (decorticate positioning)	3
	Abnormal extension (decerebrate positioning)	2
	None	1

The Glasgow Coma Scale is graded on a scale of 3–15.
- The lower the score, the lower the level of consciousness
- 8 or lower indicates a coma
- 15 indicates fully awake

Note. Reprinted with permission from the American Society of PeriAnesthesia Nurses (ASPAN). *2024 Redi-Ref for Perianesthesia Practices*. ASPAN: 2024.

Advanced Practice Considerations

Imaging Studies

Neuroradiology studies, such as computed tomography (CT) scans and MRIs, are essential for diagnosing and monitoring ICP. Because CT scans are widely available, they are often the first imaging tool used, showing signs such as effaced sulci, compressed ventricles, and mass effect (Bhalla et al., 2024). Although noncontrast CT scans remain the gold standard for detecting cerebral bleeding, MRIs with gadolinium provide higher resolution and greater sensitivity for identifying lesions and edema (Todd et al., 2021).

Brain MRIs are especially useful in detecting tumors that disrupt the BBB. Tumor-related production of vascular endothelial growth factor inhibitor increases BBB permeability, allowing gadolinium to leak into brain tissue, highlighting tumor locations (Faraj et al., 2022). However, RT, recent surgery, steroid use, and vascular endothelial growth factor inhibitor therapy can alter BBB integrity, potentially misleading the interpretation of MRI results (Dixit & Kumthekar, 2020). High-dose gadolinium with postcontrast fluid–attenuated inversion recovery is an MRI sequence that can help distinguish small metastases from other lesions (Kaidar-Person et al., 2020). Positron-emission tomography scans, often combined with CT, provide metabolic and perfusion data, helping differentiate active tumors from scar tissue and improving diagnostic accuracy in both clinical and research settings (Holzgreve et al., 2021). A definitive PRES diagnosis is usually made using radiographic studies such as MRIs. Images typically reveal symmetrical white matter edema, traditionally found in the posterior cerebrum (Zelaya & Al-Khoury, 2024). Appropriate nursing and medical staff should accompany patients who are clinically unstable with increased ICP to the procedure.

Lumbar Puncture

Lumbar puncture is the definitive test for diagnosing leptomeningeal metastasis through the detection of malignant cells in the CSF (liquid biopsies preferred). When a lumbar puncture is performed in combination with imaging studies, such as a CT scan, MRI, or positron-emission tomography–CT scan, it can identify malignancies or infections, including meningitis or carcinomatosis meningitis (Ozcan et al., 2023). However, it is contraindicated in patients with elevated ICP because of the risk of worsening pressure (Sexton & Richie, 2024). Although malignant cells in CSF confirm cancer, other findings suggest infections in the absence of cytology, such as high protein, low glucose, elevated opening pressures, and increased white blood cells (Neiderhuber et al., 2020). Flow cytometry aids in diagnosing leukemic meningitis, and laboratory technologies enhance blast detection in low-volume CSF samples. Performing a lumbar puncture in patients with increased ICP, particularly those with carcinomatous meningitis or a space-occupying lesion, can lead to brain stem compression, herniation, or death. If monitoring is available, an ICP reading greater than 20 mm Hg for more than five minutes indicates IH and requires aggressive treatment (Pinto & Adeyinka, 2025).

Laboratory Studies

Assessment of a complete blood count and chemistries is vital to evaluate chemical etiologies of increased ICP. Elevated serum white blood cells and blood cultures may be diagnostic for an existing or impending infection, such as meningitis or encephalitis. Significant anemia, a hemoglobin level between 7–10 g/dl, should be treated. In contrast, serum chemistries can detect sodium imbalances (e.g., syndrome of inappropriate antidiuretic hormone), hyperosmolarity (e.g., hyperglycemia), and hyperammonemia. These studies are used in conjunction with neurologic examination and other, more specific diagnostic tests to define the most likely etiologies of elevated ICP. Laboratory tests include the following (Niederhuber et al., 2020):

- Comprehensive metabolic panel
- Complete blood count
- Prothrombin time
- Partial prothrombin time
- International normalized ratio
- Serum and urine osmolality

Treatment Modalities

Treatment for increased ICP should begin aggressively when the first signs or symptoms of neurologic deterioration appear. Serial neurologic assessments identify these early changes and prevent the compensatory mechanisms from progressing to decompensation. Successfully addressing increased ICP requires treatment of underlying causes while monitoring cerebral hemodynamics, maintaining adequate cerebral oxygenation, and preventing seizures. Reestablishing normal CSF flow allows for the control of CNS inflammation, cerebral vasogenic edema, and palliation of symptoms (Todd et al., 2021).

Elevation of the Head of the Bed

For patients with increased ICP, the head of the bed should be elevated to 30°–45°, with the neck in a midline position to improve venous drainage from the brain and promote jugular venous drainage. The venous system within the brain has no valves, so gravity will help to increase venous drainage. Maintaining head elevation also helps preserve an appropriate intravascular volume, which is crucial for adequate brain perfusion (Bhalla et al., 2024).

Blood Pressure Maintenance

Hypotension can lead to cerebral ischemia and secondary brain injury. In contrast, hypertension does not increase the cerebral blood flow. Maintaining MAP between 70–90 mm Hg at all times will limit hypotension, which can cause reactive cerebral vasodilation and increased ICP. If hypotension does occur, careful hemodynamic monitoring, electrolyte maintenance, and strict intake and output should be ongoing. To maintain the cerebral perfusion pressure between 70–90 mm Hg, inotropes and vasopressors may be given in addition to carefully administered IV fluids, but the use of albumin is contraindicated (Liebman & Makic, 2022; Saha & Tapuria, 2024). The treatment goal for patients with intracerebral hemorrhage is to prevent and manage hypertension. The level of ICP determines target blood pressures, generally maintained below 160/90 mm Hg, with a MAP of less than 110 mm. Furosemide or other diuretics can be administered to improve central perfusion pressure in patients with volume overload or increased central venous pressure (Liebman & Makic, 2022; Saha & Tapuria, 2024).

Body Temperature Control

Maintaining normothermia (hypothermia is preferred) can raise cerebral blood flow. An increase of one degree in body temperature will raise the cerebral blood flow by 5%–6%. Increased cerebrovascular blood flow can also increase cerebral metabolic rate with a concomitant increase in ICP (Hickey & Strayer, 2019; Pandhi et al., 2020). An ideal body temperature of 98.6°F (37°C) or lower should be maintained using a combination of antipyretics and external cooling methods when necessary (Hickey & Strayer, 2019; Pandhi et al., 2020).

Intracranial Pressure Monitoring

Direct ICP monitoring can be performed via a transducer placed in the subarachnoid space (a subarachnoid bolt), a catheter placed in the subdural space, or a catheter placed in the cerebral ventricle (intraventricular catheter). For patients who require an extraventricular drain (EVD) for pressure monitoring and CSF drainage, a small catheter is placed in a ventricle to divert CSF from the ventricles of the brain. The derived ICP readings can guide interventions, such as draining additional CSF. The EVD should be leveled, and fluid must be drained based on set parameters, which guide how much CSF is emptied. Unless patients have ventriculitis, the primary purpose of the drain is to maintain a normal ICP and CSF equilibrium. Trends in ICP fluctuations can be followed and correlated with neurologic symptoms to evaluate treatment effectiveness. Patients with ICP monitoring require close observation in a neurologic intensive care unit (Faraj et al., 2022; Jeffcote et al., 2024; Pandhi et al., 2020). Clinical studies support the efficacy of this strategy for enhancing patient outcomes (Jeffcote et al., 2024). Noninvasive technologies using ocular pressure and sonographic assessment of cerebral blood flow are under investigation (Jeffcote et al., 2024; Saha & Tapuria, 2024).

Fluid and Electrolyte Management

Preserving normal fluid and electrolyte balance for patients can eliminate the risk of increased ICP in the setting of dehydration and life-threatening sodium imbalances (Tran et al., 2025). Hypotension and dehydration can result in decreased CPP and cerebral ischemia. Hyperosmotic therapy using mannitol 0.25–1 g/kg or hypertonic saline (dose depends on concentration) may be administered to reduce ICP in patients with an intact BBB (Bhalla et al., 2024). Because hyponatremia can increase ICP by causing an osmotic shift, leading to cerebral edema and increased risk of seizures, it is suggested that hypertonic saline be given with extreme caution in the critical care setting for initial sodium replacement to correct hyponatremia (serum osmolality and sodium concentration should be 10 points higher than baseline and closely monitored). In extreme circumstances, hypertonic saline is used as an adjunct to manage increased ICP. Osmotic demyelination syndrome is a rare risk of hyperosmotic therapy, particularly in the setting of rapid infusion of hypertonic saline (Nickson, 2025). If hypertonic saline is given, serum sodium levels should be checked every four to six hours to avoid overcorrection (Bhalla et al., 2024).

Hyperventilation

In patients with increased ICP nearing the range of herniation (> 22 mm Hg for adults, > 20 mm Hg for pediatrics), endotracheal intubation with mechanical ventilation may be considered (Bhalla et al., 2024). For patients who have not responded to other more conservative management techniques, hyperventilation to induce cerebral vasoconstriction may be performed only in true emergencies. This controversial procedure offers short-term benefit, typically lasting up to six hours, by reducing cerebral blood flow. As a final-tier strategy to manage increased ICP, mild to moderate hypocapnia (targeting $PaCO_2$ levels of 32–35 mm Hg) may be induced through controlled hyperventilation, ideally in conjunction with brain tissue oxygen monitoring to ensure safety and effectiveness (Bhalla et al., 2024). Hyperventilation reduces arterial carbon dioxide levels, causing cerebral vasoconstriction. By reducing blood flow to the brain, cerebral vasoconstriction immediately decreases ICP, but it can consequently induce cerebral hypoxia. Thus, this technique must be used cautiously (Hickey & Strayer, 2019; Pandhi et al., 2020).

Analgesics and Sedation

Pain, restlessness, and anxiety can exacerbate elevated ICP. Adequate sedation with agents such as propofol can help mitigate these effects by reducing the cerebral metabolic rate of oxygen and cerebral blood volume, which may subsequently decrease ICP (Bhalla et al., 2024; Liebman & Makic, 2022). Common sedatives include benzodiazepines, ketamine, dexmedetomidine, and barbiturates (e.g., pentobarbital). These agents are titrated to control agitation, pain, and coughing, as well as to maintain target ICP levels (Bhalla et al., 2024; Liebman & Makic, 2022). Propofol is often the drug of choice because of its short-acting profile and ease of reversibility. In cases of delirium, drugs such as haloperidol, olanzapine, and quetiapine (neuroleptics) can be used to stabilize patients. Benzodiazepines such as lorazepam should only be used to sedate patients who are delirious and may be a danger to themselves. Still, this drug class can potentially delay the problem and may ultimately cause worsening delirium. Melatonin at night with sunlight and stimulation during the day may also help to manage delirium (Rai et al., 2021). One study examining the effects of periodic wakeups found that agitation during arousal can transiently increase ICP. Therefore, minimizing noxious stimuli is essential, as it can help prevent Valsalva-like responses and support ICP normalization (Hickey & Strayer, 2019; Pandhi et al., 2020).

Mannitol

Mannitol is an osmotic diuretic that does not cross the BBB. It is used to draw water from the extracellular space in edematous brain tissues by altering the osmotic pressure gradient. The normal dose of mannitol is a bolus of 0.25–0.5 g/kg, up to 1 g/kg every three to six hours. In the case of emergent herniation syndrome, the initial dose is 1–15 g/kg (Kim et al., 2023). The peak effect of mannitol occurs within 15–30 minutes after administration, with a duration of action lasting one to three hours. It is usually administered after an initial dose of hypertonic saline. A rebound effect with an increase in ICP may be seen one to three hours after administration; however, it can be managed with furosemide, a potent loop diuretic. Adverse effects of mannitol include dehydration and electrolyte imbalance with hyponatremia and hypokalemia (Kim et al., 2023). If mannitol or hypertonic saline is ordered, they must be administered over 10 minutes at a minimum to avoid the cardioinhibitory Bezold-Jarisch reflex, a combination of bradycardia, vasodilation, and hypotension. If the cardiac muscle gets stretched too quickly or if blood volume changes too dramatically, asystole can occur. Rapid infusion of hypertonic saline may cause demyelination syndrome (Nickson, 2025).

Seizure Control

Many factors may cause seizures in patients with cancer, including meningitis and encephalitis from an opportunistic infection, primary or metastatic brain tumor, delayed effects of cranial irradiation, paraneoplastic limbic encephalopathy, toxicities related to chemotherapy or immunosuppressive therapy, and profound electrolyte abnormalities (Rees, 2022; Velasco et al., 2023). Seizures increase the cerebral metabolic rate of oxygen and can result in increased ICP (Rai et al., 2021; Rees, 2022).

Patients with a known primary or metastatic brain tumor may or may not receive prophylactic anticonvulsants. All antiepileptics have adverse effects, and seizure prophylaxis has not always proven beneficial to patients (Rees, 2022). Clinicians may institute seizure prophylaxis for patients with brain tumors accompanied by increased ICP or for those with a history of seizures. Antiepileptics such as levetiracetam and lacosamide do not require strict therapeutic monitoring. However, it is crucial to know their correct dosing intervals and any food or drug interactions, including for generic versions. For instance, levetiracetam comes in an extended-release formulation typically taken every 24 hours, whereas the generic version is taken every 12 hours. Phenytoin sodium provides the benefit of time-released medication, whereas generic phenytoin does not. Liquid phenytoin is poorly absorbed in the presence of food. Seizure precautions include padded bedrails, frequent neurologic assessments, avoidance of oral temperature measurement, airway equipment with available oxygen, suction, and an oral airway (Rees, 2022).

Intrathecal Therapies

Patients with leptomeningeal carcinomatosis, also referred to as leptomeningeal disease or metastases, are treated with systemic and intrathecal agents designed to cross the BBB. Intrathecal chemotherapy is delivered via lumbar puncture. An Ommaya reservoir can be used cautiously for increased ICP and allows access to CSF. Agents must be water-soluble and BBB-penetrant to reduce complications (e.g., arachnoiditis). Common intrathecal drugs are methotrexate, cytarabine, liposomal cytarabine, thiotepa, and rituximab. These have short CSF half-lives and limited tissue penetration. Bacterial, viral, and fungal infections may be treated intraventricularly with corticosteroids, antimicrobials, or antifungals. For symptom relief from increased ICP, CSF shunting using a ventriculoperitoneal shunt or intracranial drug implants may be used.

Radiation Therapy

RT is commonly used for inoperable brain tumors and tumor bed follow-up; it can cause acute and delayed reactions, such as inflammation or radiation necrosis, both of which can increase ICP. Acute reactions may appear weeks to months after therapy, causing neurologic deterioration, including headache and somnolence (Ahmed et al., 2021; Patel et al., 2023). Radiation necrosis, a less common complication, typically manifests six months to three years post-treatment and ranges from asymptomatic white matter lesions to progressive neurologic dysfunction (Ahmed et al., 2021; Patel et al., 2023). Stereotactic radiosurgery, a targeted radiation technique, may be used alone or with surgical debulking to optimize tumor removal and reduce ICP (Achrol et al., 2019; Kaidar-Person et al., 2020; Rashidi et al., 2025; Yust-Katz et al., 2020).

Surgical Intervention

Surgery may be indicated in some instances to manage increased ICP, including evacuation of a cerebral hematoma, placement of a shunt for hydrocephalus (e.g., ventriculoperitoneal, lumbarperitoneal), an EVD, or resection of a penetrating object or tumor. In high-grade gliomas, resection of the lesion is an essential first step in controlling increased ICP (Dorsey et al., 2020). Maximal resection of all visible tumor (≥ 90%) is reported to have a statistically significant positive impact on survival (Faraj et al., 2022). Craniotomy is the most common surgical technique and allows complete access for optimal tumor resection. Surgical debulking followed by standard biotherapy, chemotherapy, or RT is often used for the treatment of most intracranial tumors (Dorsey et al., 2020). As a last resort for patients at risk for brain herniation, a decompression craniotomy may be attempted (Bhalla et al., 2024; Pandhi et al., 2020).

Nursing Management

Nursing management of patients with increased ICP requires preventive interventions and strategies, careful symptom assessment, identification of changes in physical findings, and rapid clinical interventions. Continuous patient monitoring is vital, focusing on neurologic baseline assessments, fine motor skills evaluation, and regular checks of level of consciousness. Nurses need to have a clear understanding of the severity of both treatment-related toxicities and increased ICP. Early symptom recognition and management can significantly improve patient outcomes.

Evaluation Tools

Nurses should initially assess appearance, behavior, mood, level of consciousness, short- and long-term memory loss, and attention span by a quick evaluation. An assessment of the visual system is vital for identifying increased ICP or leptomeningeal disease. Key ocular markers include changes in the pupil based on light and focus (e.g., dilated unreactive, mid-position fixed, pinpoint pupils), eye movement deficits (e.g., "down and out" orientation or ptosis), and impaired upward gaze in severe cases. Behavioral shifts, such as altered consciousness (e.g., irritability, drowsiness), sudden confusion, and lethargy, further signal neurologic decline and are often accompanied by physical indicators, which may include projectile vomiting, gait ataxia, and abnormal posturing (decorticate or decerebrate). In advanced stages, observing agonal breathing serves as a critical warning of brainstem pressure and impending crisis (Olaru et al., 2024). For patients who are alert and able to speak, this initial assessment is followed by asking simple questions to evaluate increased ICP. Patient appearance is also an important indicator of neurologic function, such as whether a patient is well-kept and groomed and oriented to person, place, and time.

To assess higher-level neurologic function, nurses should consider asking patients what a phrase such as "all is well that ends well" means. Once the initial neurologic assessment is completed, more in-depth tools can be used.

For example, the GCS is frequently used to assess the severity of an individual's response to a change in neurologic status. This scale looks at three clinical dimensions: ocular, verbal, and motor responses. The maximum possible score is 15, with a minimum possible score of 3. The correlation between the GCS score and the severity of brain injury is the following (Hickey & Strayer, 2019; Hinkle et al., 2021; Schnur, 2022):

- Severe injury: GCS score 3–8
- Moderate injury: GCS score 9–12
- Mild injury: GCS score 13–15

The lower the GCS score, the greater the risk of mortality and poor prognosis.

Neurologic assessment includes observations and evaluates orientation, speech flow, attention span, memory, visual acuity, and ability to follow commands. This quick examination can usually be performed within a few minutes and is most helpful with people who have some ability to follow commands.

For minimally responsive patients with decreased responsiveness to external stimuli, the full outline of unresponsiveness (FOUR) scale can be used (Anestis et al., 2020; Camp-Sorrell et al., 2022; Patel et al., 2023) (see Table 7-6).

Finally, for patients receiving CAR T-cell therapy, the immune effector cell–associated encephalopathy assessment tool and the ICANs grading tool can be used to evaluate immune effector cell therapy–associated increased ICP. For patients undergoing immune effector cellular therapies, ICANS grading is based on the following clinical neurologic manifestations (Buitrago et al., 2019; Herr et al., 2020):

- Grade 1: mild confusion, disorientation
- Grade 2: moderate deficits, including language disturbance or attention deficits
- Grade 3: severe deficits; may include seizures (> 5 min) or focal motor weakness
- Grade 4: unresponsive, comatose state, or abnormal posturing

Nursing Interventions

Nurses should take an active role in preventing increased ICP through careful patient monitoring, prompt identification of early signs and symptoms of neurologic changes, and timely interventions aimed at minimizing its impact. They need to have a deep understanding of the severity of toxicities associated with antineoplastic therapies that

TABLE 7-6
Full Outline of Unresponsiveness Scale

Points	Eye Response	Motor Response	Brain Stem Reflexes	Respiration
4	Eyelids open or opened, tracking, or blinking to command	Thumbs-up, fist, or peace sign	Pupil and corneal reflexes present	Not intubated, regular breathing pattern
3	Eyelids open but not tracking	Localizing to pain	One pupil wide and fixed	Not intubated, Cheyne–Stokes breathing pattern
2	Eyelids closed but open to loud voice	Flexion response to pain	Pupil or corneal reflexes absent	Not intubated, irregular breathing pattern
1	Eyelids closed but open to pain	Extension response to pain	Pupil and corneal reflexes absent	Breathing pattern above ventilator rate
0	Eyelids remain closed with pain	No response to pain or generalized myoclonus status	Absent pupil, corneal, and cough reflex	Breathing pattern at ventilator rate or apnea

Note. Based on information from Anestis et al., 2020; Patel et al., 2023.

can increase ICP, such as immune effector cells and immunotherapies. The potentially devastating consequences of failing to recognize and address them promptly can result in neurologic deterioration. Early intervention can significantly improve patient outcomes. Continuous patient monitoring should focus on neurologic baseline assessments, fine motor skills evaluation, and regular checks of level of consciousness.

Symptom management of increased ICP focuses on interventions that help reduce pressure. Headaches caused by increased ICP often do not respond to analgesics but improve with corticosteroids, particularly dexamethasone, which reduces vasogenic edema linked to tumoral lesions. Nausea, vomiting, and photophobia from tumor-related increased ICP also respond well to steroids; prednisolone may be used for long-term therapy (Dixit & Kumthekar, 2020).

Seizure prophylaxis may be needed in patients with primary or metastatic brain tumors, as they can occur with increased ICP (Kaidar-Person et al., 2020). If a seizure occurs, nursing care must prioritize safety, airway management, and observation of seizure characteristics (Hickey & Strayer, 2019; Kaidar-Person et al., 2020). Postictal care includes oxygen, vital signs, neurologic monitoring, glucose checks, and hydration, especially following prolonged seizures that deplete energy stores (Dixit & Kumthekar, 2020). Motor weakness should be managed with passive range-of-motion exercises and careful positioning, provided these do not increase ICP.

Although these states and actions are not included in many evaluation tools, monitoring them should be part of the ongoing nursing assessment in the setting of increased ICP.

Emergency Management of Increased Intracranial Pressure

Establishing a baseline neurologic assessment allows nurses to gauge the improvement or decline of neurologic status. The healthcare team needs to gather information about the patient, including age, underlying cause for the increased ICP, medical history (e.g., prior treatments, comorbidities), coagulopathies, and any past treatments that may worsen ICP (Bhalla et al., 2024). Although increased ICP and IH may occur independently of one another, prevention of sustained or increasing ICP of greater than 20 mm Hg while maintaining the cerebral perfusion pressure within a narrow range (55–60 mm Hg) is essential. If measures to control ICP are unsuccessful, respiratory distress syndrome with a concomitant decline in brain tissue oxygen partial pressure may occur, requiring the initiation of emergency protocols. If ICP becomes uncontrolled, nurses' priority should shift to maintaining a patent airway, closely monitoring respiratory and cardiac status, tracking vital signs, and initiating resuscitation measures as needed (Bhalla et al., 2024; Hickey & Strayer, 2019; Pandhi et al., 2020).

Prevention of emergencies includes the following guidance (Bhalla et al., 2024; Dixit & Kumthekar, 2020; Hickey & Strayer, 2019; Pandhi et al., 2020):

- Maintain a patent airway; promote effective ventilation and adequate circulation.
- Avoid any stimuli that will elevate ICP (e.g., suctioning).
- Provide enough sedation to allow for neurologic assessments while minimizing the risk of increasing ICP.
- Maintain normothermia through targeted temperature management using a temperature feedback device, if available.
- Ensure that the head is elevated to a 30°–45° angle and kept midline to promote venous drainage. When a head or neck injury is present, the head of the bed may be elevated to 15°–45°.
- IV fluids should be isosmotic or hyperosmotic.
- Correct hyponatremia (sodium < 135 mmol/L) using hypertonic saline.
- High-dose corticosteroids should be avoided, except for cases of vasogenic edema from brain tumors, abscesses, bacterial or tuberculosis meningitis, or noninfectious neuroinflammatory disease.
- Head CT scans should only be attempted if patients can be safely positioned for the scan.

Patient and Caregiver Education

Educating patients with cancer at risk for increased ICP, along with their caregivers, is essential because of the potential for neurologic or cognitive impairments. Nurses should focus their teaching on recognizing early warning signs (e.g., headache, nausea, visual or mental status changes) and include clear guidance for maintaining safety. This includes modifying the home environment to prevent falls, ensuring proper follow-up with scheduled appointments and provider contact information, and understanding the benefits of physical, occupational, and speech therapy to preserve function after neurologic events.

Nurses also must instruct patients and caregivers to promptly report new or worsening symptoms to the appropriate specialist, especially in cases of primary or metastatic brain lesions with edema (Pinto & Adeyinka, 2025). During acute care, education should also explain increased ICP, monitoring tools (e.g., EVDs, bolt catheters), potential deficits (e.g., aphasia, hemiparesis), and available support services. After discharge, instructions should include medication use and side effects (e.g., steroids, antiepileptics), seizure risks, and strategies to support mobility and communication. Emotional support and resources should be provided continuously to improve safety, adherence, and long-term outcomes.

Summary

Increased ICP is an oncologic emergency requiring rapid and accurate neurologic assessments and interventions. Nurses are often the first healthcare professionals that patients will meet during their clinical care experience. With their ability to accurately identify patients at risk for increased ICP and recognize the alterations in physical and cognitive functioning that often accompany neurologic decline, oncology nurses are uniquely positioned to improve clinical outcomes for patients with cancer and increased ICP. Prompt assessment and treatment of increased ICP can prevent permanent neurologic deficits, preserve quality of life, and reduce mortality. Successfully managing and treating this oncologic emergency in an efficient and timely manner requires collaboration between nursing, medical, surgical, and critical care team members. Accurate identification and ongoing evaluation of this complex condition necessitate that oncology nurses assume a central role in coordinating interprofessional care and follow-up to mitigate devastating physical and psychological consequences.

The authors would like to acknowledge Brenda K. Shelton, DNP, APRN-CNS, RN, CCRN, AOCN®, Janice Skinner, RN, MS, MSN, CRNP, and Moira Baynes, RN, MSN, for their contribution to this chapter that remains unchanged from the previous edition of this book.

References

Achrol, A.S., Rennert, R.C., Anders, C., Soffietti, R., Ahluwalia, M.S., Nayak, L., … Chang, S.D. (2019). Brain metastases. *Nature Reviews. Disease Primers, 5*(1), 5. https://doi.org/10.1038/s41572-018-0055-y

Ahmed, A., UlHaq, M.U., Mustansar, Z., Shaukat, A., & Margetts, L. (2021). How growing tumour impacts intracranial pressure and deformation mechanics of brain. *Royal Society Open Science, 8*(9), 210165. https://doi.org/10.1098/rsos.210165

Al-asady, A.Q., Alshuqayfi, K.M., AlObaidy, M.H., Ahmed, F.O., Idris, O.S., Muthana, A., & Al-Sharee, A.H. (2024). Infectious diseases of the brain. In S. Hozer, A.H. Al-Sharee, M. Ismail, A.A. Dolachee,

O. Elamin, O. Atallah, & M. Delawan (Eds.), *Neuroradiology board's favorites: 100 MRI-based pathology-proven cases supplied with 170 MCQs* (pp. 131–155). Springer Nature.

Altabakhi, I.W., Babiker, H.M., & Lui, F. (2024). Paraneoplastic limbic encephalitis. In *StatPearls*. StatPearls Publishing. https://www.ncbi.nlm.nih.gov/books/NBK519523

Anestis, D.M., Tsitsopoulos, P.P., Tsonidis, C.A., & Foroglou, N. (2020). The current significance of the FOUR score: A systematic review and critical analysis of the literature. *Journal of Neurological Sciences, 409,* 116600. https://doi.org/10.1016/j.jns.2019.116600

Arjarquah, A.K., Obodai, E., Anie, H.A., Osei, M.A., Odoom, J.K., Bonney, J.H.K., ... Quaye, O. (2022). Occurrence of influenza and bacterial infections in cancer patients receiving radiotherapy in Ghana. *PLOS ONE, 17*(7), e0271877. https://doi.org/10.1371/journal.pone.0271877

Asioli, G.M., Castioni, C.A., Zinzani, P.L., Casadio, M.C., Pierucci, E., Casadei, B., ... Bonifazi, F. (2024). Intracranial pressure management in fulminant cerebral edema after CAR T-cell therapy: Not all is lost! *British Journal of Haematology, 204*(3), 1109–1113. https://doi.org/10.1111/bjh.19270

Balasubaramaniam, D., Singh, S., Qamarruddin, F.A., & Saravanamuthu, K. (2023). Bilateral large orbital lymphoma with proptosis. *Cureus, 15*(3), e36548. https://doi.org/10.7759/cureus.36548

Bangolo, A., Amoozgar, B., Mansour, C., Zhang, L., Gill, S., Ip, A., & Cho, C. (2025). Comprehensive review of early and late toxicities in CAR T-cell therapy and bispecific antibody treatments for hematologic malignancies. *Cancers, 17*(2), 282. https://doi.org/10.3390/cancers17020282

Bhalla, P., Dingman, J.S., & Aysenne, A. (2024). *Emergency Neurological Life Support® intracranial hypertension and herniation protocol Version 6.0.* https://www.neurocriticalcare.org/Portals/0/ENLS%205.0/ENLS%206.0/Protocol%20V6_0_Intracranial%20Hypertension%20and%20Herniation.pdf?ver=oGpOZQ2sI6-mgzJhEgTtTg%3d%3d

Bouché, M., Dong, Y.C., Sheikh, S., Taing, K., Saxena, D., Hsu, J.C., ... Cormode, D.P. (2021). Novel treatment for glioblastoma delivered by a radiation responsive and radiopaque hydrogel. *ACS Biomaterials Science and Engineering, 7*(7), 3209–3220. https://doi.org/10.1021/acsbiomaterials.1c00385

Buitrago, J., Adkins, S., Hawkins, M., Iyamu, K., & van Oort, T. (2019). Adult survivorship: Considerations following CAR T-cell therapy. *Clinical Journal of Oncology Nursing, 23*(2), 42–48. https://doi.org/10.1188/19.CJON.S1.42-48

Burleson, S.L., Butler, J., Gostigian, G., Parr, M.S., & Kelly, M.P. (2023). A rare cause of headache and an unorthodox transfer: A case report. *Clinical Practice and Cases in Emergency Medicine, 7*(1), 24–28. https://doi-org.ezp.twu.edu/10.5811/cpcem.2022.10.57491

Camp-Sorrell, D., Hawkins, R.A., & Cope, D.G. (2022). *Clinical manual for the oncology advanced practice nurse* (4th ed.). Oncology Nursing Society.

Davidson, C.L., & Kumar, A. (2024). Intracranial hypertension. In *StatPearls*. StatPearls Publishing. http://www.ncbi.nlm.nih.gov/books/NBK507811

Delawan, M., Al-Badri, S.G., Aynona, A.M., Alduraibi, L., Muthana, A., Dolachee, A.A., & AL-Sharee, A.H. (2024). Cranial oncology. In S. Hoz, A.H. AL-Sharee, M. Ismail, A.A. Dolachee, O. Elamin, O. Atallah, & M. Delawan (Eds.), *Neuroradiology board's favorites: 100 MRI-based pathology-proven cases supplied with 170 MCQs* (pp. 31–93). Springer. https://doi.org/10.1007/978-3-031-64261-6_2

Dixit, K.S., & Kumthekar, P.U. (2020). Optimal management of corticosteroids in patients with intracranial malignancies. *Current Treatment Options in Oncology, 21*(9), 77. https://doi.org/10.1007/s11864-020-00771-7

Dorsey, J.F., Salinas, R.D., Dang, M., Alonso-Basanta, M., Judy, K.D., Maity, A., ... Pruitt, A.A. (2020). Cancer of the central nervous system. In J.E. Niederhuber, J.O. Armitage, M.B. Kastan, J.H. Doroshow, & J.E. Tepper (Eds.), *Abeloff's clinical oncology* (6th ed., pp. 906–967.e12). Elsevier. https://doi.org/10.1016/b978-0-323-47674–4.00063-3

Faraj, C.A., Snyder, R.I., & McCutcheon, I.E. (2022). Intracranial emergencies in neurosurgical oncology: Pathophysiology and clinical management. *Emergency Cancer Care, 1*(1), 13. https://doi.org/10.1186/s44201-022-00013-6

Farkas, J. (2022, June 12). Brain abscess. *The Internet Book of Critical Care.* https://emcrit.org/ibcc/ba

Freifeld, A.G., & Kaul, D.R. (2020). Infection in the patient with cancer. In J.E. Niederhuber, J.O. Armitage, M.B. Kastan, J.H. Doroshow, & J.E. Tepper (Eds.), *Abeloff's clinical oncology* (6th ed., pp. 544–564.e6). Elsevier. https://doi.org/10.1016/B978-0-323-47674-4.00034-7

Ghandour, F., Squassina, A., Karaky, R., Diab-Assaf, M., Fadda, P., & Pisanu, C. (2021). Presenting psychiatric and neurological symptoms and signs of brain tumors before diagnosis: A systematic review. *Brain Sciences, 11*(3), 301. https://doi.org/10.3390/brainsci11030301

Godase, K.S., Mohite, U.S., Gosavi, V.S., & Kulkarni, M. (2024). Foster Kennedy syndrome: A case report. *International Journal of Innovative Science and Research Technology, 9*(5), 1410–1412. https://doi.org/10.38124/ijisrt/ijisrt24may691

Guevara, N., Akande, A., Chang, M.F., Atallah, J., & Epstein, C. (2022). A case report of a brain herniation secondary to cryptococcal meningitis with elevated intracranial pressure in a patient with human immunodeficiency virus/acquired immunodeficiency syndrome (HIV/AIDS). *IDCases, 29*, e01554. https://doi.org/10.1016/j.idcr.2022.e01554

Gwak, H.-S. (2023). Molecular biology of brain metastases. *Brain Tumor Research and Treatment, 11*(1), 8–15. https://doi.org/10.14791/btrt.2022.0045

Hall, W.A., & De Jesus, O. (2025). Ommaya reservoir. In *StatPearls*. StatPearls Publishing. http://www.ncbi.nlm.nih.gov/books/NBK559011

Herr, M.M., Chen, G.L., Ross, M., Jacobson, H., McKenzie, R., Markel, L., ... McCarthy, P.L. (2020). Identification of neurotoxicity after chimeric antigen receptor (CAR) T cell infusion without deterioration in the immune effector cell–associated encephalopathy (ICE) score. *Biology of Blood and Marrow Transplantation, 26*(11), e271–e274. https://doi.org/10.1016/j.bbmt.2020.07.031

Hickey, J.V., & Strayer, A.L. (2019). *The clinical practice of neurological and neurosurgical nursing* (8th ed.). Wolters Kluwer.

Hinkle, J.L., Cheever, K.H., & Overbaugh, K. (2021). *Brunner and Suddarth's textbook of medical–surgical nursing* (15th ed.). Wolters Kluwer.

Hladky, S.B., & Barrand, M.A. (2024). Alterations in brain fluid physiology during the early stages of development of ischaemic edema. *Fluids and Barriers of the CNS, 21*(1), 51. https://doi.org/10.1186/s12987-024-00534-8

Holzgreve, A., Albert, N.L., Galldiks, N., & Suchorska, B. (2021). Use of PET imaging in neuro-oncological surgery. *Cancers, 13*(9), 2093. https://doi.org/10.3390/cancers13092093

Javed, K., Reddy, V., & Lui, F. (2023). Neuroanatomy, choroid plexus. In *StatPearls*. StatPearls Publishing. https://www.ncbi.nlm.nih.gov/books/NBK538156

Jeffcote, T., Lu, K.-Y., Lewis, P., Gantner, D., Battistuzzo, C.R., & Udy, A.A. (2024). Brain tissue oxygen monitoring in moderate-to-severe traumatic brain injury: Physiological determinants, clinical interventions and current randomised controlled trial evidence. *Critical Care and Resuscitation, 26*(3), 204–209. https://doi.org/10.1016/j.ccrj.2024.05.003

Jeffus, S.K., Sturgis, C.D., McHugh, K.E., Verret, M., Ooms, K., Vestal, S., ... Shah, A.A. (2024). The spectrum of malignant diagnoses in cerebrospinal fluid cytology from an adult population: A multi-institutional retrospective review. *Journal of the American Society of Cytopathology, 13*(2), 141–148. https://doi.org/10.1016/j.jasc.2023.11.003

Jung, J.W., Kang, I., Park, J., Lee, S., & Jeon, S.-B. (2024). Intracranial pressure trends and clinical outcomes after decompressive hemicraniectomy in malignant middle cerebral artery infarction. *Annals of Intensive Care, 14*(1), 176. https://doi.org/10.1186/s13613-024-01412-0

Kaidar-Person, O., Cools, M., & Zagar, T. (2020). Brain metastases and neoplastic meningitis. In J.E. Niederhuber, J.O. Armitage, M.B. Kastan, J.H. Doroshow, & J.E. Tepper (Eds.), *Abeloff's clinical oncology* (6th ed., pp. 794–808.e3). Elsevier. https://doi.org/10.1016/B978-0-323-47674-4.00055-4

Kannan, N., Dass, J., Viswanathan, G.K., Khokhar, P., & Aggarwal, M. (2023). Acute promyelocytic leukemia masquerading as myeloid maturation arrest—A case report. *Journal of Clinical and Experimental Hematopathology, 63*(3), 193–196. https://doi.org/10.3960/jslrt.23030

Kareemi, H., Pratte, M., English, S., & Hendin, A. (2023). Initial diagnosis and management of acutely elevated intracranial pressure. *Journal of Intensive Care Medicine, 38*(7), 643–650. https://doi.org/10.1177/08850666231156589

Khaddam, D., McRae, H.L., Schwarz, N., Oldenburg, J., Pötzsch, B., Rühl, H., & Reda, S. (2024). High prevalence of F2 20210G > A in splanchnic vein thrombosis and cerebral venous sinus thrombosis: A retrospective cohort study of patients with thrombosis in atypical sites. *Hämostaseologie*. https://doi.org/10.1055/a-2329-1798

Khorchid, Y.M., & Malkoff, M. (2020). Intracranial hemorrhage focused on cancer and hemato-oncologic patients. In J.L. Nates & K.J. Price (Eds.), *Oncologic critical care* (pp. 381–394). Springer. https://doi.org/10.1007/978-3-319-74588-6_40

Khosla, A.A., Saxena, S., Ozair, A., Venur, V.A., Peereboom, D.M., & Ahluwalia, M.S. (2023). Novel therapeutic approaches in neoplastic meningitis. *Cancers, 15*(1), 119. https://doi.org/10.3390/cancers15010119

Kim, J.H., Jeong, H., Choo, Y.-H., Kim, M., Ha, E.J., Oh, J., ... Lee, S. (2023). Optimizing mannitol use in managing increased intracranial pressure: A comprehensive review of recent research and clinical experiences. *Korean Journal of Neurotrauma, 19*(2), 162–176. https://doi.org/10.13004/kjnt.2023.19.e25

Knox, A., Wang, T., Shackleton, M., & Ameratunga, M. (2024). Symptomatic brain metastases in melanoma. *Experimental Dermatology, 33*(4), e15075. https://doi.org/10.1111/exd.15075

Lamba, N., Catalano, P.J., Whitehouse, C., Martin, K.L., Mendu, M.L., Haas-Kogan, D.A., ... Aizer, A.A. (2021). Emergency department visits and inpatient hospitalizations among older patients with brain metastases: A dual population- and institution-level analysis. *Neuro-Oncology Practice, 8*(5), 569–580. https://doi.org/10.1093/nop/npab029

Liebman, E., & Makic, M.B.F. (2022). Care of the perioperative patient at risk for increased intracranial pressure. *Journal of PeriAnesthesia Nursing, 37*(2), 274–276. https://doi.org/10.1016/j.jopan.2021.12.011

Louis, D.N., Perry, A., Wesseling, P., Brat, D.J., Cree, I.A., Figarella-Branger, D., ... Ellison, D.W. (2021). The 2021 WHO classification of tumors of the central nervous system: A summary. *Neuro-Oncology, 23*(8), 1231–1251. https://doi.org/10.1093/neuonc/noab106

Mayo, Z.S., Halima, A., Broughman, J.R., Smile, T.D., Tom, M.C., Murphy, E.S., ... Chao, S.T. (2023). Radiation necrosis or tumor progression? A review of the radiographic modalities used in the diagnosis of cerebral radiation necrosis. *Journal of Neuro-Oncology, 161*(1), 23–31. https://doi.org/10.1007/s11060-022-04225-y

Mendoza Vasquez, L.E., Payne, S., & Zamper, R. (2023). Intracranial pressure monitoring in the perioperative period of patients with acute liver failure undergoing orthotopic liver transplantation. *World Journal of Transplantation, 13*(4), 122–128. https://doi.org/10.5500/wjt.v13.i4.122

Monro, A. (1783). Observations on the structure and functions of the nervous system, illustrated with tables. *London Medical Journal, 4*(2), 113–135.

Morrison, C., Bhalla, P., Ruzas, C.M., Tran, D.S., & Qualls, S. (2022). *Emergency neurological life support: Intracranial hypertension and herniation protocol, version 5.0.* https://www.neurocriticalcare.org/Portals/0/ENLS%205.0/ENLS%205.0%20Protocol%20- %20ICP.pdf

National Cancer Institute Surveillance, Epidemiology and End Results Program. (2025). *Cancer stat facts: Brain and other nervous system cancer.* https://seer.cancer.gov/statfacts/html/brain.html

Nguyen, A., Nguyen, A., Dada, O.T., Desai, P.D., Ricci, J.C., Godbole, N.B., ... Lucke-Wold, B. (2023). Leptomeningeal metastasis: A review of the pathophysiology, diagnostic methodology, and therapeutic landscape. *Current Oncology, 30*(6), 5906–5931. https://doi.org/10.3390/curroncol30060442

Nguyen, T., Mueller, S., & Malbari, F. (2022). Review: Neurological complications from therapies for pediatric brain tumors. *Frontiers in Oncology, 12,* 853034. https://doi.org/10.3389/fonc.2022.853034

Nickson, C. (2025, June 11). Central pontine myelinolysis. *Life in the Fast Lane.* https://litfl.com/central-pontine-myelinolysis

Niederhuber, J.E., Armitage, J.O., Doroshow, J.H., Kastan, M.B., & Tepper, J.E. (Eds.). (2020). *Abeloff's clinical oncology* (6th ed.). Elsevier.

Nolan, N.S., Kim, M.J., & Liang, S.Y. (2021). Infectious disease. In K.H. Todd, C.R. Thomas, & K. Alagappan (Eds.), *Oncologic emergency medicine* (2nd ed., pp. 501–512). Springer. https://doi.org/10.1007/978-3-030-67123-5_38

Odom-Forren, J. (2024). *Drain's perianesthesia nursing: A critical care approach* (8th ed.). Elsevier.

Olaru, C., Langberg, S., & McCoin, N.S. (2024). A review of the clinical presentation, causes, and diagnostic evaluation of increased intracranial pressure in the emergency department. *Western Journal of Emergency Medicine, 25*(6), 1003–1010. https://doi.org/10.5811/westjem.18500

Owusu, A., & Abebrese, J.K. (2023). Factors affecting HIV clients' exposures and adherence to toxoplasmosis preventive measures at the individual, interpersonal, community and institutional levels: A literature review. *Journal of Engineering Applied Science and Humanities, 8*(3), 179–201. https://doi.org/10.53075/Ijmsirq/65887879876

Ozcan, G., Singh, M., & Vredenburgh, J.J. (2023). Leptomeningeal metastasis from non–small cell lung cancer and current landscape of treatments. *Clinical Cancer Research, 29*(1), 11–29. https://doi.org/10.1158/1078–0432.CCR-22-1585

Pandhi, A., Krishnan, R., Goyal, N., & Malkoff, M. (2020). Increased intracranial pressure in critically ill cancer patients. In J.L. Nates & K.J. Price (Eds.), *Oncologic critical care* (pp. 395–407). Springer. https://doi.org/10.1007/978-3-319-74588-6_36

Patel, S., Maria-Rios, J., Parikh, A., & Okorie, O.N. (2023). Diagnosis and management of elevated intracranial pressure in the emergency department. *International Journal of Emergency Medicine, 16*(1), 72. https://doi.org/10.1186/s12245-023-00540-x

Pinto, V.L., & Adeyinka, A. (2025). Increased intracranial pressure. In *StatPearls*. StatPearls Publishing. http://www.ncbi.nlm.nih.gov/books/NBK482119

Qdaisat, A., Yeung, S.-C.J., Rojas Hernandez, C.H., Samudrala, P., Kamal, M., Li, Z., & Wechsler, A.H. (2022). Characteristics and outcomes of intracranial hemorrhage in cancer patients visiting the emergency department. *Journal of Clinical Medicine, 11*(3), 643. https://doi.org/10.3390/jcm11030643

Rai, P., Shivaprasad, A., Tremont-Lukats, I.W., & Tummala, S. (2021). Central nervous system. In K.H. Todd, C.R. Thomas, Jr., & K. Alagappan (Eds.), *Oncologic emergency medicine* (2nd ed., pp. 207–223). Springer. https://doi.org/10.1007/978-3-030-67123-5_16

Rashidi, F., Habibi, M.A., Karami, S., Mirjani, M.S., Maleki, S., Bahri, A., & Iranmehr, A. (2025). Gamma knife application for optic/hypothalamic pathway glioma: A systematic review. *Egyptian Journal of Neurosurgery, 40,* 45. https://doi-org.ezp.twu.edu/10.1186/s41984-025-00368-y

Rees, J.H. (2022). Management of immune effector cell–associated neurotoxicity syndrome (ICANS). In N. Kröger, J. Gribben, C. Chabannon, I. Yakoub-Agha, & H. Einsele (Eds.), *The EBMT/EHA CAR-T cell handbook* (pp. 141–145). Springer. https://doi.org/10.1007/978-3-030-94353-0_27

Rezaei, N., & Hanaei, S. (Eds.). (2023). *Human brain and spinal cord tumors: From bench to bedside. Volume 2: The path to bedside management.* Springer. https://doi.org/10.1007/978-3-031-23705-8

Saha, D., & Tapuria, P. (2024). Cerebrospinal fluid dynamics. In H. Prabhakar, V. Singhal, K.G. Zirpe, & H. Sapra (Eds.), *Principles and practice of neurocritical care* (pp. 27–42). Springer Nature. https://doi.org/10.1007/978-981-99-8059-8_3

Santomasso, B.D., Gust, J., & Perna, F. (2023). How I treat unique and difficult-to-manage cases of CAR T-cell therapy–associated neurotoxicity. *Blood, 141*(20), 2443–2451. https://doi.org/10.1182/blood.2022017604

Saria, M.G., & Kesari, S. (2021). Increased intracranial pressure: The use of an individualized ladder approach. *Seminars in Oncology Nursing, 37*(2), 151133. https://doi.org/10.1016/j.soncn.2021.151133

Schnur, M.B. (2022). Assessing level of consciousness. *Nursing Blog | Lippincott® NursingCenter®.* https://www.nursingcenter.com/blogs-plus/blogs/blogs-post#/post/level-of-consciousness

Seano, G. (Ed.). (2021). *Brain tumors.* Springer. https://doi.org/10.1007/978-1-0716-0856-2

Sexton, D.J., & Richie, M. (2024). Lumbar puncture: Technique, contraindications, and complications in adults. In R.P. Goddeau, Jr. (Ed.), *UpToDate.* Retrieved October 29, 2025, from https://www.uptodate.com/contents/lumbar-puncture-technique-contraindications-and-complications-in-adults

Shalabi, H., Martin, S., Yates, B., Wolters, P.L., Kaplan, C., Smith, H., ... Shah, N.N. (2022). Neurotoxicity following CD19/CD28ζ CAR T-cells in children and young adults with B-cell malignancies. *Neuro-Oncology, 24*(9), 1584–1597. https://doi.org/10.1093/neuonc/noac034

Sobti, R.C., Ganguly, N.K., & Kumar, R. (2024). *Handbook of oncobiology: From basic to clinical sciences.* Springer. https://doi.org/10.1007/978-981-99-6263-1

Tawfik, O., Hassan, A., Mohamed, W., Essmyer, C., Ewing, E., Lem, V., ... Akhtar, N. (2022). Disseminated opportunistic infections masquerading as central nervous system malignancies. *Human Pathology Reports, 28,* 300629. https://doi.org/10.1016/j.hpr.2022.300629

Tcyganov, E.N., Hanabuchi, S., Hashimoto, A., Campbell, D., Kar, G., Slidel, T.W.F., ... Grabilovich, D.I. (2021). Distinct mechanisms govern populations of myeloid-derived suppressor cells in chronic viral infection and cancer. *Journal of Clinical Investigation, 131*(16), e145971. https://doi-org.ezp.twu.edu/10.1172/JCI145971

Todd, K.H., Thomas, C.R., Jr., & Alagappan, K. (Eds.). (2021). *Oncologic emergency medicine: Principles and practice* (2nd ed.). Springer. https://doi.org/10.1007/978-3-030-67123-5

Tran, V., Flores, J., Sheldon, M., Pena, C., & Nugent, K. (2025). Fluid and electrolyte disorders in traumatic brain injury: Clinical implications and management strategies. *Journal of Clinical Medicine, 14*(3), 756. https://doi.org/10.3390/jcm14030756

Velasco, R., Mussetti, A., Villagrán-García, M., & Sureda, A. (2023). CAR T-cell–associated neurotoxicity in central nervous system hematologic disease: Is it still a concern? *Frontiers in Neurology, 14,* 1144414. https://doi.org/10.3389/fneur.2023.1144414

Wang, L., Fei, Y., Qu, H., Zhang, H., Wang, Y., Wu, Z., & Fan, G. (2024). Five years of safety profile of bevacizumab: An analysis of real-world pharmacovigilance and randomized clinical trials. *Journal of Pharmaceutical Health Care and Sciences, 10,* 1. https://doi.org/10.1186/s40780-023-00314-w

Wilcox, J.A., Estrera, R., & Boire, A. (2023). The spectrum of headache in leptomeningeal metastases: A comprehensive review with clinical management guidelines. *Current Pain and Headache Reports, 27*(11), 695–706. https://doi.org/10.1007/s11916-023-01180-9

Wilcox, J.A., Li, M.J., & Boire, A.A. (2022). Leptomeningeal metastases: New opportunity in the modern era. *Neurotherapeutics, 19*(6), 1782–1798. https://doi.org/10.1007/s13311-022-01261-4

Yanagida, M., Hosoi, Y., Kawano, T., Otake, Y., Yamanaka, Y., Baba, T., & Ito, M. (2024). Noniatrogenic meningitis caused by *Streptococcus salivarius* associated with early esophageal cancer and early gastric cancer. *Internal Medicine, 63*(3), 457–460. https://doi-org.ezp.twu.edu/10.2169/internalmedicine.1304-22

Yiangou, A., Weaver, S.R.C., Thaller, M., Mitchell, J.L., Lyons, H.S., Tsermoulas, G., ... Sinclair, A.J. (2024). The impact of Valsalva manoeuvres and exercise on intracranial pressure and cerebrovascular dynamics in idiopathic intracranial hypertension. *Neuro-Ophthalmology, 48*(2), 122–133. https://doi.org/10.1080/01658107.2023.2281433

Yust-Katz, S., Khagi, S., & Gilbert, M.R. (2020). Neurologic complications. In J.E. Niederhuber, J.O. Armitage, J.H. Doroshow, M.B. Kastan, & J.E. Tepper (Eds.), *Abeloff's clinical oncology* (6th ed., pp. 688–706.e7). Elsevier. https://doi.org/10.1016/B978-0-323-47674-4.00045-1

Zaky, M.Y., Lamloum, N.S., Yassin, N.Y.S., & Ahmed, O.M. (2024). Brain tumors: Types, diagnostic biomarkers, and new therapeutic approaches. In R.C. Sobti, N.K. Ganguly, & R. Kumar (Eds.), *Handbook of oncobiology: From basic to clinical sciences* (pp. 533–553). Springer Nature. https://doi.org/10.1007/978-981-99-6263-1_21

Zelaya, J.E., & Al-Khoury, L. (2024). Posterior reversible encephalopathy syndrome. In *StatPearls.* StatPearls Publishing. https://www.ncbi.nlm.nih.gov/books/NBK554492

Zinserling, V. (2022). *Infectious lesions of the central nervous system.* Springer Nature. https://doi.org/10.1007/978-3-030-96260-9

Zoghbi, M., Moussa, M.J., Dagher, J., Haroun, E., Qdaisat, A., Singer, E.D., ... Chaftari, P. (2024). Brain metastasis in the emergency department: Epidemiology, presentation, investigations, and management. *Cancers, 16*(14), 2583. https://doi.org/10.3390/cancers16142583

SECTION II

METABOLIC EMERGENCIES

Cindy Stern, MSN, RN, CCRP,
and Liffy I. Cherian, MSN, APRN, AGCNS-BC, OCN®

CHAPTER 8

Hypercalcemia of Malignancy

FAST FACTS

- **Description:** Hypercalcemia of malignancy is a complex metabolic disorder that is defined as total serum calcium exceeding 10.2 mg/dl (2.2 mmol/L) or ionized serum calcium exceeding 5.6 mg/dl (1.4 mmol/L). Four underlying pathologic mechanisms cause hypercalcemia of malignancy, including the humoral, osteolytic, tumor production of calcitriol, and ectopic production of parathyroid hormone by the tumor.
- **Incidence:** Hypercalcemia of malignancy occurs in approximately 20%–30% of patients with solid tumors and hematologic malignancies, most often with advanced disease. Multiple myeloma, breast cancers, and squamous cell cancers account for the most common cases.
- **Clinical Manifestations:** The rate of development and the degree of the calcium elevation influence the signs and symptoms of hypercalcemia of malignancy. Body systems most affected are renal, gastrointestinal, and neurologic.
- **Risk Factors and Etiology:** Calcium homeostasis serves an essential role in many of the body's physiologic activities. Nonmalignant and malignant etiologies can lead to disturbances in calcium homeostasis as a result of alterations in hormones, bone metabolism, intestinal calcium absorption, and renal excretion.
- **Pathophysiology and Patient Evaluation:** Although the specific underlying mechanisms vary among tumor types, hypercalcemia of malignancy develops when cancer cells produce hormones and other substances that interfere with healthy body processes for bone and calcium homeostasis. Evaluation of hypercalcemia involves a thorough review of medical and family history, cancer status, medications, diet, and potential benign causes.
- **Advanced Practice Considerations:** Diagnostic evaluation includes biochemical testing to identify the underlying mechanism and contributing factors across different cancer types. In some situations, such as low albumin levels, a standardized formula is recommended to estimate the corrected value for ionized calcium. Renal function tests are mandatory because of the crucial role of the kidneys in maintaining calcium homeostasis.
- **Treatment Modalities:** IV isotonic saline administration to correct dehydration is the cornerstone of treatment. Loop diuretics may be added for patients at increased risk or with signs of fluid overload. In addition, denosumab or a bisphosphonate is administered for acute management. Long-term therapy includes management of the underlying malignancy and ongoing administration of denosumab or bisphosphonate therapy.
- **Nursing Management:** Patient care consists of baseline and ongoing assessment of neurologic, renal, gastrointestinal, and fluid and electrolyte status. Additional nursing interventions focus on the implementation of safety measures, symptom management, evaluation of hypercalcemia of malignancy treatment outcomes, education, and emotional support for patients and caregivers.
- **Outcomes:** The success of therapeutic interventions depends on the underlying malignancy, early recognition, additional precipitating factors, and prompt initiation of care.

Although hypercalcemia of malignancy is not entirely preventable, patients at increased risk may benefit from denosumab or bisphosphonates. National oncology nursing and medical guidelines support the provision of symptom palliation and end-of-life care to improve outcomes such as quality of life for this patient population.

Introduction

Hypercalcemia is one of the most common and potentially life-threatening complications of cancer. Hypercalcemia of malignancy (HCM) is classified both as a paraneoplastic syndrome and a metabolic oncologic emergency. A paraneoplastic syndrome is a group of disorders in patients with cancer, not caused by tumor invasion, tumor compression, or metastasis. Hormones and other substances produced by the tumor or by the body's responses to tumor activity cause abnormalities that overcome healthy body feedback mechanisms (Gould Rothberg et al., 2022).

HCM most often develops in patients with advanced cancer, especially those associated with extensive bone metastasis. Depending on the underlying malignancy and other health issues, survival time is limited. However, survival time for patients with HCM has improved in those with solid tumors because of newer approaches to cancer treatment (Gupta et al., 2023; Mc Donald et al., 2023).

The diagnosis of hypercalcemia may be delayed or unrecognized when calcium levels are mildly elevated, symptoms are nonspecific, or the onset is slow (Almuradova & Cicin, 2023). Signs and symptoms are primarily related to the severity of hypercalcemia, rapidity of onset, and the underlying malignancy (Mc Donald et al., 2023). Common symptoms may include lethargy, weakness, changes in mood or mild confusion, anorexia, nausea, and constipation. When calcium levels are markedly elevated, vomiting, dehydration, renal damage, electrocardiogram (ECG) abnormalities, arrhythmias, diminished mental status, headaches, seizures, or coma may occur (Almuradova & Cicin, 2023; Walker & Shane, 2022). Therapy is individualized based on the extent of serum calcium elevation and the speed with which it develops. The primary approach to treatment focuses on rehydration and management of factors contributing to rising calcium levels. Knowledge of the types of malignancies commonly associated with an increased risk for HCM, an understanding of the underlying pathophysiology, and alertness to the early manifestations will guide oncology nurses in the prevention, recognition, and implementation of approaches for patient care. Timely initiation of appropriate management strategies and symptom palliation will enhance patients' quality of life and may help prolong survival (Liu et al., 2024; Sullivan & Slatore, 2020).

Incidence

HCM occurs in approximately 20%–30% of all patients at some point during their cancer journey (Bartkiewicz et al., 2024; Chakhtoura & El-Hajj Fuleihan, 2021; Guise & Wysolmerski, 2022; Hu, 2021). Although HCM may occur in any cancer, it is most often experienced by patients with advanced cancers, such as multiple myeloma and breast, non-small cell lung, renal, and squamous cell cancers of any origin (Frost, 2022; Goltzman, 2023; Guise & Wysolmerski, 2022). Less commonly, HCM is associated with lymphoma and some forms of leukemia. Figure 8-1 provides an overview of the incidence of HCM by cancer site. Benign causes of hypercalcemia, such as primary hyperparathyroidism, must be assessed as they contribute to elevated calcium levels in patients with HCM.

Clinical Manifestations

Signs and symptoms of HCM (see Table 8-1) are related to the severity of hypercalcemia, the rapidity of the calcium level increase, and the presence of bone metastasis (El-Hajj Fuleihan et al., 2020). Manifestations of HCM involve the gastrointestinal (GI), renal, neurologic, cardiologic, and musculoskeletal systems. Signs and symptoms are characterized by alterations in muscle contraction, nerve conductivity, intracellular signaling, bone formation, cell membrane permeability, electrolyte regulation, and acid-base balance. Early in the development of HCM, signs and symptoms may be vague and difficult to distinguish from the sequela of advanced disease, side effects of cancer treatments, general debilitation, and chronic concurrent diseases (Marshall et al., 2023).

Patients with HCM often have greater symptomatology than those with benign causes. Nonmalignant-related hypercalcemia tends to develop slowly and is usually

FIGURE 8-1. Frequency of Hypercalcemia of Malignancy by Cancer Site

Common	Multiple myeloma
	Breast without bone metastasis
	Breast with bone metastasis
	Squamous lung, head and neck, esophagus, urothelial
	Non-small cell lung adenocarcinoma
	Non-Hodgkin and Hodgkin lymphoma
	Renal
	Ovarian, endometrial, cervical
	Pancreatic
	Liver
Less Common	Parathyroid

Although hypercalcemia of malignancy has been reported in many cancers, it is most commonly associated with multiple myeloma, breast cancer (with or without metastasis), and squamous cell cancers occurring in any site.

Note. Based on information from Almuradova & Cicin, 2023; Guise & Wysolmerski, 2022.

TABLE 8-1
Signs and Symptoms of Hypercalcemia of Malignancy

Organ System	Onset	Manifestations
Neurologic	Early	May be vague; drowsiness, lethargy, weakness, decreased deep tendon reflexes, depression, restlessness, irritability, confusion, personality changes
	Late	Cognitive dysfunction, disorientation, delirium, psychotic behavior, visual disturbances, seizures, stupor, coma
Musculoskeletal	Early	Muscle weakness, fatigue, hypotonia, bone pain, osteopenia/osteoporosis
	Late	Ataxia, pathologic fractures
Cardiovascular	Early	Rare manifestations
	Late	Abnormal electrocardiogram tracings (prolonged PR interval, shortened QT interval, widened QRS, low amplitude T-wave, ST-segment elevation, atrioventricular blockade) Arrhythmias (bradycardia, tachycardia. ventricular fibrillation or tachycardia, cardiac arrest
Gastrointestinal	Early	Vague; anorexia, nausea, vomiting, constipation, abdominal pain
	Late	Obstipation, ileus, peptic ulcers, acute pancreatitis
Renal	Early	Polyuria, polydipsia, nocturia, dehydration, decreased glomerular filtration, hypercalciuria
	Late	Renal damage and insufficiency, renal failure, nephrolithiasis

Elevated calcium levels alter normal physiologic activities, such as muscle contraction, nerve conductivity, intracellular signaling, hormone production, bone formation, cell membrane permeability, electrolyte regulation, and acid-base balance. The results are manifested by signs and symptoms involving multiple organ systems. Early in the development of hypercalcemia of malignancy, signs and symptoms may be vague and difficult to recognize or distinguish from the sequela of advanced disease, side effects of cancer treatments, general debilitation, and chronic concurrent diseases.

Note. Based on information from Almuradova & Cicin, 2023; Bartkiewicz et al., 2024; Goltzman, 2023; Tiwari et al., 2022; Tonon et al., 2022; Walker & Shane, 2022.

first identified while patients are undergoing evaluation for other issues (Pokhrel et al., 2024). In addition, calcium levels of HCM tend to be higher than those related to benign etiologies (El-Hajj Fuleihan et al., 2020).

Gastrointestinal Signs and Symptoms

GI symptoms such as constipation, anorexia, nausea, and vomiting occur because of decreased smooth muscle tone or abnormal autonomic function, causing delayed gastric emptying and slowing in the GI tract. Complete ileus can occur with extremely high calcium levels. GI symptoms may easily be mistaken for the side effects of cancer treatments or advanced disease. Although rare, patients may present with pancreatitis and peptic ulcer disease thought to be caused by calcium deposits in the pancreatic duct and calcium activation of pancreatic enzymes (Mederos et al., 2021; Tiwari et al., 2022).

Renal Signs and Symptoms

Impaired renal function associated with HCM further contributes to elevated calcium levels (Tonon et al., 2022) (see Figure 8-2). For example, patients with HCM

FIGURE 8-2. Renal Pathophysiology in Hypercalcemia of Malignancy

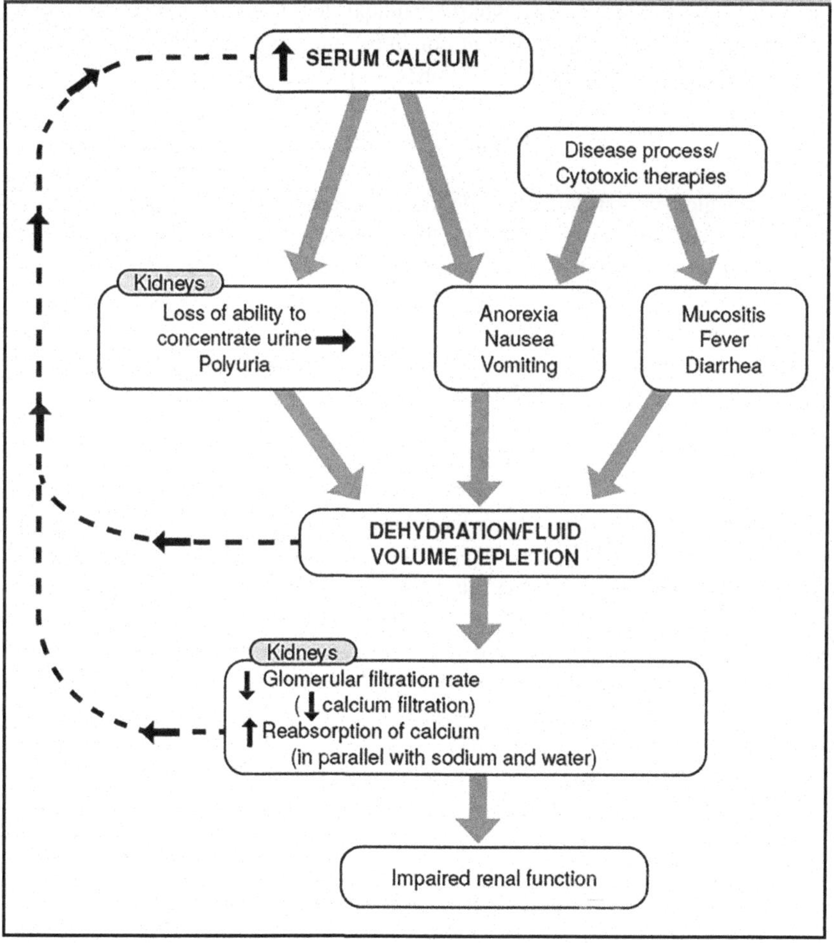

Note. From "Hypercalcemia of Malignancy: A Review of Advances in Pathophysiology," by M. Kaplan, 1994, *Oncology Nursing Forum, 21*(6), p. 1044. Copyright 1994 by Oncology Nursing Society. Adapted with permission.

may develop acquired nephrogenic diabetes insipidus, a reversible condition in which the kidneys do not respond appropriately to antidiuretic hormone (Christ-Crain et al., 2021). As a result, the kidneys are not able to regulate fluid balance. In addition, elevated calcium levels cause renal arteriole vasoconstriction, resulting in subsequent diminished renal blood flow and glomerular filtration rate (GFR); both contribute to decreased renal excretion of calcium (Tonon et al., 2022). Infrequently, prolonged hypercalcemia may lead to renal damage because calcium is deposited in the renal tubules and parenchyma (Almuradova & Cicin, 2023).

Unregulated fluid balance and the inability to concentrate urine lead to dehydration and electrolyte imbalances. Excess fluid losses alter the ratio of fluid to sodium so that the volume of fluid is less than the body's sodium content, causing sodium levels to rise (Frost, 2022). In addition, excess urine output is associated with decreased serum potassium, magnesium, and chloride and phosphate levels while urinary levels of these electrolytes are elevated (Bokhari & Zulfiqar, 2023). Disease and ongoing cancer treatment–related GI symptoms, common in patients with cancer, may contribute to volume depletion and electrolyte imbalances in patients with HCM.

Neurologic Effects

Neurologic symptoms reflect the depressant effect of hypercalcemia on the central nervous system and nerve conductivity. Early symptoms may include fatigue, anxiety, apathy, lethargy, and changes in behavior, mood, or concentration. As calcium levels rise, symptoms progress to altered mental status, confusion, and eventually coma. Neurologic testing may reveal hyporeflexia. In rare cases, patients may develop posterior reversible leukoencephalopathy syndrome, characterized by headaches, seizures, and imaging findings of subcortical edema (Almuradova & Cicin, 2023).

Cardiac Effects

Symptoms of hypercalcemia vary based on the level of calcium in the blood. However, in severe cases, patients may experience ventricular arrhythmias (e.g., ventricular tachycardia) and ECG changes, such as ST-segment depression, a shortened QT interval, and prolonged PR and QRS intervals (Almuradova & Cicin, 2023; Tonon et al., 2022). At concentrations beyond 15 mg/dl, hypercalcemia depresses the strength of myocardial contraction. Additionally, accompanying electrolyte imbalances can heighten the risk of cardiac arrhythmias (Bartkiewicz et al., 2024). Extremely high blood calcium levels can induce conditions that mimic ST-segment elevation associated with myocardial infarction. In these instances, coronary artery catheterization typically fails to reveal significant changes, and correction of electrolyte disturbances usually alleviates these ECG abnormalities (Bartkiewicz et al., 2024).

Musculoskeletal Effects

Elevated serum calcium levels decrease neuromuscular excitability, causing hypotonicity of smooth and striated muscle. Clinical manifestations include myalgia, arthralgia, muscle weakness, and easy fatigability (Hu, 2021; Tonon et al., 2022). Prolonged bed rest, immobility, and lack of weight-bearing activities caused by extreme muscle weakness, debilitation, impaired mobility, or pain further contribute to muscle atrophy and calcium loss from bones (Asonitis et al., 2019; Gilson, 2024). Bone pain is commonly related to bone metastasis and increased bone remodeling (Ansoria et al., 2024; Haroun et al., 2023). Pathologic fractures may develop with progressive disease, especially with widespread bone involvement (Almuradova & Cicin, 2023).

Risk Factors and Etiology

Calcium homeostasis serves an essential role in many physiologic activities, including muscle contraction, nerve conductivity, intracellular signaling, hormone production, bone and teeth formation, cell membrane permeability, electrolyte regulation, acid-base balance, coagulation, and enzymatic activities (Matikainen et al., 2021; Walker & Shane, 2022). Approximately 99% of calcium in the body is stored in the bones and teeth. Serum calcium exists in three forms: protein bound, ionized, and chelated (biochemical bond to other molecules). Ionized or free calcium, which accounts for approximately 51% of serum calcium, is the form of calcium required for many physiologic activities (Yu & Sharma, 2023). Although there may be a slight variation among laboratory facilities, normal serum calcium levels are 8.8–10.2 mg/dl or 2.2–2.5 mmol/L (Guise & Wysolmerski, 2022).

Chelated calcium, such as calcium phosphate, accounts for 9% of serum calcium and promotes calcium transport and absorption by tissues throughout the body. The remainder of serum calcium is not available for use by body tissues because it is bound to proteins (e.g., albumin).

The maintenance of calcium homeostasis is dependent on several body feedback mechanisms that respond to fluctuations in normal calcium levels. Calcium-sensing receptors located in various organ tissues recognize variations in calcium levels and promote the release of hormones and cytokines to maintain serum calcium values within an acceptable range (Hannan et al., 2019; Matikainen et al., 2021). Hormones such as parathyroid hormone (PTH), calcitriol, and calcitonin orchestrate interaction between signaling pathways, bones, intestines, and the kidneys to support calcium homeostasis (Al-Bari & Al Mamun, 2020; Matikainen et al., 2021) (see Figure 8-3).

The Role of Bones in Calcium Homeostasis

Skeletal bone is a dynamic organ that serves as a reservoir for 99% of total body calcium and plays a role in body structure and physiology. Although relatively low in volume, osteocytes, osteoblasts, and osteoclasts are types of bone cells essential for bone health and calcium homeostasis (Šromová et al., 2023). These bone cells are involved in bone formation and resorption (degradation) through a process called bone remodeling (Bringhurst et al., 2025). Numerous cytokines, cell membrane proteins, hormones, and cells that originate in the bone marrow contribute to the process of bone remodeling. This process prevents the accumulation of damaged bone through

FIGURE 8-3. Normal Homeostasis of Blood Calcium Levels

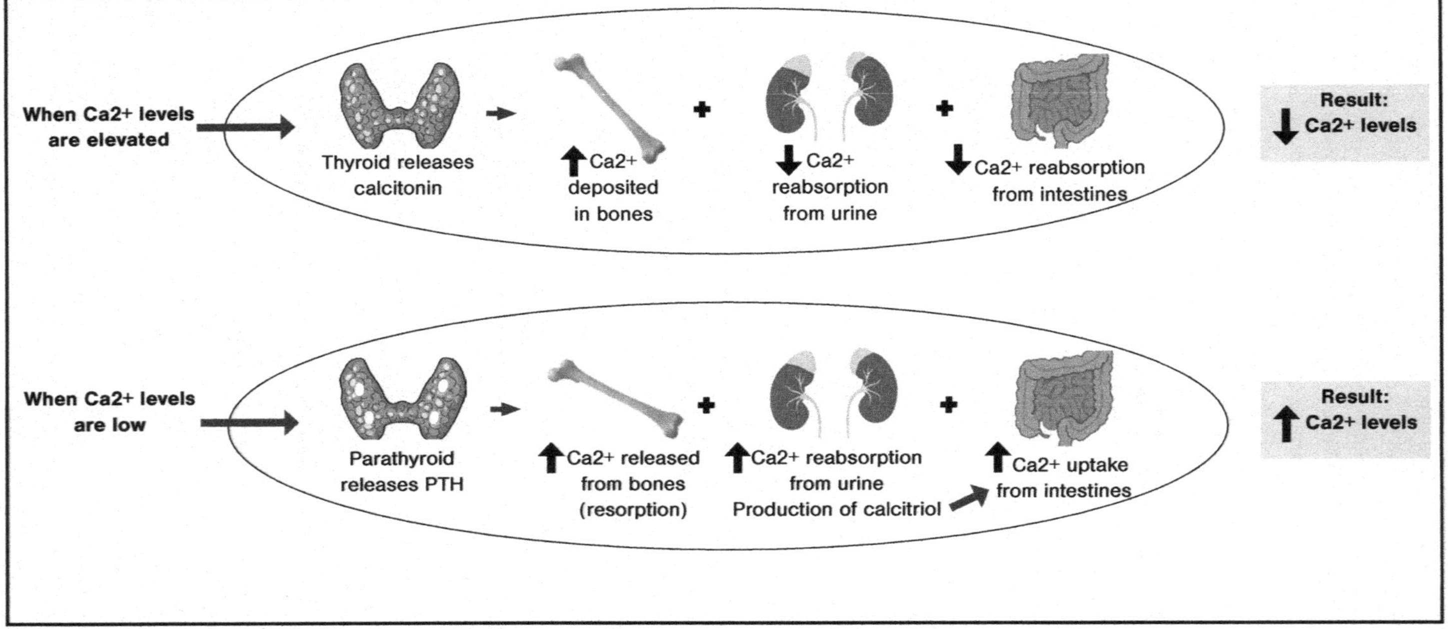

Ca^{2+}—calcium ion; PTH—parathyroid hormone

Calcium homeostasis is maintained through negative feedback mechanisms and the interaction of multiple processes involving the parathyroid and thyroid glands, bones, kidneys, and intestines. Receptors, hormones, and signaling pathways facilitate communication and management of calcium levels.

Note. Based on information from Bartkiewicz et al., 2024; Goltzman, 2021; Grunbaum & Kremer, 2022; Guise & Wysolmerski, 2022; Hu, 2021; Kim et al., 2020; Matikainen et al., 2021; Menefee et al., 2024; Tonon et al., 2022; Yu & Sharma, 2023.

resorption, maintains bone strength through bone formation, and preserves calcium, phosphate, and magnesium equilibrium (Al-Bari & Al Mamun, 2020; Bringhurst et al., 2025; Kim et al., 2020; Walker & Shane, 2022).

Osteoblasts are bone-forming cells that help to synthesize the collagen matrix on the bone surface. As the osteoblast and bone matrix calcify, it develops into an osteocyte, the most common and mature type of bone cell (Delgado-Calle & Bellido, 2022; Menefee et al., 2024). Normal system feedback processes activate osteoblast-mediated bone formation as a mechanism to lower serum calcium levels.

Osteoclasts are responsible for bone resorption through the secretion of acid and enzymes that dissolve collagen and other components of the bone matrix (Menefee et al., 2024). Osteoclast-mediated bone resorption is a mechanism by which bones release calcium to elevate serum calcium levels in response to normally functioning feedback mechanisms.

In the process of remodeling, osteoclasts and osteoblasts function in a coordinated manner so that the cycle of osteoclast-mediated bone resorption and osteoblast-mediated bone formation occurs at relatively equal rates (Park-Min & Lorenzo, 2022). Mounting data suggest that osteoclasts have numerous functions beyond bone resorption, including regulation of osteoblast formation and function (Park-Min & Lorenzo, 2022).

Bone Remodeling Pathway

Although many factors contribute to bone remodeling, an essential complex process involves hormones, cytokines, and the interaction between three components: receptor activator of nuclear factor kappa-B (RANK), RANK ligand (RANKL), and osteoprotegerin (OPG) (Y. Zhang et al., 2022). RANKL is a structure formed by osteoblasts that binds to the RANK receptor on the surface of osteoclast precursors. This initiates a cascade of activity that leads to the formation of mature osteoclasts and accelerated bone resorption (Šromová et al., 2023; Y. Zhang et al., 2022). PTH release increases the activity of RANKL, leading to bone resorption and increased calcium levels. Osteoblasts also produce OPG, another receptor for RANKL. When RANKL binds with OPG, it is prevented from binding with RANK, resulting in decreased maturation of osteoclasts and diminished bone resorption (Rowe & Koller, 2023).

The Role of Hormones and Cytokines in Calcium Homeostasis

Parathyroid Hormone

PTH plays a primary role in the regulation of blood calcium levels. When calcium levels fall, the parathyroid gland releases PTH, inhibiting osteoblast-mediated bone formation and facilitating a needed rise in serum calcium levels. PTH hormone also stimulates osteoclast activity, resulting in bone resorption and calcium release from bone into the bloodstream. In response to low calcium levels, PTH enhances renal reabsorption of calcium. It continues to contribute to an increase in serum calcium by stimulating the kidneys to release calcitriol, which enhances intestinal absorption of calcium from dietary intake. As calcium levels normalize, PTH production and release are inhibited, as are renal calcium reabsorption and calcitriol production (Goltzman, 2021).

Calcitonin

Elevated calcium levels stimulate the thyroid parafollicular cells to release calcitonin, which helps to lower serum calcium levels by stimulating osteoblast bone formation and inhibiting osteoclast-mediated bone resorption. Calcitonin also targets the kidneys to increase urinary calcium excretion. The effect of calcitonin on the intestines is to decrease absorption of dietary calcium (Goltzman, 2021).

In response to PTH and processes initiated in the liver and subsequently the kidneys, a bioactive form of vitamin D, calcitriol (1,25-dihydroxycholecalciferol), is synthesized. Calcitriol contributes to the maintenance of optimal blood calcium levels primarily by promoting intestinal absorption of dietary calcium, and to some extent, renal calcium reabsorption and bone resorption.

The Role of Kidneys in Calcium Homeostasis

The kidneys play a key role in calcium homeostasis by regulating calcium reabsorption and excretion. Under the influence of PTH, the kidneys reabsorb about 98% of filtered calcium, primarily in the proximal tubule and loop of Henle. PTH increases calcium reabsorption and promotes activation of calcitriol, which enhances intestinal calcium absorption. Together, these actions help maintain stable blood calcium levels.

The Role of the Intestines in Calcium Homeostasis

The amount of intestinal calcium absorption is closely linked to the activity of the bones, kidneys, hormonal influences, and the body's need for calcium, such as during pregnancy, lactation, and growth (Matikainen et al., 2021). When calcium levels are low, PTH release promotes renal production of calcitriol, promoting intestinal calcium absorption. In response to elevated calcium levels, body feedback mechanisms limit PTH, calcitriol production, and intestinal calcium absorption.

Pathophysiology and Patient Evaluation

HCM development is the result of cancer-associated factors that work in tandem with cytokines and other substances to overwhelm healthy body mechanisms for calcium and bone homeostasis. Although HCM, is most often caused by increased bone resorption, four underlying mechanisms have been identified: humoral, osteolytic, calcitriol (1,25-dihydroxyvitamin D) mediated, and ectopic production of PTH (Guise & Wysolmerski, 2022). Further study, including biochemical testing of patients with HCM, is needed to develop an updated understanding of the occurrence and underlying pathophysiology of HCM both overall and by specific cancer sites (Sheehan et al., 2021).

Humoral Hypercalcemia of Malignancy

Humoral-mediated processes are the underlying cause for about 80% of patients with HCM (Almuradova & Cicin, 2023; Grunbaum & Kremer, 2022; Gupta et al., 2023; Hu, 2021). Humoral HCM results from tumor cell secretion of parathyroid hormone–related protein (PTHrP) that is biologically similar to PTH. Tumor secretion of PTHrP undermines healthy calcium homeostasis by targeting tissue receptors in the bones, intestines, and kidneys (Guise & Wysolmerski, 2022; Walker & Shane, 2022). The result is increased bone resorption, excess renal calcium reabsorption, and increased intestinal absorption of dietary calcium. PTHrP stimulates osteoclast activity but suppresses osteoblast formation so that the balance between bone formation and resorption is altered (Hu, 2021). Squamous cell (e.g., head and neck, esophageal, cervical, colon), breast, kidney, bladder, endometrial, ovarian, and hematologic cancers (e.g., lymphoma, chronic myeloid leukemia) have been associated with humoral HCM (Almuradova & Cicin, 2023; Gould Rothberg et al., 2022; Hu, 2021). Patients with humoral HCM typically have few or no bone metastases (Guise & Wysolmerski, 2022).

Osteolytic Hypercalcemia of Malignancy

Osteolytic processes, accounting for about 20% of cases of HCM, occur in the setting of extensive bone metastasis (Anastasopoulou & Mewawalla, 2023; Guise & Wysolmerski, 2022). Although the most common underlying malignancies are multiple myeloma, metastatic breast cancer, renal cancer, and lung cancer, osteolytic HCM may be associated with other cancers (Hu, 2021). Cancer cells from bone metastases release cytokines and hormone-like substances that foster osteoclast proliferation and activation, resulting in increased bone resorption. For example, cancer cells that metastasize to bone produce PTHrP, which promotes osteoclast formation, bone resorption, and calcium release. Additional cytokines supporting osteoclast development include interleukins, tumor necrosis factor, macrophage–colony-stimulating factor, and prostaglandins (Riffel et al., 2022).

The RANKL–RANK–OPG triad is also disrupted in osteolytic HCM because cancer cells often overexpress RANKL. The increased levels of RANKL lead to increased binding between RANKL and the receptor RANK, resulting in increased osteoclast formation, activity, bone resorption, and calcium release. Metastatic bone cells produce PTHrP and other cytokines that block the production of OPG, inhibiting osteoblast formation and activity and allowing osteoclast-mediated bone resorption to exceed normal bone homeostasis mechanisms. The balance between bone formation and resorption is lost, and the increased calcium level is much greater than the amount that the kidneys can excrete. Growth factors, released by osteolytic bone metastasis, enter the bone marrow, resulting in increased cancer cell growth and subsequently PTHrP production (Clézardin et al., 2021). Increased RANKL–RANK binding promotes bone invasion, migration of cancer cells, and interaction with substances that can increase cancer growth and the risk of recurrence (De Leon-Oliva et al., 2023).

Calcitriol-Mediated Hypercalcemia of Malignancy

Tumor cell synthesis of calcitriol has been associated with less than 1% of HCM cases (Guise & Wysolmerski, 2022). Elevated levels of calcitriol lead to increased intestinal absorption of calcium and elevated serum levels. Historically, calcitriol-mediated HCM was thought to occur only in lymphomas; however, emerging data suggest other factors contribute to HCM in patients with lymphoma (Shallis et al., 2018). Additionally, in rare instances, calcitriol-mediated HCM is associated with solid organ tumors (Charoenngam et al., 2021).

Parathyroid Hormone–Mediated Hypercalcemia of Malignancy

PTH-mediated HCM, experienced by less than 1% of patients with cancer, occurs most commonly with parathyroid cancer and less often in other types of malignancies, such as multiple endocrine neoplasia syndromes (Asonitis et al., 2019). These syndromes, caused by germline variants, are associated with parathyroid, gastroentero-pancreatic, and anterior pituitary gland tumors and, less commonly, with tumors of the adrenal cortical gland, thymus, bronchi, and other nonendocrine tumors (Goltzman, 2021; Silva-Figueroa & Perrier, 2021). Ectopic PTH production disrupts calcium homeostasis through several mechanisms, including stimulation of osteoclast-mediated bone resorption, inhibition of osteoblastic bone formation, increased renal production of calcitriol, increased intestinal calcium absorption, and excess renal reabsorption of calcium (Goltzman, 2021).

Nonmalignant Sources of Hypercalcemia

In patients with HCM, it is important to consider benign etiologies not related to an underlying malignancy that may be the cause or contribute to elevated calcium levels. In the general population, 90% of individuals with hypercalcemia have either primary hyperparathyroidism or cancer (Walker & Shane, 2022). Benign etiologies of hypercalcemia include the following (English et al., 2024; Goltzman, 2021; Paterson, 2021; Rout et al., 2024; Walker & Shane, 2022):

- Endocrine disorders
- Hyperparathyroidism (the most common cause of hypercalcemia)
- Benign hyperplasia (adenoma) of one or more parathyroid glands
- Hyperthyroidism or thyroid toxicosis
- Hypoadrenalism
- Cancer treatment–induced or naturally occurring menopause; osteoporosis
- Excess vitamin or calcium intake
  - Vitamin A and D
  - Milk-alkali syndrome (excess intake of calcium or antacids containing calcium carbonate)
- Germline genetic abnormalities (inherited genetic variants)
  - Multiple endocrine neoplasia types (multiple forms)
  - Hyperparathyroidism jaw tumor syndrome

- Sporadic somatic abnormalities (noninherited genetic variants)
  - Familial hypocalciuric hyperthyroidism types 1–3
  - Familial isolated hyperparathyroidism
- Pharmacologic agents
  - Thiazide diuretics
  - Elevated lithium levels
  - Angiotensin-converting enzyme inhibitors
  - Nonsteroidal anti-inflammatory agents
  - Aminophylline, theophylline
  - Calcitriol
  - Teriparatide, abaloparatide
  - Rebound after discontinuation of denosumab
- Granulomatous disease
  - Inflammatory disorders (e.g., sarcoidosis, granulomatosis with polyangiitis [previously referred to as Wegener granulomatosis]), Crohn disease
  - Infections (e.g., tuberculosis, histoplasmosis)
  - Foreign bodies (e.g., silicosis, talc, berylliosis)
  - Renal impairment
  - Prolonged immobility

Patient Assessment

The evaluation of hypercalcemia includes a thorough patient and family medical history, status of the underlying cancer and treatment approaches, review of medications and supplements, assessment of benign causes of hypercalcemia, dietary review, evaluation of patient and caregiver health literacy, assessment of education needs, identification of barriers to care, and treatment adherence (see Table 8-2). A thorough review of systems and physical examination includes the assessment of signs and symptoms associated with HCM. For patients presenting with hypercalcemia without a known underlying malignancy, the evaluation focuses on signs, symptoms, physical assessment findings, and other diagnostic procedures indicative of cancer. The assessment also includes cancer risk factors such as tobacco use, alcohol consumption, and genetic predisposition.

Advanced Practice Considerations

Calcium Level Measurement

Serum calcium concentration can be measured using three approaches: total serum calcium, estimated corrected ionized calcium concentration, and ionized calcium concentration (see Figure 8-4). Total serum calcium reflects both ionized (or free) calcium and calcium bound to proteins such as albumin. The accuracy of total serum calcium measurement is impacted by low levels of albumin, commonly associated with cancer treatments or advanced disease. Other factors that alter the accuracy of total

TABLE 8-2
Components of Patient Assessment in Hypercalcemia of Malignancy

Components	Key Areas of Assessment Focus
Health history	Prior history and status of chronic illness and treatment approaches; includes benign etiologies of hypercalcemia Family history and known germline variants associated with disorders of calcium homeostasis Participation in cancer screening practices Allergies
Cancer history	Cancer risks related to lifestyle and health practices Family history of cancer or germline variants associated with cancer predisposition Known germline variants associated with cancer predisposition; management strategies if appropriate Cancer diagnoses (stage, grade, histology, bone involvement); prior or current treatment strategies • Toxicity experience and status with current (or recent) cancer treatments • Most recent cancer diagnostic procedures (e.g., imaging procedures, cancer marker status, organ function) • Known somatic variants associated with cancer diagnoses • Need for additional diagnostic procedures, especially important if no prior cancer diagnosis
Current medications and supplements	Medications and supplements associated with an increased risk of hypercalcemia Medications with potential for renal, cardiac, neurologic, and musculoskeletal impairment
Dietary review	Practices regarding the ability to access and maintain adequate nutritional intake Factors associated with impaired nutritional status
Hypercalcemia	Signs and symptoms overall, as well as those associated with hypercalcemia of malignancies; includes the date of onset and the speed with which symptoms developed and progressed Prior episodes of hypercalcemia of malignancy; previous treatment and response
Patient support and educational needs	See Table 8-7. Hypercalcemia of Malignancy: Nursing Care

Assessment of patients with hypercalcemia of malignancy focuses on the patient and family's health history, prior cancer diagnosis and risk factors, signs and symptoms at presentation, factors that contribute to hypercalcemia of malignancy, and the patient and caregiver needs for support and education.

Note. Based on information from Almuradova & Cicin, 2023; Bartkiewicz et al., 2024; English et al., 2024; Frost, 2022; Goltzman, 2021; Hu, 2021; Klein & Vanek, 2021; National Comprehensive Cancer Network, 2025b; Oncology Nursing Society, 2022; Pokhrel et al., 2024; Sadiq et al., 2022.

FIGURE 8-4. Distribution of Body Calcium and Measurement of Calcium Levels

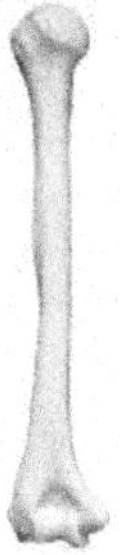

99% of calcium is stored in bones.

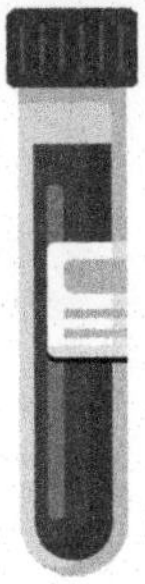

1% of calcium is in blood.

- About 50% is ionized (free).
- About 10% exists as biochemically bound molecules:
  - Calcium phosphate, calcium carbonate, calcium oxalate
- About 40% is bound to protein.
  - 70%–80% is bound to albumin.

Total Serum Level Includes

- Ionized calcium (free)
- Calcium bound to albumin

Ionized Calcium Level

- Does not include albumin-bound calcium
- Often used when albumin levels are low

Corrected Calcium Level

- A formula is used to assess calcium levels for patients with low albumin.

In healthy individuals who have normal albumin levels, total serum calcium is used to assess serum calcium concentration. However, a formula is used routinely to estimate corrected ionized calcium concentration for patients with hypercalcemia and low levels of albumin. Direct measurement of ionized calcium concentration is not routinely performed because of the availability, expense, and requirement of specialized equipment and procedures.

Note. Based on information from Desgagnés et al., 2025; Hamroun et al., 2020; Yu & Sharma, 2023.

serum calcium measurement include thrombocytosis, acid-base imbalance, elevated immunoglobulin M levels, abnormal serum proteins, multiple myeloma, and use of protein-bound drugs (Bancal et al., 2023; Tonon et al., 2022). In patients with low albumin, direct measurement of ionized calcium is considered the most accurate method for assessing calcium concentration in HCM (Bancal et al., 2023). However, measurement of ionized calcium concentration is not routinely used because of barriers such as cost, specific requirements for specimen collection and processing, and factors that contribute to variations in ionized calcium levels.

Routinely, clinicians use a formula to estimate the corrected ionized calcium concentration for patients with HCM and low albumin levels (see Figure 8-5). Although several studies have suggested that the formula does not correlate well with total or ionized calcium measurement (Kenny et al., 2021), it continues to be used widely because alternative options are not feasible or available (Bancal et al., 2023; Desgagnés et al., 2025; Hamroun et al., 2020; Yu & Sharma, 2023).

The Endocrine Society clinical practice guidelines describe HCM as mild, moderate, or severe based on calcium levels and associated symptoms (El-Hajj Fuleihan et al., 2022) (see Table 8-3). An alternative definition of hypercalcemia severity is provided

FIGURE 8-5. Corrected Ionized Calcium Formula

Corrected calcium (mg/dl) = total serum calcium (mg/dl) + [0.8 × (4 − albumin level (g/dl)]

Example:
Total serum calcium level: 10.5 mg/dl
Albumin level: 2.5 g/dl

Steps		Calculations
1	Identify the total serum calcium level.	10.5 mg/dl
2	Subtract the serum albumin level from 4.	4 − 2.5 = 1.5
3	Multiply the result of Step 2 by 0.8.	0.8 × 1.5 = 1.2
4	Add the result of Step 3 to the total serum calcium level.	10.5 + 1.2 = 11.7
5	The corrected ionized calcium level is the result of Step 4.	11.7 mg/dl

Low levels of albumin, associated with advanced cancer or cancer treatments, alter the accuracy of total serum calcium measurement. Other conditions that may alter the accuracy of total serum calcium measurement include multiple myeloma, macroglobulinemia, thrombocytosis, hyperproteinemia, and hypoproteinemia. The Payne formula is routinely used in clinical practice to estimate ionized calcium values for patients with hypercalcemia of malignancy in the setting of low albumin levels.

Note. Based on information from Desgagnés et al., 2025; Payne et al., 1973; Tonon et al., 2022.

by the National Cancer Institute Cancer Therapy Evaluation Program's (2017) *Common Terminology Criteria for Adverse Events* (see Table 8-4). This documentation was developed to provide standardization and consistency for grading abnormal signs and symptoms associated with cancer treatments. It is most frequently used to assist in the management of cancer treatment and the setting of clinical trials. Nurses should always reference the version of this documentation used by their institutions or protocols.

Measurement of Mediators

In addition to the measurement of calcium levels, evaluation of patients with known malignancy consists of measuring both PTH and PTHrP levels. Although similar in structure, PTH and PTHrP will not rise simultaneously unless there is more than one cause of elevated calcium levels. In most cases of HCM, serum PTH levels appear to be low or normal. High-normal PTH levels in the setting of hypercalcemia suggest the presence of PTH-mediated hypercalcemia or parathyroid carcinoma. If PTHrP levels are low, calcitriol levels are assessed to screen for calcitriol-mediated HCM. Osteolytic metastases are considered the cause of HCM in patients with low levels of PTH, PTHrP, and calcitriol (Almuradova & Cicin, 2023).

Serum and Urine Chemistry Assessment

Serum and urine chemistry assessment for HCM includes measurement of electrolytes and other substances in the blood or urine. These tests facilitate a differential

TABLE 8-3
Calcium Level Severity and Examples of Associated Signs and Symptoms of Hypercalcemia of Malignancy

Calcium Level	Musculoskeletal	Gastrointestinal	Neurologic	Renal	Cardiac
Mild[a]: 10–< 12 mg/dl (3 mmol/L)[b] Ionized: 5.6–8 mg/dl (1.4–2 mmol/L)	Fatigue	Constipation	Anxiety Depression	Polyuria Polydipsia	Rare
Moderate: 12–13.9 mg/dl (3–3.5 mmol/L) Ionized: > 10 mg/dl (2.5 mmol/L)	Muscle weakness Bone pain	Constipation Anorexia Nausea Vomiting	Cognitive dysfunction Hyporeflexia	Nephrogenic diabetes insipidus Dehydration Renal insufficiency (acute kidney injury)	Shortened QT interval Prolonged PR interval Widened QRS complex Arrhythmia (bradycardia or tachycardia)
Severe: > 14 mg/dl (> 3.5 mmol/L) Ionized: 10–12 mg/dl (2.5–3 mmol/L)	As above	As above Obstipation Ileus Pancreatitis	As above Confusion Stupor Coma	As above Nephrocalcinosis	As above Cardiac arrest

[a]Patients with mild hypercalcemia of malignancy may be asymptomatic or have nonspecific symptoms often attributed to other clinical issues or antineoplastic therapy.

[b]The parameters for serum calcium levels may vary slightly among laboratory facilities.

Although the manifestations of hypercalcemia of malignancy may differ among individuals, signs and symptoms are related to the severity of the blood calcium elevation and the speed with which hypercalcemia of malignancy develops.

Note. Based on information from Almuradova & Cicin, 2023; Anastasopoulou & Mewawalla, 2023; Dickens et al., 2023; El-Hajj Fuleihan et al., 2022; Hu, 2021; Walker & Shane, 2022.

TABLE 8-4
Common Terminology Criteria for Adverse Events

Grade	Parameters
1	Ionized calcium > ULN - 1.5 mmol/L or Corrected serum calcium of > ULN - 11.5 mg/dl (> ULN - 2.9 mmol/L)
2	Ionized calcium > 1.5–1.6 mmol/L; symptomatic or Corrected serum calcium of > 11.5–12.5 mg/dl (> 2.9–3.1 mmol/L)
3	Ionized calcium > 1.6–1.8 mmol/L; hospitalization indicated or Corrected serum calcium of > 12.5–13.5 mg/dl (> 3.1–3.4 mmol/L)
4	Ionized calcium > 1.8 mmol/L; life-threatening consequences or Corrected serum calcium of > 13.5 mg/dl (> 3.4 mmol/L)
5	Death

ULN—upper limit of normal

The National Cancer Institute provides grading criteria for abnormal clinical findings (referred to as adverse events) associated with antineoplastic therapies. The grading system provides standardization for the definition of treatment-related toxicity. The *Common Terminology Criteria for Adverse Events* is used for the management of chemotherapy administration and dosing and for monitoring toxicity associated with investigational therapies in clinical trials.

Note. From *Common Terminology Criteria for Adverse Events* [v.5.0], by National Cancer Institute Cancer Therapy Evaluation Program, 2017 (https://dctd.cancer.gov/research/ctep-trials/for-sites/adverse-events/ctcae-v55x7.pdf). In the public domain.

diagnosis to identify whether other conditions exist or are contributing to HCM. A differential diagnosis is important to distinguish between primary hyperparathyroidism and HCM in patients without a prior cancer diagnosis who present with elevated calcium levels (see Table 8-5). In addition, serum and urine chemistry measurement facilitates evaluation of organ function, metabolic status, other diseases, and responses to treatment.

For patients with HCM, evaluation of renal function is crucial at initial presentation, during treatment, and periodically thereafter. Renal assessment is necessary because dehydration, moderate and severely elevated calcium levels, and treatment with bisphosphonates are associated with potential renal impairment. Serum creatinine, GFR or estimated GFR, and urinary calcium clearance are routinely assessed to gauge renal status. Patients with HCM are monitored for elevated serum bicarbonate levels and metabolic alkalosis linked to polyuria and renal hydrogen ion loss.

Additional electrolyte imbalances associated with HCM mediators and renal injury are important to assess. Serum levels of phosphate are most often low in patients with HCM because of inhibition of phosphate reabsorption in the renal tubules. However, calcitriol-mediated HCM is considered if phosphate levels are elevated, as often seen in lymphoma (Hu, 2021). Elevated serum chloride, often seen in PTH- and PTHrP-mediated HCM, is associated with dehydration and disturbances in renal concentration abilities.

TABLE 8-5
Laboratory Values in Primary Hyperparathyroidism and Hypercalcemia of Malignancy

Laboratory Value	Primary Hyperparathyroidism	Hypercalcemia of Malignancy
Serum Value Assessment		
Albumin	N/A	Not affected by HCM, but necessary to interpret calcium levels
Alkaline phosphatase	Elevated	Elevated, especially in osteolytic HCM
Bicarbonate	Low	Elevated
Blood urea nitrogen	Elevated in cases of nephrocalcinosis or nephrolithiasis	Elevated, especially with renal impairment
Calcium	Normal or mild elevation	Elevated to a greater extent in HCM than with primary hyperparathyroidism
Chloride	High	Elevated in PTH and PTHrP-mediated HCM
Creatinine	May be elevated in cases of nephrocalcinosis or nephrolithiasis	Elevated, especially with renal impairment
1,25-Dihydroxyvitamin D_3 (calcitriol)	Low	Elevated in calcitriol-mediated HCM Low in other forms of HCM
Magnesium	Normal	Low or normal
Osmolarity	Elevated	Elevated
PTH	Normal or elevated	Elevated only in parathyroid cancer
PTHrP	Undetectable	Elevated in humoral-mediated HCM Low in other forms of HCM
pH	Metabolic acidosis	Metabolic alkalosis
Phosphate	Normal or low	Low with humoral HCM Normal or elevated with osteolytic HCM Elevated in calcitriol–mediated HCM
Potassium	Normal	Low
Sodium	Normal	Low

(Continued on next page)

TABLE 8-5
Laboratory Values in Primary Hyperparathyroidism and Hypercalcemia of Malignancy *(Continued)*

Laboratory Value	Primary Hyperparathyroidism	Hypercalcemia of Malignancy
Urine Value Assessment		
Phosphate	Elevated	Normal or elevated
24-hour urinary calcium	Normal or elevated	Higher than with primary hyperparathyroidism

HCM—hypercalcemia of malignancy; PTH—parathyroid hormone; PTHrP—parathyroid hormone–related protein

Serum and urine chemistry assessments help to establish a differential diagnosis to identify whether other conditions exist or are contributing to HCM, especially for patients who have yet to have a cancer diagnosis. Serum and urine chemistry measurements also provide an assessment of organ function, metabolic status, and responses to treatment.

Note. Based on information from Almuradova & Cicin, 2023; Bilezikian, 2022; El-Hajj Fuleihan et al., 2020; Pokhrel et al., 2024; Walker & Shane, 2022.

Other electrolytes (e.g., magnesium, potassium) are monitored, as these may be elevated or decreased depending on symptoms, extent of dehydration, treatment with aggressive fluid hydration, or deterioration of the patient's general condition.

Electrocardiography

An ECG is performed to identify arrhythmias or abnormalities in conduction patterns associated with moderate and severe HCM (Almuradova & Cicin, 2023; Tonon et al., 2022).

Imaging Studies

Although there is no specific imaging test to definitively diagnose hypercalcemia, a variety of modalities can be employed to detect the presence of malignancy, recurrence, progression, and metastatic bone disease. Nuclear bone scans and computed tomography scans are common imaging procedures used for cancer assessment.

Treatment Modalities

The overall goals of treatment for HCM are correction of volume depletion–related dehydration, inhibition of bone resorption, and management of the underlying malignancy, whenever feasible (Frost, 2022; Guise & Wysolmerski, 2022). The management of HCM is based on the presence of signs and symptoms, the rate at which calcium levels are elevated, and the severity of the calcium values. Neurologic impairment, such as confusion, rapid elevation of calcium levels, and calcium levels higher than

14 mg/dl (> 3.5 mmol/L), necessitates rapid intervention to prevent fatal outcomes (Almuradova & Cicin, 2023; Guise & Wysolmerski, 2022). When determining a treatment plan, physicians consider comorbidities, the type and status of the underlying malignancy, benign causes of hypercalcemia, and the adverse event profiles of medications (Mc Donald et al., 2023).

Patients Who Are Asymptomatic

Patients who are asymptomatic with mild hypercalcemia (calcium < 12 mg/dl) may only require outpatient observation while diagnostic tests are pending (Bartkiewicz et al., 2024). Mild calcium elevation is often an incidental finding before a cancer diagnosis (Frost, 2022). Management focuses on preventing dehydration, promoting oral fluid intake to enhance renal calcium excretion, and initiating symptom control for nausea, vomiting, and constipation. Patients are encouraged to engage in safe weight-bearing activities to minimize bone resorption, and pain is managed to support mobility and quality of life. Medications and supplements that can worsen hypercalcemia should be avoided if possible. In calcitriol-mediated cases, calcium restriction is unnecessary but intake should not exceed 1,000 mg/day (Gupta et al., 2023; Walker & Shane, 2022). Regular monitoring of symptoms and calcium levels remains essential.

Moderate or Severe Hypercalcemia of Malignancy

Patients with moderate or severe HCM are usually symptomatic and require prompt treatment. Management includes treatment of the underlying malignancy, when possible, along with IV hydration, antiresorptive therapy, and other medications. Table 8-6 outlines treatment strategies for moderate and severe HCM.

Intravenous Hydration

An initial goal of therapy for moderate to severe HCM is to correct volume depletion, promote calcium excretion, and prevent renal damage. Symptoms from advanced cancer and its treatment overlap with those associated with HCM, contributing to poor oral intake and dehydration. The development of nephrogenic diabetes insipidus further escalates fluid losses.

Isotonic crystalloid solution, such as normal saline, is used to restore hydration, improve renal perfusion, increase GFR, and enhance calcium excretion (Bartkiewicz et al., 2024). The infusion rate, typically 200–500 ml/hour, is based on the severity of dehydration and hypercalcemia, electrolyte and acid-base imbalances, and comorbidities, especially cardiovascular and renal disease (El-Hajj Fuleihan et al., 2022; Tonon et al., 2022). Once hydrated, the rate is reduced to 100–150 ml/hour to maintain urine output of 100–150 ml/hour (Anastasopoulou & Mewawalla, 2023; Frost, 2022; Mc Donald et al., 2023).

Although loop diuretics (e.g., furosemide) were routinely added after hydration, evidence does not support this practice. Diuretics are now reserved for patients with volume overload or at high risk of developing it, and only after hydration is restored (Chakhtoura & El-Hajj Fuleihan, 2021; Guise & Wysolmerski, 2022; LeGrand et al., 2008; Tonon et al., 2022).

TABLE 8-6
Overview of Treatment for Moderate and Severe Hypercalcemia of Malignancy

Treatment Approaches	Rationale	Dose	Potential Adverse Events
IV isotonic saline infusion	Decreased volume depletion Increased glomerular filtration rate Increased calcium excretion	200–500 ml/hr until hydration status is normalized; then 100–150 ml/hr titrated to urine output	Volume overload, especially in the setting of cardiac or renal disease Decreased sodium, potassium, and magnesium
Loop diuretics: used only for patients at increased risk of fluid overload	Increased calcium excretion	20–40 mg after normal fluid status has been restored	Decreased sodium, potassium, and magnesium Risk of renal impairment
Calcitonin: due to rapid onset of action; may be used in conjunction with other agents that have a longer onset of action	Decreased osteoclast activity and bone resorption Increased renal calcium excretion	4 IU/kg subcutaneously or intramuscularly every 12 hours May increase to 8 IU/kg subcutaneously or IM every 6 hours Discontinued after 48 hours due to tachyphylaxis	Hypersensitivity Injection site inflammation Anorexia, nausea Diarrhea Abdominal pain Tingling of the palms and soles Rashes
Bisphosphonates Zoledronate[a] Pamidronat	Target osteoclasts Decreased bone resorption	4 mg IV over 15 minutes 60–90 mg IV over 2 hours	Nephrotoxicity Bone pain, myalgia Flu-like symptoms Decreased calcium and phosphorus Uveitis, scleritis Rare: osteonecrosis of the jaw, atrial fibrillation

(Continued on next page)

TABLE 8-6
Overview of Treatment for Moderate and Severe Hypercalcemia of Malignancy *(Continued)*

Treatment Approaches	Rationale	Dose	Potential Adverse Events
Denosumab	Binds with receptor activator of nuclear factor kappa-B ligand Inhibits osteoclast activity and bone resorption	120 mg subcutaneously; repeat at 1, 2, and 4 weeks; monthly thereafter	Injection site inflammation Decreased calcium levels Bone pain Nausea, diarrhea Shortness of breath Rare: osteonecrosis of the jaw, atypical fractures
Glucocorticoids[b] Hydrocortisone	Limits calcitriol production and intestinal calcium absorption	200–400 mg/day for 3–5 days, followed by 60 mg/day for 10 days or 10–20 mg/day for 7 days	Hyperglycemia Hypertension Mood alterations Myopathy
Prednisolone Prednisone		Orally, 30 mg twice daily, then titrate up to a maximum dose of 60–90 mg for 3–4 times daily to achieve normal calcium level	
Cinacalcet: recommended for persistent or refractory hypercalcemia despite denosumab or bisphosphonates; used in the setting of parathyroid cancer	Decreased parathyroid protein secretion Binds to calcium-sensing receptors on parathyroid glands and kidneys Blocks renal tubular reabsorption of calcium	–	Anorexia, nausea, vomiting Headache Decreased calcium Fractures

(Continued on next page)

TABLE 8-6
Overview of Treatment for Moderate and Severe Hypercalcemia of Malignancy *(Continued)*

Treatment Approaches	Rationale	Dose	Potential Adverse Events
Dialysis (peritoneal or hemodialysis): useful for life-threatening hypercalcemia of malignancy and for patients who cannot tolerate aggressive hydration due to advanced renal or cardiac disease	Rapid, but transient removal of calcium	–	Fluid and electrolyte imbalance

[a]Superior efficacy compared to pamidronate in reducing calcium levels and in duration of response

[b]First-line treatment of calcitriol-mediated hypercalcemia of malignancy

Several factors are considered in the development of treatment plans for hypercalcemia of malignancy, such as calcium level, signs and symptoms, underlying malignancy, mediator of calcium elevation, concurrent history of chronic diseases, organ function, and non-cancer–related contributing causes. As available, treatment for the underlying malignancy is provided. In the absence of signs and symptoms, mild or early hypercalcemia of malignancy may be monitored without IV fluids or pharmacologic agents.

Note. Based on information from Almuradova & Cicin, 2023; Bartkiewicz et al., 2024; El-Hajj Fuleihan et al., 2022; Frost, 2022; Guise & Wysolmerski, 2022; Mc Donald et al., 2023; Walker & Shane, 2022.

Bisphosphonates

Bisphosphonates, including pamidronate and zoledronate, inhibit osteoclast activity and bone resorption—the primary cause of HCM, especially in patients with extensive bone metastasis. In addition to IV hydration, bisphosphonates are first-line therapy for HCM (Guise & Wysolmerski, 2022). Zoledronate is the preferred bisphosphonate because of its superior efficacy and longer-lasting calcium reduction compared to pamidronate (El-Hajj Fuleihan et al., 2022; Major et al., 2001). Clinical response typically occurs within 24–72 hours, with normalization of calcium levels occurring in two to six weeks (El-Hajj Fuleihan et al., 2022; Tonon et al., 2022; Walker & Shane, 2022). For ongoing control, especially with bone metastasis, zoledronate is given every three to four weeks (Van Poznak et al., 2017). In refractory cases, redosing may be considered, with a second dose as soon as seven days after the initial treatment.

Because of the risk of nephrotoxicity, particularly in patients with renal impairment, dosing must be individualized, with baseline and ongoing renal function monitoring (Almuradova & Cicin, 2023; Walker & Shane, 2022). Common adverse effects include bone pain and flu-like symptoms. Rare but serious complications are osteonecrosis of the jaw, especially with long-term use, invasive dental procedures, and poor oral hygiene (Almuradova & Cicin, 2023; Terpos et al., 2021). Atypical fractures are also rare, occurring with long-term use of bisphosphonates (Mc Donald et al., 2023). In some instances, patients can also develop atrial fibrillation one to two days after administration (Frost, 2022).

Denosumab

Denosumab is a monoclonal antibody that inhibits RANKL, blocking osteoclast maturation and reducing bone resorption and calcium release (Guise & Wysolmerski, 2022). The Endocrine Society recommends denosumab or an IV bisphosphonate for treating symptomatic moderate to severe HCM; however, evidence favoring denosumab over bisphosphonates remains limited (El-Hajj Fuleihan et al., 2022). Treatment decisions should consider patients' medical history, comorbidities, cancer type, calcium level, symptoms, and potential adverse effects (Mc Donald et al., 2023).

Denosumab is often used as a second-line treatment for bisphosphonate-resistant HCM. In the acute phase of HCM, the standard dose is 120 mg via subcutaneous injection, repeated weekly for up to a month if needed (Frensius Kabi, 2025a, 2025b; Mc Donald et al., 2023; Tonon et al., 2022). Unlike bisphosphonates, denosumab is not renally excreted, making it safer for patients with renal impairment (Almuradova & Cicin, 2023). However, because of its high potency, hypocalcemia is a concern, especially in those with renal failure and calcitriol deficiency, requiring close calcium monitoring.

Common side effects are injection site reactions, bone pain, nausea, diarrhea, shortness of breath, and, in rare instances, osteonecrosis of the jaw and atypical fractures (Almuradova & Cicin, 2023; Frensius Kabi, 2025a, 2025b).

Ongoing use of denosumab or bisphosphonates is recommended in cancers with high bone involvement risk to prevent skeletal-related events, such as bone metastases, fractures, spinal cord compression, and cancer treatment–induced bone loss (Alzahrani et al., 2022; Coleman et al., 2020; National Comprehensive Cancer Network, 2025a; Park & Wong, 2022; Saylor et al., 2020; Zhu et al., 2024). Skeletal-related events increase morbidity and mortality, decrease quality of life, and raise healthcare costs (D'Oronzo et al., 2021; Ryan et al., 2022). Denosumab 120 mg every four weeks has shown greater effectiveness than zoledronic acid 4 mg IV in preventing skeletal-related events in metastatic bone disease (Cadieux et al., 2022; D'Oronzo et al., 2021).

Calcitonin

Calcitonin, a thyroid-derived hormone, inhibits osteoclast activity and enhances renal calcium excretion. The pharmaceutical form, derived from salmon and now synthetically manufactured, is more potent than human calcitonin (McLaughlin et al., 2023). It serves as an adjunctive treatment for severe HCM because of its rapid onset, providing temporary calcium reduction while waiting for agents such as bisphosphonates or denosumab to take effect (Guise & Wysolmerski, 2022; Mc Donald et al., 2023).

Calcitonin is administered intramuscularly or subcutaneously at 4 IU/kg every 12 hours, with dosing increased to 8 IU/kg every six hours if needed. Serum calcium levels are rechecked four to six hours postadministration to assess response (Bartkiewicz et al., 2024). However, its efficacy diminishes after 48 hours because of tachyphylaxis, limiting long-term use (Almuradova & Cicin, 2023; Frost, 2022).

Adverse effects include hypersensitivity reactions, injection site reactions, nausea, decreased appetite, diarrhea, abdominal pain, pruritus, tingling in extremities, increased diuresis, and, rarely, maculopapular rashes and urticaria (McLaughlin et al., 2023). Skin testing is recommended for patients with fish allergies because of increased hypersensitivity risk (McLaughlin et al., 2023; Mylan Institutional, 2021). Clinicians are advised to use caution in patients with bipolar disorder who are receiving lithium because calcitonin may lower serum lithium levels (SteriMax, 2024).

Glucocorticoids

Glucocorticoids reduce calcium levels by inhibiting calcitriol production, thereby decreasing intestinal calcium absorption (Vieth, 2020). They are the first-line treatment for calcitriol-mediated HCM, commonly associated with lymphoma and ovarian germ cell tumors (Bartkiewicz et al., 2024; Mc Donald et al., 2023). Additionally, glucocorticoids suppress tumor-derived cytokines, reducing osteoclast-mediated bone resorption (Almuradova & Cicin, 2023).

In patients with both elevated PTHrP and calcitriol, glucocorticoids may enhance response when antiresorptive therapy alone is insufficient (Guise & Wysolmerski, 2022). Common agents include IV hydrocortisone and oral prednisone (Bartkiewicz et al., 2024). Hydrocortisone is typically given at 200–400 mg/day for three to five days, followed by prednisone 10–20 mg/day for seven days or 60 mg/day for 10 days (Almuradova & Cicin, 2023; El-Hajj Fuleihan et al., 2022). If the response is seen after 10 days, treatment should be discontinued.

Patients require close monitoring for adverse effects, such as hyperglycemia, hypertension, myopathy, infection, and psychiatric symptoms (Bartkiewicz et al., 2024; Walker & Shane, 2022).

Calcimimetics

Calcimimetics, such as cinacalcet, lower serum calcium by reducing PTH secretion and inhibiting renal calcium reabsorption through activation of calcium-sensing receptors in the parathyroid glands and kidneys (Guise & Wysolmerski, 2022). The Endocrine Society recommends oral cinacalcet for hypercalcemia associated with resected or unresectable parathyroid cancer (El-Hajj Fuleihan et al., 2022).

Treatment typically begins at a dose of 30 mg twice daily, titrated every two to four weeks to 60 mg, then 90 mg twice daily, with some cases requiring up to 90 mg three to four times daily to maintain normal calcium levels (Junaid & Patel, 2024). Cinacalcet is also helpful in cases of refractory hypercalcemia unresponsive to bisphosphonates and denosumab, including those related to non-small cell lung, neuroendocrine, breast, and renal cancers (El-Hajj Fuleihan et al., 2022; Guise & Wysolmerski, 2022).

Common side effects are anorexia, nausea, vomiting, headache, and bone fractures. Patients should be monitored for hypocalcemia symptoms such as paresthesia, muscle cramps, mood changes, seizures, and prolonged QT intervals, particularly in those with impaired cardiac function (Junaid & Patel, 2024).

Dialysis

Hemodialysis or peritoneal dialysis is considered in acute HCM when IV hydration is contraindicated because of severe cardiac or renal impairment (Guise & Wysolmerski, 2022). Dialysis may also be used emergently for patients with life-threatening arrhythmias due to severe HCM. It provides a rapid but temporary reduction in serum calcium levels, requiring careful monitoring for hypocalcemia.

Mobilization

Decreased weight-bearing activity, such as limited ambulation, increases osteoclast activity and bone resorption, contributing to elevated calcium levels (Kanduri et al., 2024). Although immobility is not the primary cause of HCM, addressing contributing factors plays a role in prevention. Historically, healthcare providers have hesitated to encourage physical activity in patients with advanced cancer or bone metastasis because of concerns about pain, pathologic fractures, and spinal cord compression. However, a systematic review involving patients with bone metastases found that supervised aerobic or resistance exercise at least once weekly did not increase the risk of pathologic fracture, pain, or pain medication use (Weller et al., 2021).

The International Bone Metastases Exercise Working Group, the American College of Sports Medicine, and the National Comprehensive Cancer Network support exercise for patients with cancer (American Cancer Society, 2022; Campbell et al., 2019, 2022; National Comprehensive Cancer Network, 2025c). Although its direct impact on HCM prevention is unknown, physical activity offers proven benefits, such as reducing bone loss, improving quality of life, lowering recurrence risk, enhancing strength, managing fatigue, enhancing psychosocial health, and improving treatment adherence (Guinan et al., 2022; Thomas et al., 2021).

Before recommending exercise programs, clinicians should assess cancer type, sites of metastasis, mobility, fall risk, comorbidities, treatment side effects, and patient willingness to exercise. Referrals should be made to exercise professionals with oncology-specific training (Schmitz et al., 2020).

Dietary Calcium

Dietary calcium restriction is generally unnecessary in patients with HCM, as intestinal calcium absorption is often diminished in this setting (Klein & Vanek, 2021). However, in patients with calcitriol-mediated hypercalcemia, where GI absorption is increased, a dietary calcium intake of less than 1,000 mg/day is recommended (Gupta et al., 2023; Walker & Shane, 2022).

Nursing Management

Regardless of the care setting, nurses play a significant role in patient-centered management of HCM. Oncology nurses can effectively manage patient care through the prevention and recognition of signs and symptoms of HCM. Understanding the types of malignancies linked to increased risk for HCM, the underlying pathophysiology, and being alert to early manifestations facilitates patient care.

Nursing care focuses on patient and caregiver education, administration of medical therapies as per provider orders, monitoring responses to treatment, implementation of symptom management interventions, initiation of advocacy and support measures, and ongoing communication with other members of the healthcare team. Additional details regarding nursing management of patients with HCM can be found in Table 8-7.

Patients at risk for HCM require close monitoring, including ongoing evaluation of new or existing symptoms and physical assessment with particular focus on

TABLE 8-7
Hypercalcemia of Malignancy: Nursing Care

Focus	Strategies
At-risk populations	Recognize at-risk populations. • Cancers with a high incidence of bone metastasis • Cancers associated with calcitriol-mediated hypercalcemia of malignancy • Cancer treatment approaches associated with hypercalcemia • Benign etiologies of hypercalcemia • Patients with ongoing immobility
Proactive prevention measures	Implement preventive measures. • Educate patients and caregivers about risks, signs, and symptoms associated with hypercalcemia of malignancy, oral fluid hydration, needed mobility, safe approaches to weight-bearing mobility (especially in light of neurologic impairment), physical impairment, pain, adherence to medical regimens, and information to report to the care team in a time-sensitive manner. • To minimize the risk of bisphosphonate- or denosumab-associated osteonecrosis of the jaw, patients at increased risk for hypercalcemia are advised to complete required dental work prior to treatment. In addition, patients are advised to avoid dental extractions during treatment, when feasible. • Education about good oral hygiene and the importance of regular dental checkups is essential. • Oral intake is at least 3 L/day. • Collaborate with physical and occupational therapy or cancer exercise specialists to develop patient-specific approaches for weight-bearing mobility with assistive devices as needed. • Implement appropriate pain control measures to promote comfort and enable improved mobility; consult with palliative care as warranted. • Collaborate with physicians to identify the need for alternatives to medications associated with hypercalcemia. • Discontinue supplemental calcitriol intake. • Monitor for signs and symptoms associated with hypercalcemia of malignancy.
Management of hypercalcemia of malignancy	Provide education for patients and caregivers. • Role and implementation of management strategies • Symptoms or changes in patient status that are to be reported to the care team in a time-sensitive manner
	Mild hypercalcemia • Implement proactive preventive measures as described previously. • Advise patients to maintain oral fluid intake of 3–4 L/day.

(Continued on next page)

TABLE 8-7
Hypercalcemia of Malignancy: Nursing Care *(Continued)*

Focus	Strategies
Management of hypercalcemia of malignancy *(Cont.)*	Moderate to severe hypercalcemia • As per provider orders, administer normal saline hydration and monitor: – Response to hydration – Fluid balance through daily weights, fluid intake and output, and cardiopulmonary and renal assessment – Serum chemistry and electrolyte levels (Administer agents to address electrolyte imbalances.) – Symptom profile • Administer pharmacologic agents as per provider orders and monitor: – Response to treatment – Serum chemistry and electrolyte levels (Address electrolyte imbalances as indicated previously.) – Renal function – Potential side effects of pharmacologic agents • Implement strategies to manage symptoms associated with hypercalcemia of malignancy and therapeutic interventions for the condition.
Advocacy and support	• Identify and address barriers to care, such as access to care, adherence to care strategies, insurance status, financial concerns, transportation, competing priorities, and caregiver support. Consult social work, oncology navigators, financial navigators, homecare personnel, pharmacists, and community support agencies as available. • Provide emotional and coping support; consult with social work or mental health professionals as warranted. • Provide education and communicate with consideration of health literacy assessment and information sharing preferences for patients and caregivers. • Share identified barriers and education and communication needs through interprofessional collaboration in the process of developing a plan of care. • Collaborate with the physician regarding goals of care discussions; consult palliative care as needed.

Nursing care, based on an understanding of cancers with an increased risk of hypercalcemia of malignancy, focuses on proactive measures, ongoing patient assessment and prompt recognition of signs and symptoms, administration of medical therapies, and symptom management. In addition, nurses should address patient and caregiver needs for education, advocacy, and support.

Note. Based on information from Almuradova & Cicin, 2023; Bartkiewicz et al., 2024; Burkett, 2024; Frost, 2022; Guise & Wysolmerski, 2022; Kanduri et al., 2024; Klein & Vanek, 2021; Maloney, 2023; National Comprehensive Cancer Network, 2025b, 2025c; Oncology Nursing Society, 2022.

hydration, neurologic, and musculoskeletal status. Close appraisal of laboratory results is important with attention to serum calcium and albumin levels, as well as renal and electrolyte status to differentiate between disease progression, treatment-related effects, preexisting chronic illness, and the manifestations of hypercalcemia. Through proactive monitoring and early intervention, nurses can contribute to improving patient outcomes and preventing complications related to HCM.

Patients with mild or asymptomatic HCM and those who have achieved normocalcemia may continue to be followed on an outpatient basis. Ongoing serial assessments are necessary for timely intervention. Nurses should provide education for patients and caregivers to facilitate their active participation in care.

Patients in the acute phase of moderate and severe HCM are most often treated on an inpatient basis for rehydration and pharmacologic intervention. In this setting, nurses should regularly monitor renal function, total or corrected serum calcium levels, cardiopulmonary status, and fluid and electrolytes until calcium levels normalize. As calcium levels are corrected with aggressive hydration, potassium, magnesium, and phosphate levels may decline rapidly, necessitating timely replacement.

For patients with moderate and severe HCM, symptom management is a priority in addition to measures directed at restoring fluid status and decreasing calcium levels. Symptom management interventions include controlling the nausea, vomiting, and constipation associated with HCM. Nurses should consider strategies that ensure the safety of patients experiencing altered mental status or impaired mobility. They also should focus on pain management, especially for patients with metastatic bone involvement, commonly experienced by patients with HCM. Nurses will need to monitor opioid-induced oversedation in patients who may already be lethargic or confused because of HCM.

Nurses should assess patients' dietary intake and daily medications to provide guidance and education about appropriate nutritional choices and medication management. Adjustments may be necessary to minimize calcium intake and avoid medications that can exacerbate hypercalcemia, such as certain diuretics or calcium-containing supplements. Nurses can also provide comfort measures, a safe environment, and emotional support to patients and caregivers who are often experiencing emotional distress related to the underlying diagnosis, treatment, uncertainty about the future, and cancer-related symptoms.

Education of patients and caregivers is based on assessment of health literacy and preferred methods for learning. The overall goal of education is to support shared decision-making and empower patients and caregivers to participate in care actively. Learning should focus on prevention strategies, early recognition and management of signs and symptoms, adherence to treatment, and ongoing communication with healthcare providers.

Nurses should collaborate with other disciplines providing oncology care to ensure that patients have an opportunity to discuss their goals of care and advance care planning. Ideally, these discussions begin early during the cancer experience, but if they do not, they take on great significance for patients with advanced cancer approaching the end of life. In the role of educator, nurses should assess patients' and caregivers' understanding of health, the underlying cancer, HCM, and treatment plans. Based on the assessment, nurses will need to address misconceptions, provide required information, and implement measures to support coping with anxiety, fears, and concerns related to the implications of HCM and advanced disease. As advocates, nurses, as well as other clinicians, must foster patient articulation of values, goals, and preferences for medical care (Boucher, 2021).

Nurses are key participants in oncology care team discussions regarding initiation or continuation of antineoplastic and HCM treatments with consideration of patient wishes, health literacy, and cultural beliefs (Boucher, 2021). Interprofessional discussions, as well as those with patients and caregivers, should attempt to balance further treatment of possibly reversible HCM symptoms with the pursuit of symptom palliation, quality of life, and a peaceful death (Ferraro & Sanchez-Reilly, 2020). It may not be feasible for patients with progressing cancer to resume an independent or symptom-free quality of life by reducing calcium levels. For these patients, HCM may represent a life-ending symptom.

Patients with HCM and their caregivers may be confronted with distressing information about their cancer diagnosis, including disease recurrence or progression, availability of viable treatment options, and disease prognosis. In addition, they may face emotionally laden choices about continuation of antineoplastic therapies if available, initiation or continuation of treatment for HCM, inpatient or home hospice care, identification of a healthcare proxy, and other decisions involving family or finances (Boucher, 2021). The information and choices become more challenging in the setting of HCM-associated symptoms, such as impaired mental status, pain, lethargy, nausea, vomiting, and weakness. If patients are not able to participate in goals of care or end-of-life care discussions, nurses should support caregivers by addressing questions, providing information, and identifying patient wishes. Nurses must remain mindful of the emotional burden of these discussions for patients and caregivers.

HCM, most often associated with advanced cancer, tends to have poor survival outcomes. Patients with advanced disease frequently have a poor performance status and experience cachexia, anorexia, weight loss, weakness, and a variety of other symptoms related to the underlying cancer or antineoplastic treatments. Those with mild HCM and options for cancer treatment may have better outcomes. However, mortality is 35%–50% at one month and up to 75% at three months after diagnosis (Mc Donald et al., 2023; Sundriyal et al., 2020; Tonon et al., 2022). Although most patients respond to treatment for HCM, it is not uncommon to see elevated calcium levels recur after the completion of antineoplastic therapy or as the underlying cancer progresses despite multiple therapeutic approaches. Ultimately, patients die from the manifestations of advanced cancer or hypercalcemia-related organ damage.

Summary

HCM, a complication seen in 20%–30% of patients with advanced cancer, is linked to a poor prognosis. Although HCM has been reported in many malignancies, it occurs most frequently in multiple myeloma, breast cancer, lung cancer, and squamous cell cancers of any origin. Increased bone resorption and calcium release, decreased renal calcium excretion, and increased intestinal calcium absorption are processes that lead to HCM. The classifications of HCM are humoral, associated with tumor production of PTHrP; osteolytic, associated with extensive bone metastases; calcitriol (1,25-dihydroxyvitamin D) mediated, associated with excess vitamin D production and increased intestinal calcium absorption; and PTH, associated with ectopic PTH production.

Management of HCM relies on the recognition of individuals at risk, identification of early and often vague signs and symptoms, and elimination of factors contributing to elevated calcium levels. In addition, prompt initiation of IV fluids to address dehydration and maintain or restore renal function is essential. If feasible, treatment of the underlying malignancy is a priority, along with measures to decrease calcium levels. Administration of pharmacologic agents to limit bone resorption and symptom management strategies are components of the standard of care.

Nurses should collaborate with other members of the healthcare team to achieve desired clinical outcomes. Nursing care incorporates ongoing assessment, administration of the therapeutic plan of care as per provider orders, monitoring responses to treatment, care team communication, symptom palliation, and facilitation of goals of care discussions. Nurses should address physical needs and patient and caregiver psychosocial concerns through education, promotion of strategies to empower participation in care, and collaboration with cancer care providers.

The authors would like to acknowledge Marcelle Kaplan, MS, RN, CNS, for her contribution to this chapter that remains unchanged from the previous edition of this book.

References

Al-Bari, A.A., & Al Mamun, A. (2020). Current advances in regulation of bone homeostasis. *FASEB BioAdvances, 2*(11), 668–679. https://doi.org/10.1096/fba.2020-00058

Almuradova, E., & Cicin, I. (2023). Cancer-related hypercalcemia and potential treatments. *Frontiers in Endocrinology, 14.* https://doi.org/10.3389/fendo.2023.1039490

Alzahrani, M., Stober, C., Liu, M., Awan, A., Ng, T.L., Pond, G., ... Clemons, M. (2022). Symptomatic skeletal-related events in patients receiving longer term bone-modifying agents for bone metastases from breast and castration resistant prostate cancers. *Supportive Care in Cancer, 30*(5), 3977–3984. https://doi.org/10.1007/s00520-021-06714-8

American Cancer Society. (2022). *Physical activity and the person with cancer.* https://www.cancer.org/cancer/survivorship/be-healthy-after-treatment/physical-activity-and-the-cancer-patient.html

Anastasopoulou, C., & Mewawalla, P. (2023). Malignancy-related hypercalcemia. In *StatPearls.* StatPearls Publishing. https://www.ncbi.nlm.nih.gov/books/NBK482423

Ansoria, A.N.M., Widyananda, M.H., Antonius, Y., Murtadlo, A.A.A., Kharisma, V.D., Wiradana, P.A., ... Zainul, R. (2024). A review of cancer-related hypercalcemia: Pathophysiology, current treatments, and future directions. *Journal of Medicinal and Pharmaceutical Chemistry Research, 6*(7), 944–952. https://doi.org/10.48309/JMPCR.2024.435280.1088

Asonitis, N., Angelousi, A., Zafeiris, C., Lambrou, G.I., Dontas, I., & Kassi, E. (2019). Diagnosis, pathophysiology and management of hypercalcemia in malignancy: A review of the literature. *Hormone and Metabolic Research, 51*(12), 770–778. https://doi.org/10.1055/a-1049-0647

Bancal, C., Salipante, F., Hannas, N., Lumbroso, S., Cavalier, E., & De Brauwere, D.-P. (2023). A new approach to assessing calcium status via a machine learning algorithm. *Clinica Chimica Acta, 539,* 198–205. https://doi.org/10.1016/j.cca.2022.12.018

Bartkiewicz, P., Kunachowicz, D., Filipski, M., Stebel, A., Ligoda, J., & Rembiałkowska, N. (2024). Hypercalcemia in cancer: Causes, effects, and treatment strategies. *Cells, 13*(12), 1051. https://doi.org/10.3390/cells13121051

Bilezikian, J.P. (2022). Primary hyperparathyroidism. In M. Donovan Walker (Ed.), *Hypercalcemia clinical diagnosis and management* (pp. 89–110). Springer. https://doi.org/10.1007/978-3-030-93182-7

Bokhari, S.R., & Zulfiqar, H. (2023). Bartter syndrome. In *StatPearls*. StatPearls Publishing. https://www.statpearls.com/point-of-care/18152

Boucher, J. (2021). Advance care planning: Having goals-of-care conversations in oncology nursing. *Clinical Journal of Oncology Nursing, 25*(3), 333–336. https://doi.org/10.1188/21.cjon.333-336

Bringhurst, F., Kronenberg, H.M., Liu, E.S., & Wein, M.N. (2025). Bone and mineral metabolism in health and disease. In D. Longo, A. Fauci, D. Kasper, S. Hauser, J. Jameson, J. Loscalzo, ... C. Langford (Eds.), *Harrison's principles of internal medicine* (22nd ed.). McGraw-Hill. https://accesspharmacy-mhmedical-com.proxy.library.upenn.edu/content.aspx?bookid=3541&sectionid=295625185

Burkett, M.S. (2024). Daily weight monitoring for inpatients receiving chemotherapy. *Nursing, 54*(6), 48–51. https://doi.org/10.1097/nsg.0000000000000012

Cadieux, B., Coleman, R., Jafarinasabian, P., Lipton, A., Orlowski, R.Z., Saad, F., ... Stopeck, A. (2022). Experience with denosumab (XGEVA®) for prevention of skeletal-related events in the 10 years after approval. *Journal of Bone Oncology, 33*, 100416. https://doi.org/10.1016/j.jbo.2022.100416

Campbell, K.L., Cormie, P., Weller, S., Alibhai, S.M., Bolam, K.A., Campbell, A., ... Goulart, J. (2022). Exercise recommendation for people with bone metastases: Expert consensus for health care providers and exercise professionals. *JCO Oncology Practice, 18*(5), e697–e709. https://doi.org/10.1200/op.21.00454

Campbell, K.L., Winters-Stone, K.M., Wiskemann, J., May, A.M., Schwartz, A.L., Courneya, K.S., ... Schmitz, K.H. (2019). Exercise guidelines for cancer survivors: Consensus statement from international multidisciplinary roundtable. *Medicine and Science in Sports and Exercise, 51*(11), 2375–2390. https://doi.org/10.1249/mss.0000000000002116

Chakhtoura, M., & El-Hajj Fuleihan, G. (2021). Treatment of hypercalcemia of malignancy. *Endocrinology and Metabolism Clinics of North America, 50*(4), 781–792. https://doi.org/10.1016/j.ecl.2021.08.002

Charoenngam, N., Ponvilawan, B., Rujirachun, P., & Wattanachayakul, P. (2021). 1,25-dihydroxyvitamin D-mediated hypercalcemia associated with solid organ malignancy: A systematic review. *Minerva Endocrinology, 50*(1), 97–104. https://doi.org/10.23736/S2724-6507.21.03508-9

Christ-Crain, M., Winzeler, B., & Refardt, J. (2021). Diagnosis and management of diabetes insipidus for the internist: An update. *Journal of Internal Medicine, 290*(1), 73–87. https://doi.org/10.1111/joim.13261

Clézardin, P., Coleman, R., Puppo, M., Ottewell, P., Bonnelye, E., Paycha, F., ... Holen, I. (2021). Bone metastasis: Mechanisms, therapies, and biomarkers. *Physiological Reviews, 101*(3), 797–855. https://doi.org/10.1152/physrev.00012.2019

Coleman, R., Hadji, P., Body, J., Santini, D., Chow, E., Terpos, E., ... Jordan, K. (2020). Bone health in cancer: ESMO Clinical Practice Guidelines. *Annals of Oncology, 31*(12), 1650–1663. https://doi.org/10.1016/j.annonc.2020.07.019

De Leon-Oliva, D., Barrena-Blázquez, S., Jiménez-Álvarez, L., Fraile-Martinez, O., García-Montero, C., López-González, L., ... Ortega, M.A. (2023). The RANK–RANKL–OPG system: A multifaceted regulator of homeostasis, immunity, and cancer. *Medicina, 59*(10), 1752. https://doi.org/10.3390/medicina59101752

Delgado-Calle, J., & Bellido, T. (2022). The osteocyte as a signaling cell. *Physiologic Reviews, 102*(1), 379–410. https://doi.org/10.1152/physrev.00043.2020

Desgagnés, N., King, J.A., Kline, G.A., Seiden-Long, I., & Leung, A.A. (2025). Use of albumin-adjusted calcium measurements in clinical practice. *JAMA Network Open, 8*(1), e2455251. https://doi.org/10.1001/jamanetworkopen.2024.55251

Dickens, L.T., Derman, B., & Alexander, J.T. (2023). Endocrine Society hypercalcemia of malignancy guidelines. *JAMA Oncology, 9*(3), 430–431. https://doi.org/10.1001/jamaoncol.2022.7941

D'Oronzo, S., Wood, S., & Brown, J.E. (2021). "The use of bisphosphonates to treat skeletal complications in solid tumours". *Bone, 147*, 115907. https://doi.org/10.1016/j.bone.2021.115907

El-Hajj Fuleihan, G., Chakhtoura, M., Cipriani, C., Eastell, R., Karonova, T., Liu, J., ... Marcocci, C. (2020). Classical and nonclassical manifestations of primary hyperparathyroidism. *Journal of Bone and Mineral Research, 37*(11), 2330–2350. https://doi.org/10.1002/jbmr.4679

El-Hajj Fuleihan, G., Clines, G.A., Hu, M.I., Marcocci, C., Murad, M.H., Piggott, T., ... Drake, M.T. (2022). Treatment of hypercalcemia of malignancy in adults: An Endocrine Society clinical practice guideline. *Journal of Clinical Endocrinology and Metabolism, 108*(3), 507–528. https://doi.org/10.1210/clinem/dgac621

English, K.A., Lines, K.E., & Thakker, R.V. (2024). Genetics of hereditary forms of primary hyperparathyroidism. *Hormones, 23*(1), 3–14. https://doi.org/10.1007/s42000-023-00508-9

Ferraro, K., & Sanchez-Reilly, S. (2020). Palliative volume resuscitation in a patient with cancer and hypercalcemia: Why bother? *Journal of Palliative Medicine, 23*(6), 871–873. https://doi.org/10.1089/jpm.2019.0343

Frensius Kabi. (2025a). *Bomyntra® (denosumab-bnht)* [Package insert]. https://www.accessdata.fda.gov/drugsatfda_docs/label/2025/761398Orig1s000lbl.pdf

Frensius Kabi. (2025b). *Conexxence® (denosumab-bnht)* [Package insert]. https://www.accessdata.fda.gov/drugsatfda_docs/label/2025/761398Orig1s000lbl.pdf

Frost, K. (2022). Onco-nephrology in the critical care setting: Recognizing and treating renal manifestations of cancer and oncological emergencies. *Critical Care Nursing Clinics of North America, 34*(4), 453–466. https://doi.org/10.1016/j.cnc.2022.07.002

Gilson, S. (2024). Deconditioning in hospitalized patients with cancer. *Seminars in Oncology Nursing, 40*(4), 151676. https://doi.org/10.1016/j.soncn.2024.151676

Goltzman, D. (2021). Pathophysiology of hypercalcemia. *Endocrinology and Metabolism Clinics of North America, 50*(4), 591–607. https://doi.org/10.1016/j.ecl.2021.07.008

Goltzman, D. (2023). Approach to hypercalcemia. In K.R. Feingold, S.F. Ahmed, B. Anawalt, M.R. Blackman, A. Boyce, G. Chrousos, ... D.P. Wilson (Eds.), *Endotext* [Internet]. MDText.com.

Gould Rothberg, B.E., Quest, T.E., Yeung, S.J., Pelosof, L.C., Gerber, D.E., Seltzer, J.A., ... Kyriacou, D.N. (2022). Oncologic emergencies and urgencies: A comprehensive review. *CA: A Cancer Journal for Clinicians, 72*(6), 570–593. https://doi.org/10.3322/caac.21727

Grunbaum, A., & Kremer, R. (2022). Parathyroid hormone-related protein (PTHrP) and malignancy. In G. Litwack (Ed.), *Parathyroid hormone* (pp. 133–177). Elsevier. https://doi.org/10.1016/bs.vh.2022.03.002

Guinan, E.M., Devenney, K., Quinn, C., Sheill, G., Eochagáin, C.M., Kennedy, M.J., ... Balding, L. (2022). Associations among physical activity, skeletal-related events, and patient-reported outcomes in patients with bone metastases. *Seminars in Oncology Nursing, 38*(2), 151274. https://doi.org/10.1016/j.soncn.2022.151274

Guise, T.A., & Wysolmerski, J.J. (2022). Cancer-associated hypercalcemia. *New England Journal of Medicine, 386*(15), 1443–1451. https://doi.org/10.1056/nejmcp2113128

Gupta, S., Rastogi, A., Singh, P., Chophy, A., Roushan, R., Krishnan, A.S., ... Gupta, M. (2023). Treatment outcomes and survival in hypercalcemia of malignancy: A grave metabolic emergency. *Cureus 15*(3). https://doi.org/10.7759/cureus.35783

Hamroun, A., Pekar, J., Lionet, A., Ghulam, A., Maboudou, P., Mercier, A., ... Glowacki, F. (2020). Ionized calcium: Analytical challenges and clinical relevance. *Journal of Laboratory and Precision Medicine, 5*, 22. https://doi.org/10.21037/jlpm-20-60

Hannan, F.M., Kallay, E., Chang, W., Brandi, M.L., & Thakker, R.V. (2019). The calcium-sensing receptor in physiology and in calcitropic and noncalcitropic diseases. *Nature Reviews Endocrinology, 15*(1), 33–51. https://doi.org/10.1038/s41574-018-0115-0

Haroun, R., Wood, J.N., & Sikander, S. (2023). Mechanisms of cancer pain. *Frontiers in Pain Research, 3*, 1–20. https://doi.org/10.3389/fpain.2022.1030899

Hu, M.I. (2021). Hypercalcemia of malignancy. *Endocrinology and Metabolism Clinics of North America, 50*(4), 721–728. https://doi.org/10.1016/j.ecl.2021.07.003

Junaid, S.Z.S., & Patel, P. (2024). Cinacalcet. In *StatPearls*. StatPearls Publishing. https://www.statpearls.com/point-of-care/40477

Kanduri, S.R., Stark, A., & Velez, J.C. (2024). Immobilization-associated hypercalcaemia in patients with malignancy in the hospital setting. *Clinical Kidney Journal, 17*(9), sfae252. https://doi.org/10.1093/ckj/sfae252

Kenny, C.M., Murphy, C.E., Boyce, D.S., Ashley, D.M., & Jahanmir, J. (2021). Things We Do for No Reason™: Calculating a "corrected calcium" level. *Journal of Hospital Medicine, 16*(8), 499–501. https://doi.org/10.12788/jhm.3619

Kim, J., Lin, C., Stavre, Z., Greenblatt, M.B., & Shim, J. (2020). Osteoblast-osteoclast communication and bone homeostasis. *Cells, 9*(9), 2073. https://doi.org/10.3390/cells9092073

Klein, R., & Vanek, C. (2021). Hypercalcemia. In L. Loriaux & C. Vanek (Eds.), *Endocrine emergencies: Recognition and treatment* (2nd ed., pp. 159–171). Springer International.

LeGrand, S.B., Leskuski, D., & Zama, I. (2008). Narrative review: Furosemide for hypercalcemia: An unproven yet common practice. *Annals of Internal Medicine, 149*(4), 259–263. https://doi.org/10.7326/0003-4819-149-4-200808190-00007

Liu, J., Cheng, W., Du, J., & Li, Y. (2024). Early palliative care in advanced non-small cell lung cancer patients: A meta-analysis. *American Journal of Hospice and Palliative Medicine, 42*(11), 1109–1119. https://doi.org/10.1177/10499091241300530

Major, P., Lortholary, A., Hon, J., Abdi, E., Mills, G., Menssen, H.D., ... Seaman, J. (2001). Zoledronic acid is superior to pamidronate in the treatment of hypercalcemia of malignancy: A pooled analysis of two randomized, controlled clinical trials. *Journal of Clinical Oncology, 19*(2), 558–567. https://doi.org/10.1200/jco.2001.19.2.558

Maloney, K. (2023). Metabolic emergencies. In S. Maloney-Newton, M. Hickey, & J.M. Brant (Eds.), *Mosby's oncology nursing advisor: A comprehensive guide to clinical practice.* Elsevier.

Marshall, E., Patel, N., & Selvaratnam, R. (2023). Oncological emergencies. *Medicine, 51*(1), 80–85. https://doi.org/10.1016/j.mpmed.2022.10.015

Matikainen, N., Pekkarinen, T., Ryhänen, E.M., & Schalin-Jäntti, C. (2021). Physiology of calcium homeostasis: An overview. *Endocrinology and Metabolism Clinics of North America, 50*(4), 575–590. https://doi.org/10.1016/j.ecl.2021.07.005

Mc Donald, D., Drake, M.T., & Crowley, R.K. (2023). Treatment of hypercalcaemia of malignancy in adults. *Clinical Medicine, 23*(5), 503–507. https://doi.org/10.7861/clinmed.2023-0227

McLaughlin, M.B., Awosika, A.O., & Jialal, I. (2023). Calcitonin. In *StatPearls.* StatPearls Publishing. https://www.ncbi.nlm.nih.gov/books/NBK537269

Mederos, M.A., Reber, H.A., & Girgis, M.D. (2021). Acute pancreatitis. *JAMA, 325*(4), 382–390. https://doi.org/10.1001/jama.2020.20317

Menefee, W., Jenks, J., Mazzasette, C., & Nguyen, K.-L. (2024). Bone structure. In *General Human Anatomy.* ASCCC Open Educational Resources Initiative. https://med.libretexts.org/@go/page/22279

Mylan Institutional. (2021). *Miacalcin® (calcitonin salmon injection, solution)* [Package insert]. https://dailymed.nlm.nih.gov/dailymed/fda/fdaDrugXsl.cfm?setid=89cd4f46-b88a-4c10-b25c-47352280dc4e

National Cancer Institute Cancer Therapy Evaluation Program. (2017). *Common terminology criteria for adverse events* [v.5.0]. https://dctd.cancer.gov/research/ctep-trials/for-sites/adverse-events/ctcae-v5-5x7.pdf 5_Quick_Reference_5x7.pdf

National Comprehensive Cancer Network. (2025a). *NCCN Clinical Practice Guidelines in Oncology (NCCN Guidelines®): Multiple myeloma* [v.2.2026]. https://www.nccn.org

National Comprehensive Cancer Network. (2025b). *NCCN Clinical Practice Guidelines in Oncology (NCCN Guidelines®): Palliative care* [v.2.2025]. https://www.nccn.org

National Comprehensive Cancer Network. (2025c). *NCCN Clinical Practice Guidelines in Oncology (NCCN Guidelines®): Survivorship* [v.2.2025]. https://www.nccn.org

Oncology Nursing Society. (2022). *Position statement from the Oncology Nursing Society regarding palliative care for people with cancer.* https://onf.ons.org/network-advocacy/position-statements/palliative-care-people-cancer

Park, J.J., & Wong, C. (2022). Pharmacological prevention and management of skeletal-related events and bone loss in individuals with cancer. *Seminars in Oncology Nursing, 38*(2), 151276. https://doi.org/10.1016/j.soncn.2022.151276

Park-Min, K.-H., & Lorenzo, J. (2022). Osteoclasts: Other functions. *Bone, 165,* 116576. https://doi.org/10.1016/j.bone.2022.116576

Paterson, A.H.G. (2021). Bone-targeted agents and skeletal-related events in breast cancer patients with bone metastases. In D. Heymann (Ed.), *Bone cancer* (3rd ed., 943–955). https://doi.org/10.1016/b978-0-12-821666-8.00001-3

Payne, R.B., Little, A.J., Williams, R.B., & Milner, J.R. (1973). Interpretation of serum calcium in patients with abnormal serum proteins. *BMJ, 4*(5893), 643–646. https://doi.org/10.1136/bmj.4.5893.643

Pokhrel, B., Leslie, S.W., & Levine, S.N. (2024). Primary hyperparathyroidism. In *StatPearls*. StatPearls Publishing. https://www.ncbi.nlm.nih.gov/books/NBK441895

Riffel, R.M., Göbel, A., & Rachner, T.D. (2022). Bone metastases: From mechanisms to treatment. *Seminars in Oncology Nursing, 38*(2), 151277. https://doi.org/10.1016/j.soncn.2022.151277

Rout, P., Hashmi, M.F., & Patel, C. (2024). Milk-alkali syndrome. In *StatPearls*. StatPearls Publishing. https://www.ncbi.nlm.nih.gov/books/NBK557500

Rowe, P., & Koller, A. (2023). Physiology, bone remodeling. In *StatPearls*. StatPearls Publishing. https://www.statpearls.com/point-of-care/18453

Ryan, C., Stoltzfus, K.C., Horn, S., Chen, H., Louie, A.V., Lehrer, E.J., ... Zaorsky, N.G. (2022). Epidemiology of bone metastases. *Bone, 158*, 115783. https://doi.org/10.1016/j.bone.2020.115783

Sadiq, M.W., Anastasopoulou, C., Patel, G., & Badireddy, M. (2022). Hypercalcemia. In *StatPearls*. StatPearls Publishing. https://www.ncbi.nlm.nih.gov/books/NBK430714

Saylor, P.J., Rumble, R.B., Tagawa, S., Eastham, J.A., Finelli, A., Reddy, P.S., ... Michalski, J.M. (2020). Bone health and bone-targeted therapies for prostate cancer: ASCO endorsement of a Cancer Care Ontario guideline. *Journal of Clinical Oncology, 38*(15), 1736–1743. https://doi.org/10.1200/jco.19.03148

Schmitz, K.H., Stout, N.L., Maitin-Shepard, M., Campbell, A., Schwartz, A.L., Grimmett, C., ... Sokolof, J.M. (2020). Moving through cancer: Setting the agenda to make exercise standard in oncology practice. *Cancer, 127*(3), 476–484. https://doi.org/10.1002/cncr.33245

Shallis, R.M., Rome, R.S., & Reagan, J.L. (2018). Mechanisms of hypercalcemia in non-Hodgkin lymphoma and associated outcomes: A retrospective review. *Clinical Lymphoma Myeloma and Leukemia, 18*(2), e123–e129. https://doi.org/10.1016/j.clml.2017.12.006

Sheehan, M.T., Li, Y.-H., Doi, S.A., & Onitilo, A.A. (2021). Evaluation of diagnostic workup and etiology of hypercalcemia of malignancy in a cohort of 167,551 patients over 20 years. *Journal of the Endocrine Society, 5*(11). https://doi.org/10.1210/jendso/bvab157

Silva-Figueroa, A., & Perrier, N.D. (2021). Diagnosis and surgical management of parathyroid carcinoma. In A.L. Shifrin, M. Raffaelli, G.W. Randolph, & O. Gimm (Eds.), *Endocrine surgery comprehensive board exam guide* (pp. 379–403). Springer. https://doi.org/10.1007/978-3-030-84737-1_15

Šromová, V., Sobola, D., & Kaspar, P. (2023). A brief review of bone cell function and importance. *Cells, 12*(21), 2576. https://doi.org/10.3390/cells12212576

SteriMax. (2024). *Calcitonin salmon injection USP* [Package insert]. https://pdf.hres.ca/dpd_pm/00075315.PDF

Sullivan, D.R., & Slatore, C.G. (2020). Association of early palliative care with survival in patients with advanced lung cancer—Reply. *JAMA Oncology, 6*(3), 443–444. https://doi.org/10.1001/jamaoncol.2019.6301

Sundriyal, D., Arya, L., Saha, R., Walia, M., & Nayak, P.P. (2020). Hypercalcemia of malignancy: Time to pull the brakes. *Indian Journal of Surgical Oncology, 13*(1), 28–32. https://doi.org/10.1007/s13193-020-01131-5

Terpos, E., Zamagni, E., Lentzsch, S., Drake, M.T., García-Sanz, R., Abildgaard, N., ... Raje, N. (2021). Treatment of multiple myeloma-related bone disease: Recommendations from the Bone Working Group of the International Myeloma Working Group. *Lancet Oncology, 22*(3), e119–e130. https://doi.org/10.1016/s1470-2045(20)30559-3

Thomas, R., Kenfield, S.A., Yanagisawa, Y., & Newton, R.U. (2021). Why exercise has a crucial role in cancer prevention, risk reduction and improved outcomes. *British Medical Bulletin, 139*(1), 100–119. https://doi.org/10.1093/bmb/ldab019

Tiwari, Q.K., Gurvachan, V., Yadav, D.P., Shukla, S.K., Das, D., Singh, G., ... Chaturvedi, V.K. (2022). Hypercalcemia—An enigmatic cause of acute pancreatitis. *Journal of Clinical and Translational Research, 8*(3), 176–180. https://doi.org/10.18053/jctres.08.202203.002

Tonon, C.R., Silva, T.A., Pereira, F.W., Queiroz, D.A., Junior, E.L., Martins, D., ... Polegato, B.F. (2022). A review of current clinical concepts in the pathophysiology, etiology, diagnosis, and management of hypercalcemia. *Medical Science Monitor, 28.* https://doi.org/10.12659/msm.935821

Van Poznak, C., Somerfield, M.R., & Moy, B. (2017). Role of bone-modifying agents in metastatic breast cancer: An American Society of Clinical Oncology–Cancer Care Ontario focused guideline update summary. *Journal of Oncology Practice, 13*(12), 822–824. https://doi.org/10.1200/jop.2017.027672

Vieth, R. (2020). Vitamin D supplementation: Cholecalciferol, calcifediol, and calcitriol. *European Journal of Clinical Nutrition, 74*(11), 1493–1497. https://doi.org/10.1038/s41430-020-0697-1

Walker, M.D., & Shane, E. (2022). Hypercalcemia. *JAMA, 328*(16), 1624–1636. https://doi.org/10.1001/jama.2022.18331

Weller, S., Hart, N.H., Bolam, K.A., Mansfield, S., Santa Mina, D., Winters-Stone, K.M., ... Campbell, K.L. (2021). Exercise for individuals with bone metastases: A systematic review. *Critical Reviews in Oncology/Hematology, 166,* 103433. https://doi.org/10.1016/j.critrevonc.2021.103433

Yu, E., & Sharma, S. (2023). Physiology, calcium. In *StatPearls.* StatPearls Publishing. https://www.ncbi.nlm.nih.gov/books/NBK482128

Zhang, Y., Liang, J., Liu, P., Wang, Q., Liu, L., & Zhao, H. (2022). The RANK/RANKL/OPG system and tumor bone metastasis: Potential mechanisms and therapeutic strategies. *Frontiers in Endocrinology, 13.* https://doi.org/10.3389/fendo.2022.1063815

Zhu, N., Ni, H., Guo, S., Shen, Y.-Q., & Chen, Q. (2024). Bone complications of cancer treatment. *Cancer Treatment Reviews, 130*(102828), 1–25. https://doi.org/10.1016/j.ctrv.2024.102828

Diane G. Cope, PhD, APRN, BC, AOCNP®,
and Chinomso Nwozichi, PhD, RN, CMSRN, OCN®, FAAN

CHAPTER 9

Syndrome of Inappropriate Antidiuretic Hormone Secretion

FAST FACTS

- **Description:** Syndrome of inappropriate antidiuretic hormone secretion is an uncommon endocrine disorder characterized by unregulated hypersecretion of antidiuretic hormone caused by malignant or nonmalignant conditions. The antidiuretic hormone helps to regulate the amount of water the body retains. With excess antidiuretic hormone secretion, the kidneys retain water, resulting in dilutional serum hyponatremia and concentrated urine.
- **Incidence:** Syndrome of inappropriate antidiuretic hormone secretion is associated mainly with small cell lung cancer but is also related to a variety of other malignant and nonmalignant conditions, such as pulmonary disorders, infections, and central nervous system disorders, as well as medications.
- **Clinical Manifestations:** Neurologic changes are most common. Syndrome of inappropriate antidiuretic hormone secretion is considered an oncologic endocrine emergency when patients present in later stages of the syndrome with central nervous system symptoms such as weakness, mental changes, and neurologic alterations that can progress to seizures, coma, and death. In early stages, symptoms may be absent or nonspecific and mimic treatment side effects.
- **Risk Factors and Etiology:** Multiple risk factors, both malignant and nonmalignant, exist for the development of syndrome of inappropriate antidiuretic hormone secretion. The most common malignant condition is small cell lung cancer. Nonmalignant risk factors include pulmonary disorders.
- **Pathophysiology and Patient Evaluation:** Water and electrolyte homeostasis is maintained through coordinated regulation by antidiuretic hormone, osmoreceptors, and baroreceptors, ensuring balance between intracellular and extracellular compartments. In syndrome of inappropriate antidiuretic hormone secretion, excessive antidiuretic hormone secretion leads to water retention, dilutional hyponatremia, and cerebral edema. Diagnosis is based on hyponatremia with low serum osmolality and inappropriately concentrated urine despite normal adrenal, thyroid, and renal function.
- **Advanced Practice Considerations:** Ongoing assessment of syndrome of inappropriate antidiuretic hormone secretion risk factors and symptoms with prompt intervention can improve patient outcomes and prevent life-threatening neurologic changes.
- **Treatment Modalities:** Treatment of the underlying cause is definitive therapy followed by fluid restriction, hypertonic saline infusion, and pharmacologic therapy options, including demeclocycline, diuretics, lithium, urea, and vaptans.

- **Nursing Management:** Oncology nurses play a key role in the assessment of risk factors, provision of symptom management, and treatment modalities. Patient and caregiver education regarding fluid restriction, medications, high-sodium diet, and safety issues is critical to promote positive patient outcomes.
- **Outcomes:** Prompt recognition of at-risk patients and the early signs of the syndrome can prevent progression of neurologic sequelae to an oncologic emergency.

Introduction

Syndrome of inappropriate antidiuretic hormone secretion (SIADH) is a rare endocrine disorder characterized by the unregulated release of arginine vasopressin (AVP), also known as antidiuretic hormone (ADH). This is caused by excessive secretion of ADH from its normal hypothalamic source or ectopic production by tumor cells, resulting in fluid and electrolyte imbalances. Excessive secretion of ADH stimulates the kidneys to conserve water, causing dilutional serum hyponatremia and resulting in plasma hyposmolality, urine hyperosmolality, and elevated urinary sodium concentrations. Patients often remain euvolemic as plasma volume remains stable despite the low serum osmolality (Tkacs & Herrmann, 2024). Clinical manifestations of SIADH arise from hyponatremia-induced cerebral edema, with early symptoms, such as nausea and malaise, typically appearing when serum sodium levels drop below 125–130 mEq/L (Yasir & Mechanic, 2023).

Although SIADH has many possible causes, the most common etiology is the ectopic production of ADH by malignant cells, such as lung cancer and cancer cells in other parts of the body (Tkacs & Herrmann, 2024). Although early symptoms of SIADH are usually mild (e.g., nausea, headache, fatigue), if left untreated, the condition can significantly worsen, leading to severe neurologic complications, including seizures, coma, and even death due to the progressively low sodium levels in the blood. Therefore, oncology nurses should be knowledgeable about SIADH to prevent this oncologic emergency through prompt recognition and intervention.

Incidence

In general, hyponatremia is the most common electrolyte imbalance, affecting more than 15% of hospitalized patients, and is linked to increased mortality and prolonged hospital stays (Warren et al., 2023). This condition is also associated with adverse clinical outcomes, further contributing to morbidity and healthcare burden (Al Yaqoubi et al., 2024). The incidence of hyponatremia in patients with cancer is estimated at 1%–40% and is dependent on the type of cancer and the designated serum sodium level parameters (Fibbi et al., 2023). In a study of 2,644 patients with malignancy, 24.8% experienced hyponatremia, with approximately 80% attributed to renal sodium wasting, which was associated with worse patient outcomes (Murashima et al., 2023). SIADH is the most prevalent etiology of hyponatremia in malignancy (Mc Donald et al., 2022). It is most frequently associated with bronchogenic cancer, especially small cell lung cancer (SCLC), which accounts for nearly 75% of all malignancy-associated SIADH cases (Fibbi et al., 2023). SIADH is a recognized complication following surgery for malignant tumors; its occurrence has been identified after pancreatic cancer resection but is underreported because of the nonspecific nature of hyponatremia symptoms (Rahnea-Nita et al., 2023).

Clinical Manifestations

Signs and symptoms of SIADH vary and depend on the severity of hyponatremia, the rate of change in plasma sodium concentration, the duration, and the osmotic gradient between intracellular and extracellular fluids (see Table 9-1). Initially, patients may be asymptomatic or have nonspecific symptoms with slight decreases in serum sodium. A diagnosis of SIADH may not be made until the hyponatremia becomes severe and causes progressive changes in central nervous system (CNS) function (Mentrasti et al., 2020). However, patients may experience symptoms even at higher plasma sodium concentrations if plasma sodium decreases rapidly.

Hyponatremia primarily affects the CNS. As the cells in the brain swell with excess free water, neurologic symptoms reflective of increasing cerebral edema and intracranial pressure are demonstrated, such as loss of appetite, headache, irritability, attention deficit, confusion, and disorientation (Mentrasti et al., 2020; Thomas, 2023). Although SIADH is characterized by water excess, patients usually do not

TABLE 9-1
Clinical Manifestations of Syndrome of Inappropriate Antidiuretic Hormone Secretion

Type	Serum Sodium Level (mEq/L)	Signs and Symptoms
Normal sodium	135–145	–
Mild hyponatremia	130–134	Nonspecific or none; or complaints of muscle cramps, anorexia, nausea, vomiting, fatigue, headache, or lethargy
Moderate hyponatremia	125–129	Irritability, disorientation, confusion, abdominal cramps, diarrhea, or extrapyramidal effects, such as changes in muscle tone, abnormal posturing, or tremors
Severe hyponatremia	< 125	Signs and symptoms related to cerebral edema, such as papilledema, delirium, hypoactive reflexes, ataxia, gait disturbance, seizures, coma, or death

Manifestations vary depending on the rate of onset of hyponatremia; signs of fluid volume depletion or overload are absent.

Note. Based on information from Kengne, 2023; Mentrasti et al., 2020; Shelton, 2022; Thomas, 2023.

exhibit clinical signs of edema. This is because the intravascular volume increases only slightly with SIADH, so signs of fluid overload, such as peripheral edema, heart failure, or ascites, typically are not present (Warren et al., 2023). With mild hyponatremia, defined as a plasma sodium concentration of 130–134 mEq/L, patients usually are asymptomatic or complain of muscle cramps, anorexia, nausea, vomiting, fatigue, headache, or lethargy (Shelton, 2022; Thomas, 2023). With moderate hyponatremia, defined as plasma sodium concentrations of 125–129 mEq/L, patients may exhibit irritability, disorientation, confusion, abdominal cramps, diarrhea, or extrapyramidal effects, such as changes in muscle tone, abnormal posturing, or tremors. With severe hyponatremia (defined as plasma sodium concentrations below 125 mEq/L), development of cerebral edema leading to increased intracranial pressure, cerebral herniation, hypoxia, seizures, coma, and possibly death can occur (Kengne, 2023; Mentrasti et al., 2020; Shelton, 2022).

Risk Factors and Etiology

Multiple risk factors, both malignant and nonmalignant, exist for the development of SIADH. These risk factors are outlined in Figure 9-1.

Malignancies

The most common malignancy associated with SIADH due to ectopic ADH secretion is SCLC, with approximately 25% of individuals with SCLC developing SIADH during the course of their illness (Workeneh et al., 2020). In many cases, ADH is synthesized in tumor tissues. Hyponatremia, a frequent complication in SCLC, can be attributed to the cancer itself, its treatments, paraneoplastic SIADH, and brain metastases (Imran et al., 2023; Yucel et al., 2022). Other malignancies associated with SIADH are non-small cell lung cancer, mesothelioma, lymphoma, breast cancer, Ewing sarcoma, thymoma, primary brain tumors, and carcinomas of the head and neck, esophagus, stomach, duodenum, colon, pancreas, ureter, bladder, prostate, ovary, and endometrium (Dang et al., 2024; Fibbi et al., 2023; Warren et al., 2023). Gastric cancer, nasal and paranasal malignant tumors, reninoma, and olfactory neuroblastoma have also been associated with the development of SIADH (Dang et al., 2024; Heiland & Heiland, 2023; Sekhon et al., 2024).

Nonmalignant Conditions

In addition to SIADH associated with malignancy, many nonmalignant conditions have been implicated in its development. Nonmalignant causes include pulmonary disorders such as infections and chronic obstructive pulmonary disease, CNS disorders, certain medications, trauma, surgery, stress, and older age (Mentrasti et al., 2020). SIADH encompasses a diverse range of etiologies, including pulmonary infections (e.g., pneumonia) and hypothalamic disorders—all characterized by the abnormal overproduction of ADH (Soleimani, 2023).

FIGURE 9-1. Risk Factors for Syndrome of Inappropriate Antidiuretic Hormone

Conditions		
• Cancers – Bladder – Brain – Breast – Carcinoid – Cervix – Colon – Duodenum – Esophagus – Hypopharynx – Leukemia – Lung (especially small cell lung cancer) – Lymphomas (Hodgkin and non-Hodgkin) – Multiple myeloma – Neuroblastoma – Ovarian – Pancreas – Prostate – Sarcomas (Ewing and mesothelioma) – Thymomas (rare)	• Nonmalignant conditions – AIDS – Asthma – Cerebral atrophy – Chronic obstructive pulmonary disease – Encephalitis – Guillain-Barré syndrome – Hypothyroidism – Lung abscess – Meningitis – Multiple sclerosis – Older age – Pneumonia – Skull fracture – Stroke – Subarachnoid hemorrhage – Subdural hematoma – Systemic lupus erythematosus – Tuberculosis	• Miscellaneous – Anxiety – Nausea – Positive end-expiratory pressure breathing devices – Severe pain – Stress – Trauma
Medications		
• Analgesics – Acetaminophen – Aspirin – Barbiturates – General anesthetics – Meperidine – Morphine – Nicotine – Nonsteroidal anti-inflammatory drugs	• Antidepressants – Imipramine – Monoamine oxidase inhibitors – Selective serotonin reuptake inhibitors	• Chemotherapy – Cisplatin – Cyclophosphamide – Docetaxel – Ifosfamide – Melphalan – Vincristine • Monoclonal antibodies – Alemtuzumab – Bevacizumab • Targeted therapies – Bortezomib – Imatinib
Other Medications		
• Bromocriptine • Carbamazepine • Chlorpropamide • Haloperidol • Thiazide diuretics		

Note. Based on information from Imran et al., 2023; Jamhour et al., 2023; Mentrasti et al., 2020; Warren et al., 2023; Yarandi & Shirali, 2023.

Pulmonary Disorders

Various pulmonary and systemic diseases can induce the ectopic release of ADH, including bacterial and viral pneumonia, lung abscesses, tuberculosis, asthma, bronchiolitis, cystic fibrosis, chronic obstructive pulmonary disease, respiratory failure, and interstitial lung disease. Additionally, COVID-19, respiratory infections, viral gastroenteritis in children, and metabolic disorders (e.g., type 1 diabetes) have been implicated in ADH dysregulation (Ali et al., 2023; Al-kuraishy et al., 2021; Maesaka et al., 2023; Paudel et al., 2024; Rawson et al., 2024; Saha et al., 2023). Although the exact pathophysiologic process causing SIADH is unknown in patients with pulmonary disease, it has been theorized that pulmonary hyperinflation and hypoxia send false volume depletion signals to the intrathoracic osmoreceptors that activate ADH secretion (Saha et al., 2023). ADH stimulates water absorption in the renal collecting ducts through the action of aquaporins in the walls of the tubules. As a result, very concentrated, high-density urine, high serum sodium concentration, a reduction in plasma osmolality, and dilutional hyponatremia occur. In addition to high urine osmolality, persistent hypernatremia in urine may indicate a poor response to fluid restriction in patients with SIADH (Lee et al., 2022).

Central Nervous System Disorders

SIADH has been associated with surgical resection of primary brain tumors, following hypophysectomy, and with CNS disorders, including infection, AIDS, meningitis, brain abscess, subdural hematomas, subarachnoid hemorrhage, cerebrovascular accident, brain tumors, head trauma, multiple sclerosis, Guillain-Barré syndrome, and traumatic brain injury (Maesaka et al., 2023; Paudel et al., 2024; Rossignon et al., 2024; Saha et al., 2023). SIADH has also been associated with Parkinson disease and Alzheimer disease (Maesaka et al., 2023; Paudel et al., 2024; Saha et al., 2023). The stimulation of AVP (the biologically active form of ADH) release from the neurohypophysis (the posterior portion of the pituitary gland) in these diseases has been theorized as the mechanism for SIADH. Patients with neurologic diseases may be more vulnerable to cerebral edema because of impaired osmoregulation. They can exhibit more aggressive cerebral edema with deterioration of clinical status and intracranial pressure compared to hyponatremic patients without CNS disorders (Al-kuraishy et al., 2021). Patients with neurologic diseases are particularly susceptible to fluid and electrolyte disturbances, such as hyponatremia and hypernatremia, which can significantly affect clinical outcomes because of their potential to exacerbate cerebral edema and intracranial pressure (Olaoye et al., 2024). The majority of SIADH cases associated with traumatic brain injury, however, are mild and transient (Petria et al., 2025).

Medications

Several antineoplastic, antidepressant, antipsychotic, and AVP analog agents have been implicated in the development of SIADH. Among antineoplastic agents, those reported to induce SIADH include cyclophosphamide, ifosfamide, vinca alkaloids (e.g., vincristine, vinblastine, vinorelbine), melphalan, methotrexate, cytarabine, fludarabine, hydroxyurea, carboplatin, and cisplatin (Mentrasti et al., 2020). Additional chemotherapy agents associated with SIADH include doxorubicin, doxycycline, and cyclophosphamide-based regimens (Imran et al., 2023; Jamhour et al., 2023).

Although not a common side effect, hyponatremia has been documented in patients receiving the proteasome inhibitor, bortezomib, and the tyrosine kinase inhibitor, imatinib (Yarandi & Shirali, 2023).

Antidepressants can also be associated with SIADH. Between 0.6% and 40% of patients taking selective serotonin reuptake inhibitors (SSRIs) for depression have been reported to develop SIADH, with older adults and those concurrently using thiazide diuretics at higher risk (Mentrasti et al., 2020). SSRIs can induce SIADH by triggering antidiuretic hormone release, leading to fluid retention and hyponatremia (Warren et al., 2023).

Various drug classes, including antipsychotics, antidepressants, anticonvulsants, and thiazide diuretics, can cause hyponatremia through intrarenal mechanisms involving aquaporin-2 upregulation, a phenomenon consistent with nephrogenic syndrome of inappropriate antidiuresis, even in the absence of elevated plasma AVP levels (Mentrasti et al., 2020).

Thiazide diuretics are particularly associated with a higher incidence of hyponatremia in the older adult population. Beyond excess ADH secretion, many patients on antidepressants experience increased thirst and fluid intake or develop self-induced water intoxication in the context of psychosis, further exacerbating hyponatremia in SIADH. Patients treated with SSRIs or serotonin-norepinephrine reuptake inhibitors may develop hyponatremia from the combined effects of excessive ADH secretion, heightened thirst, and psychiatric-related water intoxication (Zhao et al., 2023). Additionally, AVP analogs, such as desmopressin and oxytocin, can induce SIADH. Nicotine, narcotics, and nonsteroidal anti-inflammatory drugs have also been implicated (Mentrasti et al., 2020). Individuals with preexisting renal dysfunction or fluid balance disorders, such as central diabetes insipidus, may be at heightened risk of SIADH when using nonsteroidal anti-inflammatory drugs (Vishal et al., 2023).

Other Conditions

The development of SIADH has been linked to various physiologic and environmental factors, including pain, stress, nausea, and general anesthesia (Mentrasti et al., 2020). Although SIADH incidence generally increases with age, reports indicate a rising occurrence in children, particularly those hospitalized with respiratory or CNS infections, such as pneumonia or meningitis, which heighten the risk of hyponatremia (Yasir & Mechanic, 2023). Endocrine disorders, such as hypothyroidism and glucocorticoid deficiency, have also been associated with an increased risk of SIADH (Mentrasti et al., 2020). Additionally, SIADH can manifest as a hydro-saline imbalance in Cushing syndrome, potentially due to impaired glucocorticoid-mediated renal sodium reabsorption, reduced renal tubular sodium channel activity, and increased water retention driven by elevated vasopressin secretion (Pivonello et al., 2023).

Pathophysiology and Patient Evaluation

Physiology of Water Homeostasis

Understanding the physiology of fluid and electrolyte balance within body compartments provides critical context for the pathophysiology of SIADH. Water homeostasis is maintained through a complex interplay of body fluid balance, sodium and water regulation, and the renal effects of ADH. Total body water accounts for approximately 50%–70% of body weight, depending on factors such as age, gender, muscle mass, and adipose tissue composition (Tobias et al., 2022). Table 9-2 outlines key terms relevant to the physiology of SIADH. Intracellular fluid, which constitutes approximately 40% of body weight, primarily resides in the cytoplasm and provides a stable environment crucial for cellular function. It maintains a consistent osmolality to support vital biochemical reactions.

In contrast, extracellular fluid, comprising about 20% of body weight (including 5% plasma and 12% interstitial fluid), exhibits greater variability (Brinkman et al., 2023). It is further distributed between the intravascular space (plasma), which accounts for approximately 7% of total body fluid, and the interstitial space, which

TABLE 9-2
Terms Associated With Syndrome of Inappropriate Antidiuretic Hormone Secretion

Term	Definition
Antidiuretic hormone (ADH)	Hormone synthesized in the hypothalamus and released from the posterior pituitary that regulates total body water volume, in part, with renal activity and the stimulus of thirst
Aquaporin-2	A membrane protein in collecting tubules and ducts in kidney nephrons that acts as a semipermeable water channel to reabsorb water following stimulation by ADH
Arginine vasopressin	The biologically active form of ADH that is the primary controller of extracellular volume and acts to conserve fluid by decreasing urine output
Baroreceptors	Receptors located in the carotid sinus, aortic arch, and left atrium that respond to plasma volume changes to direct the release of ADH through nonosmolar control
Central pontine myelinolysis	Demyelination of neurons and the development of neurologic dysfunction, including seizures, dysphagia, dysarthria, paresis, and even death
Osmoreceptors	Receptors located in the central nervous system that respond to changes in the serum sodium concentration or plasma osmolality to direct the release of ADH through osmolar control
Osmosis	Free water movement across a semipermeable cell membrane to maintain an equal concentration of dissolved particles or solutes in the intracellular and extracellular spaces
Serum osmolality	Ratio of solute to free water in the circulation; determined by sodium, which does not freely cross the cell membrane

Note. Based on information from Kharin & Klussmann, 2024; Maesaka et al., 2023; Najem et al., 2024; Noda & Sasaki, 2021; Saha et al., 2023; Tkacs & Herrmann, 2024.

comprises about 26%. The distribution of electrolytes in intracellular and extracellular fluid is illustrated in Figure 9-2, whereas major intracellular and extracellular fluid components are detailed in Table 9-3.

FIGURE 9-2. Composition of Intracellular and Extracellular Fluid

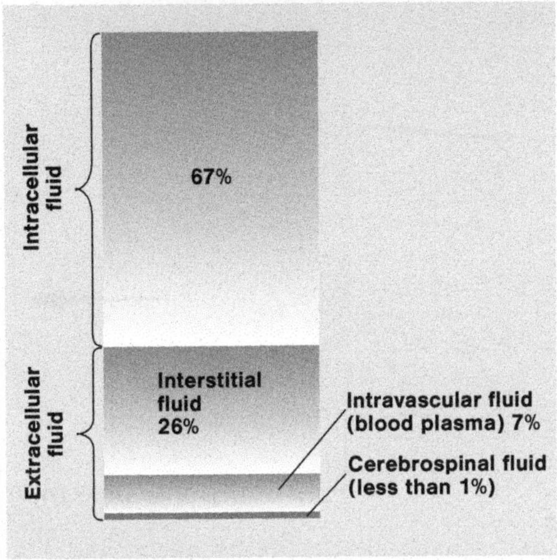

Note. From "Cellular Fluid Content," by Welcome1To1The1Jungle, 2014 (https://commons.wikimedia.org/w/index.php?curid=48498104). Licensed under CC BY-SA 4.0 (https://creativecommons.org/licenses/by-sa/4.0/deed.en).

Regulation of body water between the intracellular and extracellular compartments is achieved through osmosis (see Figure 9-3), a process in which water moves freely across a semipermeable membrane to equalize solute concentrations in both spaces. Sodium, which does not freely cross the membrane, is the primary determinant of serum osmolality, defined as the ratio of solute to free water in circulation. Normal serum osmolality ranges from 275–290 mOsm/kg and is maintained through renal water reabsorption or excretion (Najem et al., 2024). Total body water volume is regulated by ADH secretion, thirst, and renal activity. ADH, known in its

TABLE 9-3
Normal Intracellular and Extracellular Fluid Components and Concentrations

Component	Extracellular Fluid	Intracellular Fluid
Sodium (Na+)	135–145 mEq/L	~10–15 mEq/L
Potassium (K+)	3.5-5.0 mEq/L	~120–150 mEq/L
Calcium (Ca2+)	4.5–5.5 mEq/L	< 1 mEq/L
Magnesium (Mg2+)	~1.5–2.5 mEq/L	~25–30 mEq/L
Chloride (Cl–)	98–106 mEq/L	~3–4 mEq/L
Bicarbonate (HCO3–)	22–26 mEq/L	~10–12 mEq/L
Phosphates	~2–4.5 mEq/L	~75–100 mEq/L
Osmolality	~280–295 mOsm/kg	~280–295 mOsm/kg

Note. Based on information from Henderson et al., 2024; Hunt et al., 2024; Tkacs & Herrmann, 2024.

FIGURE 9-3. Effect of Osmosis Across a Semipermeable Membrane

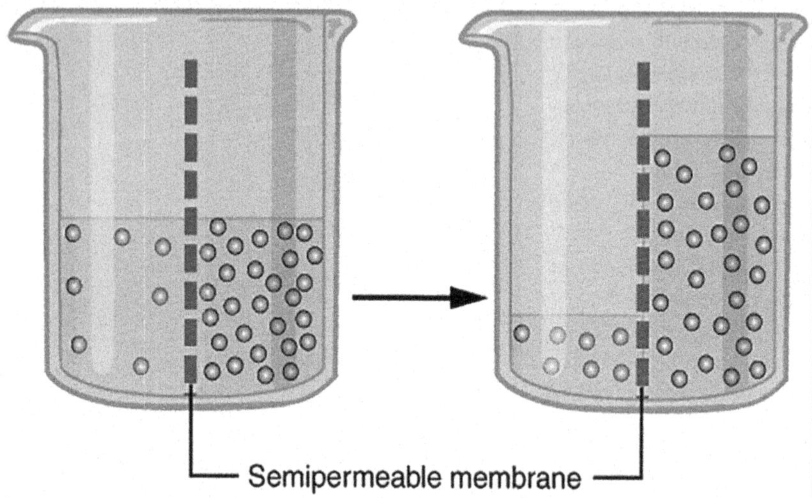

Water moves freely across a semipermeable cell membrane to maintain an equal concentration of dissolved particles in the intracellular and extracellular spaces.

Note. From "Anatomy and Physiology," by OpenStax, 2016 (https://commons.wikimedia.org/w/index.php?curid=30131189). Licensed under CC BY-SA 4.0 (https://creativecommons.org/licenses/by-sa/4.0/deed.en).

biologically active form as AVP, is the primary regulator of extracellular volume, acting to conserve fluid by reducing urine output.

Synthesized in the hypothalamus, ADH is transported to and stored in the posterior pituitary until release is triggered. Upon release, ADH binds to vasopressin receptors on kidney epithelial cells in the collecting tubules and ducts, initiating a signaling cascade that mobilizes aquaporin-2 vesicles to the plasma membrane, thereby enhancing water reabsorption in the renal medulla (Noda & Sasaki, 2021).

Two primary receptor types mediate ADH release. Osmoreceptors in the CNS regulate ADH secretion based on changes in plasma sodium concentration (plasma osmolality). Baroreceptors in the carotid sinus, aortic arch, and left atrium respond to variations in plasma volume. When these receptors detect decreased circulatory volume (e.g., dehydration) and elevated serum sodium concentration, the hypothalamus triggers thirst, and the posterior pituitary releases ADH. Additionally, reduced renal blood flow activates the renin–angiotensin–aldosterone system, which can contribute to hypertension, vasoconstriction, and vascular remodeling (Dalal et al., 2023). ADH controls the expression of aquaporins, a family of integral membrane proteins that facilitate bidirectional water transport across biological membranes (Kharin & Klussman, 2024; Wagner et al., 2022). Through the vasopressin–aquaporin signaling cascade, ADH binds to vasopressin receptor 2 (V2) on principal cells in the collecting ducts, activating the cAMP signaling pathway and promoting the insertion of aquaporin-2 into the apical membrane, enhancing water reabsorption and urine concentration (Ando et al., 2024; Cuzzo et al., 2023; Zhao et al., 2023).

Acute hyponatremia and hyposmolality result in water influx into brain cells, leading to cerebral edema. In response, an adaptive mechanism known as osmoregulation restores brain volume by initiating a compensatory loss of intracerebral fluid and electrolytes, particularly sodium and potassium. However, if severe hyposmotic hyponatremia remains untreated, the resulting cerebral edema can cause life-threatening neurologic complications, as the brain's capacity to expand within the skull is limited, and neuronal function critically depends on extracellular sodium balance (Kengne, 2023). Over the next several days, further decrease of intracerebral osmolality occurs with loss of the primary organic solutes, myo-inositol and choline compounds, and, to a lesser extent, glutamine and glutamate, facilitating plasma osmolality equilibration. Hypotonic hyponatremia, characterized by electrolyte-free water excess, results from excessive intake or inadequate renal excretion, leading to cerebral edema due to water movement into brain cells (Rondon-Berrios & Sterns, 2022). Rapid correction of hyponatremia can lead to excessive water loss from cells, resulting in cellular dehydration and central pontine myelinolysis (CPM), a demyelinating disorder characterized by myelin loss in the pons and often triggered by abrupt shifts in serum osmolality following the correction of severe chronic hyponatremia (Sun et al., 2023). This condition can cause significant neurologic dysfunction, including seizures, dysphagia, dysarthria, paresis, and, in severe cases, death. Conversely, when serum osmolality decreases and fluid volume increases, as seen in overhydration, ADH release is inhibited, reducing water reabsorption and leading to the excretion of dilute urine.

Types of Hyponatremia

Although SIADH is the most common cause of hyponatremia in patients with cancer, various types and causes exist. Understanding the underlying etiology and duration of hyponatremia is crucial for guiding appropriate therapy. Hyponatremia is classified based on chronicity as acute or chronic and by fluid volume status as hypovolemic, euvolemic, or hypervolemic. Acute hyponatremia, lasting less than 48 hours, often presents with altered mental status (Decaux, 2023). In contrast, chronic hyponatremia, persisting for more than 48 hours, can lead to neurologic and musculoskeletal complications, such as attention deficits, dizziness, gait disturbances, falls, sarcopenia, bone fractures, and osteoporosis. Notably, rather than being a direct cause of falls and fractures, hyponatremia—especially in older adults—may serve as a marker of overall unhealthy aging, confounding its association with these outcomes (Fratangelo et al., 2023).

Hyponatremia can be categorized based on fluid status. Hypovolemic hyponatremia, resulting from sodium and fluid loss due to vomiting, diarrhea, or diuretic use, is associated with hypotension and tachycardia. The body compensates by releasing ADH and renin, increasing water reabsorption and renal sodium retention in response to low urine sodium concentration, elevated urine osmolality, and reduced urine output (Ghosal et al., 2023).

Hypervolemic hyponatremia, commonly seen in refractory ascites, spontaneous bacterial peritonitis, and hepatic encephalopathy, results from excessive total body water and sodium retention, with a disproportionate increase in water due to inappropriately elevated ADH levels (Praharaj & Anand, 2022). This form of hyponatremia is frequently associated with conditions such as congestive heart failure, chronic renal insufficiency, and cirrhosis, presenting with volume overload and edema (Bhasin-Chhabra et al., 2022).

Euvolemic (normovolemic) hyponatremia, as seen in SIADH, is primarily due to water excess rather than sodium loss, driven by uncontrolled ADH secretion. SIADH can arise from nonmalignant conditions such as pneumonia or from ectopic ADH production by malignant tumors, including brain tumors, lung cancers, and hypothalamic diseases, as part of a paraneoplastic syndrome (Fibbi et al., 2023; Soleimani, 2023; Torres et al., 2023).

Paraneoplastic endocrine syndromes occur when tumors aberrantly produce hormones, hormone precursors, or hormone-like substances, often signaling disease progression or relapse (Shankar et al., 2024). These syndromes can present with endocrine, neuromuscular, cardiovascular, cutaneous, hematologic, gastrointestinal, and renal manifestations. Among paraneoplastic neurologic syndromes, Cushing syndrome caused by ectopic adrenocorticotropic hormone secretion is the most prevalent, followed by SIADH, anti–Hu-mediated chronic intestinal pseudo-obstruction, limbic encephalitis, Evans syndrome, hypercalcemia, dermatomyositis, and polycythemia (Abufaraj et al., 2024).

In patients with SIADH, certain malignant cells can synthesize, store, and produce ectopic secretion of ADH that is not affected by the negative feedback mechanisms that normally regulate the release or inhibition of ADH. Inappropriately elevated levels of circulating ADH cause reabsorption of water from the renal collecting ducts, diminished urine output, and excretion of concentrated urine (> 200 mOsm/kg), with increased urine sodium osmolality from the decreased water excretion (Warren et al., 2023). The diagnosis of the SIADH is confirmed by the presence of hyponatremia with hyposmololity (< 275 mOsm/kg), inappropriately elevated urine osmolality (> 100 mOsmol/L), and elevated urine sodium (Na+) levels (Reddy, 2023). The resulting increased amount of free water in the extracellular fluid expands the plasma volume, leading to decreased serum sodium concentration (serum hyposmolality) and dilutional serum hyponatremia. In an attempt to equalize osmotic pressure, water moves from the extracellular fluid to the intracellular fluid, causing cerebral edema and profound neurologic alterations.

Patient Assessment

Many disorders can cause hyponatremia; therefore, a thorough patient history is essential to evaluate for and diagnose SIADH. Nurses should include a family member or caregiver when obtaining the history. Patients may be experiencing neurologic symptoms associated with SIADH, such as confusion or personality changes, and may not be able to give a complete, accurate history. Nurses should assess patients for risk factors for SIADH, including oncologic and medical conditions associated with increased ADH secretion. Disorders can include a history of cardiac failure, pulmonary disease, hypothyroidism, pneumonia, tuberculosis, CNS disorders (e.g., stroke, hemorrhage, trauma, psychosis), hepatic dysfunction, adrenal insufficiency, renal disorders, recent surgery, head injury, chronic pain, smoking, weight loss, drug intake, or substance abuse (Shelton, 2022; Thomas, 2023; Yasir & Mechanic, 2023). A review of antineoplastic agents, prescription drugs, and over-the-counter medications will help to determine whether the hyponatremia is medication induced. Drugs that can be associated with hyponatremia include cyclophosphamide, vincristine, vinblastine, cisplatin, morphine, immunoglobulins, interferon, interleukin-2, levamisole, carbamazepine, and drugs classified as SSRIs, nonsteroidal anti-inflammatories, and tricyclics (Fibbi et al., 2023). Newer therapeutic oncologic agents, including targeted therapies and immune checkpoint inhibitors, can also be associated with hyponatremia due to the potential side effect of corticotropin deficiency with subsequent hypocortisolism (Mentrasti et al., 2020). Review of dietary and fluid intake, gastrointestinal losses, urinary output, and weight loss history will also assist in determining whether the hyponatremia is acute or chronic.

The most common clinical manifestations of SIADH are neurologic changes that necessitate a thorough neurologic examination. Although patients may be asymptomatic with mild hyponatremia, those with severe or acute rapid-onset hyponatremia will exhibit changes on neurologic examination that can include confusion, lethargy, disorientation, weakness, myoclonus, hyporeflexia, nystagmus, unstable gait, tremors, seizures, and coma, which require emergent treatment (Shelton, 2022; Thomas, 2023).

Assessment of hydration status is crucial to accurately diagnose the etiology of the hyponatremia and determine appropriate treatment interventions. Initially, evaluating for signs of volume depletion and volume overload can help to distinguish between SIADH and other conditions as the cause of hyponatremia. Volume depletion, associated with vomiting, diarrhea, excessive sweating, or excessive diuretic use, and volume overload, associated with edematous type conditions such as congestive heart failure, chronic renal insufficiency, or cirrhosis, can cause hyponatremia but are not linked to unregulated release of ADH and SIADH and are treated differently than SIADH (Mentrasti et al., 2020; Thomas, 2023). Findings consistent with volume depletion may include vomiting, diarrhea, orthostatic hypotension, tachycardia, decreased skin turgor, and dry mucous membranes, signifying a state of hypovolemic hyponatremia (Mentrasti et al., 2020; Thomas, 2023). Findings consistent with volume overload may include pulmonary rales, S3 gallop, hypertension, peripheral edema, and jugular distension, signifying a state of hypervolemic hyponatremia (Mentrasti et al., 2020; Thomas, 2023). Physical examination findings with SIADH, characterized by normal extracellular fluid volume, include normal blood pressure and pulse, moist mucous membranes, and the absence of peripheral edema.

Advanced Practice Considerations

Diagnostic studies performed in the SIADH workup include the following laboratory and radiographic studies (Hamrahian, 2025; Mentrasti et al., 2020; Warren et al., 2023; Yasir & Mechanic, 2023):

- Serum sodium < 135 mEq/L
- Serum hyposmolality < 275 mOsm/kg
- Urine osmolality > 100 mOsm/kg
- Urinary sodium > 40 mmol/L
- Clinical euvolemia
- Normal thyroid function
- Normal adrenal function
- Normal pituitary function
- Normal renal function
- Chest x-ray, if indicated
- Computed tomography scan of the head, if indicated

Other laboratory results that should be reviewed are serum potassium, bicarbonate levels, blood urea nitrogen, serum uric acid levels, and glucose (Thomas, 2023). Serum uric acid levels may be subnormal or low normal as a result of plasma dilution and increased excretion of nitrogen waste. Serum glucose should be evaluated because increased glucose draws water into the intravascular space by osmosis, resulting in dilutional hyponatremia. When hyperglycemia is corrected, serum sodium levels usually return to normal. Serum cortisol level may also be obtained to rule out adrenal insufficiency as the cause of SIADH (Thomas, 2023). Radiographic studies ordered may include a chest x-ray to evaluate for pulmonary disease or lung cancer and a computed tomography scan of the head to evaluate for cerebral edema, brain tumor, or brain herniation (Thomas, 2023).

Another diagnostic tool for SIADH is the water loading test, which involves massive water intake in a short period of time. Healthy patients excrete 78%–82% of the ingested water load within four hours due to AVP suppression; however, in patients with SIADH, the expected urine amount within four hours is reduced to 30%–40% (Pliquett & Obermüller, 2022). This test must be performed with extreme caution in the hospital setting and is not a safe procedure for most patients because of possible increased intravascular overhydration, increased risk of adverse effects with underlying cardiac comorbidity, and the potential to worsen hyponatremia with risk of increasing symptoms such as seizures.

Treatment Modalities

Treatment Goals

The management of hyponatremia in patients with cancer is the same as for non-oncologic patients. Once a diagnosis of SIADH has been established, the initial goal is to identify and treat the underlying cause. If the cause is malignancy related, oncologic therapy should be initiated promptly. If the cause is medication related, the causative drug should be discontinued. Treatment should be initiated for other disorders, such as hypothyroidism or pulmonary infection, if identified as the precipitating factor.

Control of the underlying malignancy is the only effective way to reverse the effects of unregulated release of ADH and SIADH. Treatment to correct the sodium–water imbalance is based on the severity and rapidity of onset of symptoms and the level of hyponatremia (Adrogué et al., 2022; Fibbi et al., 2023; Mentrasti et al., 2020; Sterns et al., 2024; Thomas, 2023; Warren et al., 2023; Yasir & Mechanic, 2023). Traditionally, interventions for SIADH have been directed at patients with severe hyponatremia who were experiencing acute, advanced symptoms, such as mental status changes or seizures. However, studies have suggested that even mild or chronic hyponatremia may predispose patients to osteoporosis and increase the risk of gait abnormalities and falls with injury, particularly hip fractures (Adams et al., 2019; Corona et al., 2018).

The principles of SIADH therapy involve fluid restriction, sodium correction, maintaining patient safety, and pharmacologic therapy. See Figure 9-4 for a summary of SIADH treatment.

Treatments Based on Serum Sodium Concentration

Mild to Moderate Hyponatremia

Mild to moderate hyponatremia is defined as plasma sodium concentrations greater than 130 mEq/L. At these sodium levels, patients may be asymptomatic or have nonspecific symptoms, such as lethargy, weakness, anorexia, and irritability. Generally, patients may be managed with fluid restriction, oral pharmacologic therapy, and close monitoring (Yasir & Mechanic, 2023).

Fluid restriction is the initial treatment for patients with mild to moderate hyponatremia caused by SIADH. The goal of fluid restriction in SIADH is to create a water–electrolyte balance by decreasing excess body water. The usual recommendation for fluid restriction is 500 ml/day less than the daily urine output, which can improve sodium levels by 2–4 mEq/L/day (Warren et al., 2023). For patients with cancer, fluid restrictions may be difficult due to the need for IV fluids with oncologic therapies. Other challenges with fluid restrictions can include poor patient adherence

FIGURE 9-4. Summary of Syndrome of Inappropriate Antidiuretic Hormone Secretion Treatment

Mild to Moderate Hyponatremia	Severe Hyponatremia
• Fluid restriction is 500 ml/day less than the daily urine output. • Review medications. • Perform a neurologic assessment. • Monitor sodium and renal function levels. • Medications include loop diuretics, salt tablets, and urea.	• Admit to the intensive care unit, as needed. • Administer hypertonic saline (3%), as ordered. • Limit sodium correction to 8–12 mEq/L in 24 hours. • Administer vaptans, as ordered. • Perform frequent neurologic assessments. • Initiate seizure precautions. • Monitor sodium and renal function levels frequently during the first 48 hours.

Note. Based on information from Adrogué et al., 2022; Danyalian & Heller, 2023; Krisanapan et al., 2023; Mc Donald et al., 2022; Mentrasti et al., 2020; Rondon-Berrios & Sterns, 2022; Shelton, 2022; Workeneh et al., 2020; Yasir & Mechanic, 2023.

to treatment and the need for ongoing fluid restriction for three to five days to show improvement in sodium levels (Mentrasti et al., 2020).

Loop diuretics and salt tablets have been used in the treatment of chronic, mild to moderate hyponatremia; however, evidence is limited regarding efficacy. Loop diuretics act by inhibiting sodium chloride reabsorption, which decreases interstitial tonicity and causes free water excretion. Salt tablets can replace diuretic-induced sodium losses and may act as an osmotic agent (Workeneh et al., 2020).

In a randomized controlled trial comparing the combination of furosemide and salt tablets plus fluid restriction with fluid restriction alone in patients with SIADH, results found that furosemide and salt tablets in addition to fluid restriction is not significantly better than fluid restriction alone in increasing sodium levels, with more patients in the furosemide group withdrawing from the study because of acute kidney injury (Krisanapan et al., 2020). Long-term use of diuretic therapy for chronic SIADH is not recommended, as continuous treatment can produce excessive loss of sodium in the urine that can worsen hyponatremia.

Spanuchart et al. (2020) conducted a retrospective study of patients with euvolemic hyponatremia. Findings suggested that the use of salt tablets was associated with a mild but significant increase in sodium levels compared to a group of patients who did not receive salt tablets.

Other oral medications that have been used for mild to moderate hyponatremia are urea and demeclocycline. Urea stimulates osmotic excretion of free water without electrolyte depletion. Dosing is 15–30 g/day or a dose of 0.25–0.50 g/kg (Wu et al., 2020). Wendt et al. (2023) conducted a systematic review investigating the use of urea for SIADH. Results suggested that urea increased serum sodium levels with a very low risk of overcorrection. Disadvantages of urea use included poor palatability and the development of azotemia at higher doses. To improve palatability and disguise the taste of urea, patients should be advised to dissolve the drug in a strong-flavored liquid such as orange juice. Demeclocycline, a semisynthetic tetracycline, acts by interfering with the vasopressin–aquaporin signaling cascade, thereby promoting water excretion. Because of the lack of clinical and economic evidence supporting the use of demeclocycline for hyponatremia secondary to SIADH, the need for complex dose adjustments, and close patient monitoring, demeclocycline is not routinely recommended (Wu et al., 2020).

Severe Hyponatremia

Severe hyponatremia is defined as plasma sodium concentrations less than 120 mEq/L. At these sodium levels, patients experience significant neurologic changes, such as seizures and coma, and need immediate treatment and hospitalization, usually in intensive care. Medical management comprises IV saline (isotonic [0.9%] or, if warranted, hypertonic [3%]), in addition to pharmacologic therapy, including anticonvulsants (Adrogué et al., 2022; Shelton, 2022). Patient safety considerations should include supplemental oxygen, close monitoring, and fall prevention. In emergent situations, airway intubation and ventilatory support may be necessary.

Saline infusions may be administered to patients with SIADH; however, rapid overcorrection of hyponatremia may place patients at risk for CPM. This disorder is caused by cellular edema that compresses nerve fiber tracts and myelin sheaths and results in demyelination. A risk factor for developing CPM is chronic hyponatremia, especially if the serum sodium is lower than 120 mmol/L, because of compensatory solute losses. The clinical presentation of CPM may vary and depends on the severity of the injury and the involved areas. The diagnosis of CPM is based on neurologic symptoms in patients following a recent overly rapid correction of hyponatremia. It can be confirmed by the presence of lesions on magnetic resonance imaging. The onset of symptoms is usually seen 1–14 days after rapid electrolyte correction (Danyalian & Heller, 2023). Acute encephalopathy and seizures are generally the initial findings that resolve once sodium levels are returned to normal. Clinical worsening can then occur three to five days later with neurologic symptoms, such as spastic quadriparesis, impairment in short-term memory, dysphagia, dysarthria, oculomotor abnormalities, ataxia, lethargy, tremors, dizziness, dystonia, tremor, and in the most severe cases, locked-in syndrome, coma, and death (Danyalian & Heller, 2023). One or two 100 ml boluses of 3% sodium chloride solution via IV infusion over 10 minutes is recommended to reverse hyponatremia promptly and reliably (Mc Donald et al., 2022; Sterns et al., 2024). Sodium chloride boluses can increase serum sodium level by 4–6 mEq/L, which is generally sufficient to arrest the progression of CPM symptoms. A third bolus should be reserved for active seizures or continuing signs of herniation (Rondon-Berrios & Sterns, 2022). Once initial, immediate therapy has been administered with an increase of sodium levels, a slow infusion rate is recommended and is adjusted based on every-two-hour plasma sodium concentration levels to maintain a rate of rise of plasma sodium of less than 1 mmol/L over an hour or 8–12 mmol over 24 hours.

Vaptans, or vasopressin receptor antagonists, a class of agents that inhibit the effects of vasopressin on water reabsorption, have been studied as a targeted treatment option for SIADH. Tolvaptan and conivaptan are available in the United States and approved for the treatment of SIADH (Krisanapan et al., 2020). Tolvaptan, an oral agent, is a selective V2 receptor antagonist, whereas conivaptan, an IV agent, blocks both the V2 and V1a receptors. The use of vaptans is controversial (Krisanapan et al., 2020). Vaptans can cause a rapid initial elevation in serum sodium over one to two hours; however, there is an increased likelihood of an excessive correction and potentially irreversible neurologic injury. If vaptan therapy is considered and administered in patients with severe hyponatremia who do not respond to other treatments, serum sodium levels should be measured immediately and after 6, 24, and 48 hours of treatment (Krisanapan et al., 2020).

Nursing Management

SIADH is an oncologic emergency when patients with cancer present with severe hyponatremia. Overall, the prognosis is poor if SIADH is related to malignancy, particularly in SCLC. Nursing management is directed toward assessment of risk factors and provision of symptom management and supportive care. Table 9-4 presents an overview of nursing interventions for this patient population.

TABLE 9-4
Nursing Management of Syndrome of Inappropriate Antidiuretic Hormone Secretion

Nursing Management	Nursing Interventions
Initial nursing assessment for early detection	Identify patients with risk factors for the development of SIADH, such as small cell lung cancer; carcinomas of the pancreas, duodenum, prostate, or lymphoid tissue; pulmonary infections; and chemotherapy treatment regimens that contain agents that cause SIADH. Review all medications to identify drugs that increase the risk of SIADH. Closely monitor serum and urine electrolytes and osmolality. Assess for early signs of hyponatremia, including headache, nausea, anorexia, generalized weakness, or muscle cramps.
Mild hyponatremia	Restrict fluids to 500 ml/day less than daily urine output. Monitor electrolyte levels frequently, especially sodium and potassium. Educate patients and caregivers about the importance of fluid restriction. Provide an easy method to measure and record oral fluid intake, including fluids from food. Discontinue medications associated with SIADH risk.
Moderate hyponatremia	Restrict fluids to 500 ml/day less than daily urine output. Monitor electrolyte levels, urine output, and renal function. Document response to treatment, including fluid weight loss and increased serum sodium and osmolality. Relieve pain, anxiety, and stress with relaxation techniques. Opioids, barbiturates, and tricyclic antidepressants increase antidiuretic hormone release and should be minimized.
Severe hyponatremia	Hospitalize patients for medication administration, and closely monitor serum and urine electrolytes and osmolality, intake and output, vital signs, and neurologic status. Administer IV hypertonic saline as ordered, using caution with the rate of administration (0.05 ml/kg/min). Possibly admit patients to the intensive care unit for monitoring of serum sodium every 1–2 hours. Administer furosemide as ordered to increase diuresis. Monitor potassium level. Institute safety measures and seizure precautions as indicated. Assess for adequate symptom management related to pain, anxiety, depression, nausea, and vomiting. Assess coping abilities.

(Continued on next page)

TABLE 9-4
Nursing Management of Syndrome of Inappropriate Antidiuretic Hormone Secretion *(Continued)*

Nursing Management	Nursing Interventions
Neurologic changes	Monitor for changes in level of consciousness and behavior. Institute seizure precautions for sodium level > 120 mEq/L. Provide safety measures and assist with daily care, including with walking, eating, self-care, and administration of medications. For generalized weakness, provide means of safety with ambulation (e.g., walker, cane).
Pain management	Assess for adequate pain control and evidence of side effects with discontinuation of medications associated with SIADH risk.
Fluid and electrolyte balance	Restrict fluids as ordered. Closely monitor electrolytes and daily weights; encourage a diet high in sodium. If loop diuretics are ordered, monitor serum sodium and potassium levels; provide a diet high in potassium. Administer hypertonic saline as ordered, using caution with the rate of administration (0.05 ml/kg/min). Watch for signs of central pontine myelinolysis, which often are delayed 2–6 days after correction of hyponatremia.
Seizure precautions	Monitor closely for seizures; institute seizure precautions for serum sodium level < 120 mEq/L. Administer anticonvulsants for seizure activity as ordered. Institute safety precautions and fall prevention measures.
Patient and caregiver education	Restrict fluids, and measure and record intake. Control thirst and dry mouth. Use ice, hard candy, artificial saliva, and artificial saliva gel; avoid alcohol-based mouthwashes. Recognize nonspecific signs of mild hyponatremia that should be promptly reported, including nausea, headache, anorexia, and muscle cramps. Provide medication instructions about the schedule and side effects of demeclocycline and furosemide. Maintain a diet high in sodium. Reinforce coping strategies related to fluid restrictions, muscle weakness, mental changes, and cancer diagnosis.

SIADH—syndrome of inappropriate antidiuretic hormone secretion

Note. Based on information from Adrogué et al., 2022; Campbell & Mortimore, 2022; Fibbi et al., 2023; Shelton, 2022; Wu et al., 2020.

Oncology nurses should be aware of high-risk malignancies and other contributing factors for SIADH and be able to perform thorough ongoing patient assessment. Specifically, reviewing patient medications may alert nurses to drugs that can increase the risk of SIADH in patients with cancer, such as SSRIs, antidepressants, narcotics, and certain antineoplastic agents (e.g., cyclophosphamide, ifosfamide, carboplatin, cisplatin, bortezomib, vincristine, vinblastine, vinorelbine). Nurses also should assess patients for narcotic use, pain, anxiety, nausea, and stress, as these are common issues for patients with cancer and are risk factors for developing SIADH.

Reviewing laboratory studies is critical in identifying potential electrolyte imbalances that may suggest SIADH. Serum sodium, blood urea nitrogen and creatinine, glucose levels, and osmolality abnormalities may necessitate closer monitoring and patient assessment. Patients identified as at risk for SIADH should be frequently assessed head-to-toe, especially noting symptoms of early hyponatremia, including generalized weakness, lethargy, anorexia, nausea, headache, and personality changes (Campbell & Mortimore, 2022). Patients with SIADH are euvolemic and therefore will have normal blood pressure and pulse without signs of volume depletion or volume overload.

Initially, patients with mild to moderate hyponatremia will be ordered to restrict fluids to 500 ml/day less than daily urine output to increase plasma osmolality and normalize the sodium level (Wu et al., 2020). This can be challenging for patients who are receiving cisplatin and are at risk for hemorrhagic cystitis without adequate hydration. Furthermore, patient adherence to fluid restrictions can be difficult. Education and emotional support should be provided to both patients and caregivers. Maintaining an accurate intake and output chart with daily weight assessment is a key nursing responsibility in the close monitoring of fluid restrictions.

Patients may experience constipation because of the decrease in fluid intake. They should be advised not to use tap water or hypotonic enemas because the fluid may be absorbed in the bowel and worsen water intoxication. Stool softeners, laxatives, or hypertonic enemas may be used to alleviate constipation.

Nurses may anticipate patient orders for IV fluid hydration. Patients may be given isotonic saline if hyponatremia is mild or hypertonic saline infusions if hyponatremia is severe (Adrogué et al., 2022; Shelton, 2022). IV fluids should be given at a slow rate to prevent rapid overcorrection of hyponatremia and decrease the risk of central pontine myelinolysis.

Patients with SIADH will experience neurologic alterations; therefore, precautions and interventions must be executed for patient safety. Weakness and gait disturbances may occur, and patients should be provided with mobility aids to prevent falls and possible fractures. Seizure precautions should be employed because the risk of seizure activity will increase with worsening hyponatremia. Caregivers should be educated about possible neurologic changes and observations to report to the healthcare professionals.

Nurses should also provide patient and caregiver education about symptom recognition, treatment plans, and prompt reporting to healthcare providers. Both verbal and written instructions should be given and explained to facilitate patient and caregiver understanding. Instructions regarding daily fluid intake and fluid restriction must also include estimated fluid from foods with high water content, such as soups and fruit. Patients should be instructed to increase dietary sodium and given a list of foods high in sodium to promote elevations in blood sodium concentrations.

Patients should be advised that high-sodium foods might cause thirst, and the importance of maintaining fluid restriction guidelines should be stressed. Measures to alleviate xerostomia or dry mouth, such as sucking on hard candy or ice, performing frequent oral care, using oral rinses without swallowing, and using artificial saliva gels, may assist patients in maintaining their fluid restrictions.

Patients with mild to moderate hyponatremia may be managed in the outpatient setting and will require frequent monitoring to ensure adherence to instructions and medications. Nurses should assist patients in understanding fluid restrictions, recording intake and output, and monitoring any change in daily weights. Charts should be developed to assist patients in accurately documenting their daily fluid status.

Symptoms of SIADH, such as weakness, fatigue, lethargy, anorexia, and mental status changes, can be frightening for patients and caregivers. Providing information about the diagnosis may allay anxiety and assist patients in adhering to the prescribed therapy. Nurses should allow time to give support and reassurance, with opportunities for patients and caregivers to discuss their fears and ask questions. Nurses should also provide safety strategies for fall precautions and seizure prevention. Furthermore, they should assess patients for possible referral to social services, home care, and support groups if further assistance is needed.

Summary

SIADH is a paraneoplastic syndrome that causes unregulated secretion of ADH and, subsequently, dilutional serum hyponatremia, serum hyposmolality, and urine hyperosmolality. Early symptoms often are nonspecific, and a diagnosis may be delayed until the condition becomes severe and presents as a life-threatening oncologic emergency.

Oncology nurses should know the physiologic mechanisms regulating water and electrolyte balance to understand and recognize the pathophysiologic processes involved in the development of SIADH. They also need to know which malignancies are associated with increased risk of SIADH so that their awareness of this condition is raised, especially for patients with SCLC. Early recognition and prompt intervention can improve patient outcomes and prevent life-threatening neurologic changes from progressing to seizures, coma, and death.

References

Abufaraj, M., Ramadan, R., & Alkhatib, A. (2024). Paraneoplastic syndromes in neuroendocrine prostate cancer: A systematic review. *Current Oncology, 31*(3), 1618–1632. https://doi.org/10.3390/curroncol31030123

Adams, A.L., Li, B.H., Bhandari, S., Kamat, S., Sundar, S., Krasa, H., ... Sim, J.J. (2019). Chronic hyponatremia and association with osteoporosis among a large racially/ethnically diverse population. *Osteoporosis International, 30*(4), 853–861. https://doi.org/10.1007/s00198-018-04832-4

Adrogué, H.J., Tucker, B.M., & Madias, N.E. (2022). Diagnosis and management of hyponatremia: A review. *JAMA, 328*(3), 280–291. https://doi.org/10.1001/jama.2022.11176

Ali, K., Najjar, Y., Mehta, S., & Faddoul, G. (2023). Syndrome of inappropriate antidiuretic hormone secretion as a presentation of untreated Parkinson's disease. *Cureus, 15*(4), e37286. https://doi.org/10.7759/cureus.37286

Al-kuraishy, H.M., Al-Gareeb, A.I., Qusti, S., Alshammari, E.M., Atanu, F.O., & Batiha, G.E.-S. (2021). Arginine vasopressin and pathophysiology of COVID-19: An innovative perspective. *Biomedicine and Pharmacotherapy, 143,* 112193. https://doi.org/10.1016/j.biopha.2021.112193

Al Yaqoubi, I.H., Al-Maqbali, J.S., Al Farsi, A.A., Al Jabri, R.K., Khan, S.A., & Al Alawi, A.M. (2024). Prevalence of hyponatremia among medically hospitalized patients and associated outcomes: a retrospective cohort study. *Annals of Saudi Medicine, 44*(5), 339–348. https://doi.org/10.5144/0256-4947.2024.339

Ando, F., Hara, Y., & Uchida, S. (2024). Identification of protein kinase A signaling molecules in renal collecting ducts. *Journal of Physiology, 602*(13), 3057–3067. https://doi.org/10.1113/JP284178

Bhasin-Chhabra, B., Veitla, V., Weinberg, S., & Koratala, A. (2022). Demystifying hyponatremia: A clinical guide to evaluation and management. *Nutrition in Clinical Practice, 37*(5), 1023–1032. https://doi.org/10.1002/ncp.10907

Brinkman, J.E., Dorius, B., & Sharma, S. (2023). Physiology, body fluids. In *StatPearls.* StatPearls Publishing. https://www.ncbi.nlm.nih.gov/books/NBK482447

Campbell, K., & Mortimore, G. (2022). The diagnosis and management of acute hyponatraemia in critical care. *British Journal of Nursing, 31*(18), 934–939. https://doi.org/10.12968/bjon.2022.31.18.934

Corona, G., Norello, D., Parenti, G., Sforza, A., Maggi, M., & Peri, A. (2018). Hyponatremia, falls and bone fractures: A systematic review and meta-analysis. *Clinical Endocrinology, 89*(4), 505–513. https://doi.org/10.1111/cen.13790

Cuzzo, B., Padala, S.A., & Lappin, S.L. (2023). Physiology, vasopressin. In *StatPearls.* StatPearls Publishing. https://www.ncbi.nlm.nih.gov/books/NBK526069

Dalal, R., Bruss, Z.S., & Sehdev, J.S. (2023). Physiology, renal blood flow and filtration. In *StatPearls.* StatPearls Publishing. https://www.ncbi.nlm.nih.gov/books/NBK482248

Dang, S., Zhang, S., Zhao, J., Li, X., & Li, W. (2024). The syndrome of inappropriate antidiuretic hormone associated with nasal and paranasal malignant tumors. *European Archives of Oto-rhino-laryngology, 281*(3), 1443–1448. https://doi.org/10.1007/s00405-023-08347-5

Danyalian, A., & Heller, D. (2023). Central pontine myelinolysis. In *StatPearls.* StatPearls Publishing. https://www.ncbi.nlm.nih.gov/books/NBK551697

Decaux, G. (2023). Morbidity associated with chronic hyponatremia. *Journal of Clinical Medicine, 12*(3), 978. https://doi.org/10.3390/jcm12030978

Fibbi, B., Marroncini, G., Naldi, L., Anceschi, C., Errico, A., Norello, D., & Peri, A. (2023). Hyponatremia and cancer: From bedside to benchside. *Cancers, 15*(4), 1197. https://doi.org/10.3390/cancers15041197

Fratangelo, L., Nguyen, S., & D'Amelio, P. (2023). Hyponatremia and aging-related diseases: Key player or innocent bystander? A systematic review. *Systematic Review, 12*(84). https://doi.org/10.1186/s13643-023-02246-w

Ghosal, A., Qadeer, H.A., Nekkanti, S.K., Pradhan, P., Okoye, C., & Waqar, D. (2023). A conspectus of euvolemic hyponatremia, its various etiologies, and treatment modalities: A comprehensive review of the literature. *Cureus, 15*(8), e43390. https://doi.org/10.7759/cureus.43390

Hamrahian, S.M. (2025). Hyponatremia workup. *Medscape.* https://emedicine.medscape.com/article/242166-workup

Heiland, L., & Heiland, K. (2023). Functional olfactory neuroblastoma inducing symptomatic SIADH. *Ear, Nose and Throat Journal, 102*(10), NP518–NP521. https://doi.org/10.1177/01455613211022102

Henderson, M.A., Gillon, S., & Al-Haddad, M. (2024). Organization and composition of body fluids. *Anaesthesia and Intensive Care Medicine, 25*(6), 432–438. https://doi.org/10.1016/j.mpaic.2024.03.014

Hunt, A., Essa, A., & Macnab, R. (2024). Regulation of fluid and electrolyte balance. *Anaesthesia and Intensive Care Medicine, 25*(5), 332–338. https://doi.org/10.1016/j.mpaic.2024.03.007

Imran, R., Zia, Z., Siddiqi, A.I., Shafiq, W., & Irfan, H. (2023). Overcoming challenges: Doxycycline as an alternative treatment for hyponatremia in managing syndrome of inappropriate secretion of antidiuretic hormone (SIADH) in small cell lung cancer (SCLC): A case report. *Cureus, 15*(7), e42102. https://doi.org/10.7759/cureus.42102

Jamhour, C., Haddad, A., & Daw, H. (2023). Severe hyponatremia during first cycle of cyclophosphamide/doxorubicin chemotherapy. *American Journal of Therapeutics, 30*(4), e369–e371. https://doi.org/10.1097/MJT.0000000000001476

Kengne, F. (2023). Adaptation of the brain to hyponatremia and its clinical implications. *Journal of Clinical Medicine, 12*(5), 1714. https://doi.org/10.3390/jcm12051714

Kharin, A., & Klussmann, E. (2024). Many kinases for controlling the water channel aquaporin-2. *Journal of Physiology, 602*(13), 3025–3039. https://doi.org/10.1113/JP284100

Krisanapan, P., Vongsanim, S., Pin-On, P., Ruengorn, C., & Noppakun, K. (2020). Efficacy of furosemide, oral sodium chloride, and fluid restriction for treatment of syndrome of inappropriate antidiuresis (SIAD): An open-label randomized controlled study (The EFFUSE-FLUID Trial). *American Journal of Kidney Diseases, 76*(2), 203–212. https://doi.org/10.1053/j.ajkd.2019.11.012

Lee, L.M.Y., Tan, S.Y.T., & Loh, W.J. (2022). High urinary sodium concentrations in severe SIADH: Case reports of 2 patients and literature review. *Frontiers in Medicine, 9,* 897940. https://doi.org/10.3389/fmed.2022.897940

Maesaka, J.K., Imbriano, L.J., Grant, C., & Miyawaki, N. (2023). Haptoglobin-related protein without signal peptide as biomarker of renal salt wasting in hyponatremia, hyponatremia-related diseases and as new syndrome in Alzheimer's disease. *Biomolecules, 13*(4), 638. https://doi.org/10.3390/biom13040638

Mc Donald, D., Sherlock, M., & Thompson, C.J. (2022). Hyponatraemia and the syndrome of inappropriate antidiuresis (SIAD) in cancer. *Endocrine Oncology, 2*(1), R78–R89. https://doi.org/10.1530/EO-22-0056

Mentrasti, G., Scortichini, L., Torniai, M., Giampieri, R., Morgese, F., Rinaldi, S., & Berardi, R. (2020). Syndrome of inappropriate antidiuretic hormone secretion (SIADH): Optimal management. *Therapeutics and Clinical Risk Management, 16,* 663–672. https://doi.org/10.2147/TCRM.S206066

Murashima, M., Ambe, K., Aoki, Y., Kasugai, T., Tomonari, T., Ono, M., ... Hamano, T. (2023). Epidemiology and predictors of hyponatremia in a contemporary cohort of patients with malignancy: A retrospective cohort study. *Clinical Kidney Journal, 16*(11), 2072–2081. https://doi.org/10.1093/ckj/sfad189

Najem, O., Shah, M.M., Zubair, M., & De Jesus, O. (2024). Serum osmolality. In *StatPearls.* StatPearls Publishing. https://www.ncbi.nlm.nih.gov/books/NBK567764

Noda, Y., & Sasaki, S. (2021). Updates and perspectives on aquaporin-2 and water balance disorders. *International Journal of Molecular Sciences, 22*(23), 12950. https://doi.org/10.3390/ijms222312950

Olaoye, O., Chamarthi, G., Rahman, M., & Bihorac, A. (2024). Bodily water and electrolyte abnormalities in neurological disease. In E. Mahanna Gabrielli, K.H. O'Phelan, M.A. Kumar, J. Levine, P. Le Roux, A. Gabrielli, & A.J. Layon (Eds.), *Textbook of neurointensive care: Volume 1: Neuroanatomy, diagnostic assessment, disease management* (3rd ed., pp. 211–231). Springer. https://doi.org/10.1007/978-3-031-62220-5_13

Paudel, S., Dhanani, M., Patel, K.H., Vakkalagadda, N.P., Sanker, V., Damera, A.R., ... Bhandari, P. (2024). Pulmonary tuberculosis in an adult presenting with severe hyponatremia: A case report and review of literature. *Clinical Case Reports, 12*(2), e8469. https://doi.org/10.1002/ccr3.8469

Petria, I., Indirli, R., Mantovani, B., Lanzi, V., Mantovani, G., & Ferrante, E. (2025). Recurrent hyponatremia due to syndrome of inappropriate antidiuresis after traumatic brain injury: Two case reports. *Frontiers in Endocrinology, 16,* 1536247. https://doi.org/10.3389/fendo.2025.1536247

Pivonello, R., Simeoli, C., Di Paola, N., Ferrigno, R., & Colao, A. (2023). Hydro-saline alterations in central adrenal insufficiency. In M. Caprio & F.L. Fernandes-Rosa (Eds.), *Hydro saline metabolism* (pp. 191–223). Springer. https://doi.org/10.1007/978-3-031-27119-9_7

Pliquett, R.U., & Obermüller, N. (2022). Endocrine testing for the syndrome of inappropriate antidiuretic hormone secretion (SIADH). In K.R. Feingold, S.F. Ahmed, B. Anawalt, M.R. Blackman, A. Boyce, G. Chrousos, ... W.W. de Herder (Eds.), *Endotext.* MDText.com. https://www.ncbi.nlm.nih.gov/books/NBK279055

Praharaj, D.L., & Anand, A.C. (2022). Clinical implications, evaluation, and management of hyponatremia in cirrhosis. *Journal of Clinical and Experimental Hepatology, 12*(2), 575–594. https://doi.org/10.1016/j.jceh.2021.09.008

Rahnea-Nita, R.-A., Stoian, A.-R., Anghel, R.-M., Rebegea, L.-F., Ciuhu, A.-N., Bacinschi, X.-E., ... Rahnea-Nita, G. (2023). The efficacy of immunotherapy in long-term survival in non-small cell lung cancer (NSCLC) associated with the syndrome of inappropriate antidiuretic hormone secretion (SIADH). *Life, 13*(6), 1279. https://doi.org/10.3390/life13061279

Rawson, A., Schwaderer, A., & Khalid, M. (2024). Acid–base and electrolyte disorders. In N. Liao, J. Mahan, S. Misra, R. Scherzer, & J. Schiller (Eds.), *Pediatric rotations* (pp. 111–127). Springer. https://doi.org/10.1007/978-3-031-59873-9_11

Reddy, P. (2023). Clinical approach to euvolemic hyponatremia. *Cureus, 15*(2), e35574. https://doi.org/10.7759/cureus.35574

Rondon-Berrios, H., & Sterns, R.H. (2022). Hypertonic saline for hyponatremia: Meeting goals and avoiding harm. *American Journal of Kidney Diseases, 79*(6), 890–896. https://doi.org/10.1053/j.ajkd.2021.07.020

Rossignon, P., Chaudhry, A., Alloum, M., Antoine-Moussiaux, T., & Soupart, A. (2024). Long-term persistence of inappropriate antidiuretic hormone secretion following minor head injury. *European Journal of Case Reports in Internal Medicine, 11*(12), 005028. https://doi.org/10.12890/2024_005028

Saha, S., Saha, T., Sharma, S., & Mahmood, N. (2023). An unusual association of idiopathic syndrome of inappropriate antidiuretic hormone secretion (SIADH) with interstitial lung disease (ILD). *Cureus, 15*(11), e48304. https://doi.org/10.7759/cureus.48304

Sekhon, S., Taha, K., Kim, L., Humphreys, R., Patel, T., Andrews, A., ... Abdulhussein, F. (2024). A pediatric case of reninoma presenting with paraneoplastic syndrome of inappropriate antidiuretic hormone secretion. *Hormone Research in Paediatrics, 97*(5), 515–522. https://doi.org/10.1159/000533521

Shankar, S., Sundar, S.S., Vaishnav, M.S., Thummala, K., Lekkala, L., Srikanta, S., ... Chitra, M.D. (2024). 7901 Clinical challenges of paraneoplastic endocrine metabolic syndromes: An illustrative example. *Journal of the Endocrine Society, 8*(Suppl. 1), bvae163.1037. https://doi.org/10.1210/jendso/bvae163.1037

Shelton, G. (2022). Syndrome of inappropriate antidiuretic hormone. In D. Camp-Sorrell, R.A. Hawkins, & D.G. Cope (Eds.), *Clinical manual for the oncology advanced practice nurse* (4th ed., pp. 749–753). Oncology Nursing Society.

Soleimani, M. (2023). Acid base homeostasis and serum bicarbonate concentration in syndrome of inappropriate antidiuretic hormone secretion (SIADH) with hyponatremia. *Frontiers in Endocrinology, 14,* 1321338. https://doi.org/10.3389/fendo.2023.1321338

Spanuchart, I., Watanabe, H., Aldan, T., Chow, D., & Ng, R.C.K. (2020). Are salt tablets effective in the treatment of euvolemic hyponatremia? *Southern Medical Journal, 113*(3), 125–129. https://doi.org/10.14423/SMJ.0000000000001075

Sterns, R.H., Rondon-Berrios, H., Adrogué, H., Berl, T., Burst, V., Cohen, D., ... Verbalis, J. (2024). Treatment guidelines for hyponatremia: Stay the course. *Clinical Journal of the American Society of Nephrology, 19*(1), 129–135. https://doi.org/10.2215/CJN.0000000000000244

Sun, W.-P., Wang, Y.-D., Gao, S., Wang, Y.-F., & Li, D.-W. (2023). A rare presentation of central pontine myelinolysis secondary to hyperglycaemia. *BMC Endocrine Disorders, 23*(1), 106. https://doi.org/10.1186/s12902-023-01361-y

Thomas, C.P. (2023, July 12). Syndrome of inappropriate antidiuretic hormone secretion (SIADH). *Medscape.* https://emedicine.medscape.com/article/246650-overview

Tkacs, N.C., & Herrmann, L.L. (2024). *Advanced physiology and pathophysiology: Essentials for clinical practice.* Springer.

Tobias, A., Ballard, B.D., & Mohiuddin, S.S. (2022). Physiology, water balance. In *StatPearls.* StatPearls Publishing. https://www.ncbi.nlm.nih.gov/books/NBK541059

Torres, N., Rios, H., Rios, G., Medina, Y., Valerio, L., Rosa, S., & Ortiz, A. (2023). FRI357: A rare case of paraneoplastic syndrome of inappropriate secretion of antidiuretic hormone in oropharyngeal squamous cell carcinoma. *Journal of the Endocrine Society, 7*(Suppl. 1). https://doi.org/10.1210/jendso/bvad114.1290

Vishal, M., Mohit, K., & Anil, V. (2023). A case of acute symptomatic hyponatremia secondary to aceclofenac-induced syndrome of inappropriate antidiuretic hormone. *Indian Journal of Pharmacology, 55*(3), 196–197. https://doi.org/10.4103/ijp.ijp_281_23

Wagner, K., Unger, L., Salman, M.M., Kitchen, P., Bill, R.M., & Yool, A.J. (2022). Signaling mechanisms and pharmacological modulators governing diverse aquaporin functions in human health and disease. *International Journal of Molecular Sciences, 23*(3), 1388. https://doi.org/10.3390/ijms23031388

Warren, A.M., Grossmann, M., Christ-Crain, M., & Russell, N. (2023). Syndrome of inappropriate antidiuresis: From pathophysiology to management. *Endocrine Reviews, 44*(5), 819–861. https://doi.org/10.1210/endrev/bnad010

Wendt, R., Fenves, A.Z., & Geisler, B.P. (2023). Use of urea for the syndrome of inappropriate secretion of antidiuretic hormone: A systematic review. *JAMA Network Open, 6*(10), e2340313. https://doi.org/10.1001/jamanetworkopen.2023.40313

Workeneh, B.T., Jhaveri, K.D., & Rondon-Berrios, H. (2020). Hyponatremia in the cancer patient. *Kidney International, 98*(4), 870–882. https://doi.org/10.1016/j.kint.2020.05.015

Wu, R., Li, C., Wang, Z., Fan, H., Song, Y., & Liu, H. (2020). A narrative review of progress in diagnosis and treatment of small cell lung cancer patients with hyponatremia. *Translational Lung Cancer Research, 9*(6), 2469–2478. https://doi.org/10.21037/tlcr-20-1147

Yarandi, S., & Shirali, A. (2023). Onconephrology: Core curriculum. *American Journal of Kidney Diseases, 82*(6), 743–761. https://doi.org/10.1053/j.ajkd.2023.04.014

Yasir, M., & Mechanic, O.J. (2023). Syndrome of inappropriate antidiuretic hormone secretion. In *StatPearls*. StatPearls Publishing. https://www.ncbi.nlm.nih.gov/books/NBK507777

Yucel, D., Mekheal, E., Kania, B., Aron, P., Kapoor, A., Tailor, R.P., & Maroules, M. (2022). A rare case of paraneoplastic syndrome of inappropriate secretion of antidiuretic hormone in cervical squamous cell carcinoma: A case report and literature review. *Journal of Community Hospital Internal Medicine Perspectives, 12*(5), 119–123. https://doi.org/10.55729/2000-9666.1109

Zhao, Z., Zhao, F., Jin, P., Hu, X., Tian, C., Liu, D., & Zhang, Y. (2023). SSRI/SNRI-induced hyponatremia: A case series of 26 patients in a single institution from 2018 to 2020. *Psychiatric Quarterly, 94*(2), 113–125. https://doi.org/10.1007/s11126-023-10018-x

Colleen McCracken, MSN, RN, CMSRN, CHPN, OCN®, NPD-BC,
and Hamza Abid, MS, APRN-CNS, AOCNS®, OCN®

CHAPTER 10

Tumor Lysis Syndrome

FAST FACTS

- **Description:** Destruction or lysis of large numbers of cancer cells following cytotoxic therapies (e.g., chemotherapy, biotherapy, radiation therapy) causes the release of potassium, phosphorus, and uric acid into the systemic circulation. This can result in hyperkalemia, hyperuricemia, and hyperphosphatemia with secondary hypocalcemia. Tumor lysis syndrome can also occur spontaneously (primary) or because of surgery.
- **Incidence:** Tumor lysis syndrome is the most common oncologic emergency in hematologic malignancies with a large tumor burden and high proliferative rate (e.g., Burkitt lymphoma, acute lymphoblastic leukemia). It can also occur, though less frequently, in other rapidly proliferating, highly chemosensitive and radiosensitive malignancies (e.g., small cell lung cancer). The most significant risk occurs within the first few days after starting cytotoxic therapy.
- **Clinical Manifestations:** The syndrome is often asymptomatic initially. Blood chemistry shows hyperkalemia, hyperphosphatemia, hypocalcemia, and hyperuricemia. Nonspecific manifestations include confusion, agitation, nausea, vomiting, muscle cramps, tetany, paresthesia, fluid overload, renal failure, lethargy, seizures, cardiac arrhythmias, and sudden death within one to five days of initiating cytotoxic therapy.
- **Risk Factors and Etiology:** Risk factors for tumor lysis syndrome include patient-related risk factors such as large tumor burden, elevated white blood cell count, and extensive lymphadenopathy, as well as treatment-related risk factors, such as chemotherapy, monoclonal antibodies, and corticosteroids.
- **Pathophysiology and Patient Evaluation:** Tumor lysis syndrome occurs when the rapid destruction of malignant cells releases intracellular components (e.g., potassium, phosphate, nucleic acids) into the systemic circulation. Laboratory studies include complete blood count, metabolic panel, total and ionized calcium, phosphorus, uric acid, lactate dehydrogenase, and urinalysis.
- **Advanced Practice Considerations:** A comprehensive history, physical examination, and baseline laboratory assessment should be performed for all patients at risk for tumor lysis syndrome. The Cairo-Bishop system should be used to diagnose tumor lysis syndrome.
- **Treatment Modalities:** Prevention and management are similar and include frequent monitoring of laboratory values; aggressive hydration and diuresis before, during, and after cancer treatments; and pharmacologic prophylaxis. Medical management involves treatment with allopurinol, febuxostat (outside the United States), or rasburicase. Additional treatment is based on specific metabolic disturbances.
- **Nursing Management:** The nursing role includes prompt identification of at-risk patients, especially those early in treatment for hematologic malignancies, to implement critical prevention strategies.

- **Outcomes:** Prompt recognition, diagnosis, and treatment are essential to preventing the metabolic changes related to tumor lysis syndrome. Nurses caring for patients with hematologic malignancies must maintain a high index of suspicion for this potentially life-threatening oncologic emergency.

Introduction

Tumor lysis syndrome (TLS) is a critical metabolic oncologic emergency that occurs from the rapid destruction of malignant cells, most commonly after the initiation of cytotoxic therapy. The abrupt release of intracellular ions and metabolites, including potassium, phosphate, and nucleic acids, can overwhelm the body's healthy homeostatic mechanisms, resulting in hyperkalemia, hyperuricemia, and hyperphosphatemia with secondary hypocalcemia. These metabolic derangements can lead to serious complications, most notably, acute kidney injury (AKI) through uric acid and calcium phosphate crystal deposition, and other life-threatening complications, such as cardiac arrhythmias, seizures, and multiorgan failure (Barbar & Jaffer Sathick, 2021; Howard et al., 2024). Nurses play a critical role in the prevention, early recognition, and timely management of TLS.

Incidence

The incidence of TLS varies greatly depending on the tumor type, disease burden, and treatment modality. TLS is the most common oncologic emergency in hematologic malignancies with high proliferative rates and large tumor burdens, such as acute lymphoblastic leukemia, acute myeloid leukemia, and high-grade non-Hodgkin lymphomas (particularly Burkitt lymphoma) (Barbar & Jaffer Sathick, 2021; Delaney, 2023; Olsen et al., 2023; Rahmani et al., 2019; Webster & Kaplow, 2021) (see Figure 10-1). In these high-risk populations, TLS can be seen in up to 42% of patients, with clinically significant cases occurring in a smaller proportion (Barbar & Jaffer Sathick, 2021; Howard et al., 2024). Pediatric patients are at increased risk due to the higher prevalence of chemosensitive hematologic malignancies and larger relative tumor burdens (Olsen et al., 2023).

TLS is less common in solid tumors because of a general slower growth rate and lower chemosensitivity (Alqurashi et al., 2022). However, it has been reported in tumors with high proliferative rates or large tumor burdens, and the incidence of TLS may be rising with the increase of newer, more aggressive cytotoxic and targeted therapies (Alqurashi et al., 2022; Webster & Kaplow, 2021). Most solid tumors associated with TLS are highly chemosensitive, but cases have also been described in tumors with moderate or low chemosensitivity (Alqurashi et al., 2022; Greguska, 2021; Rahmani et al., 2019; Webster & Kaplow, 2021).

The occurrence of acute, spontaneous TLS is a rare but serious event. Spontaneous development of TLS is fulminant at its onset with severe metabolic abnormalities, but as with other causes of TLS, it often is reversible. This can occur in a variety of

FIGURE 10-1. Malignancies Associated With Tumor Lysis Syndrome

Frequently Associated Malignancies	Occasionally or Infrequently Associated Malignancies
• Acute myeloid leukemia • Acute lymphoid leukemia • Chronic lymphocytic leukemia • Chronic myeloid leukemia • Hodgkin lymphoma • Myeloproliferative diseases • High-grade non-Hodgkin lymphomas, especially Burkitt lymphoma and diffuse large B-cell lymphoma	• Breast cancer • Colorectal cancer • Gastric cancer • Germ cell tumor • Gestational trophoblastic neoplasia • Head and neck cancer • Hepatoblastoma • Hepatocellular cancer • Leiomyosarcoma • Medulloblastoma • Melanoma • Merkel cell carcinoma • Metastatic prostate cancer • Multiple myeloma • Neuroblastoma • Non-small cell lung cancer • Ovarian cancer • Prostate cancer • Renal cell carcinoma • Rhabdomyosarcoma • Sarcoma • Seminoma • Small cell lung cancer • Testicular cancer • Thymoma • Transitional cell carcinoma • Vulvar cancer

Note. Based on information from Alqurashi et al., 2022; Barbar & Jaffer Sathick, 2021; Delaney, 2023; Olsen et al., 2023; Rahmani et al., 2019; Webster & Kaplow, 2021.

tumor types, including hematologic and solid tumors (Barbar & Jaffer Sathick, 2021; Greguska, 2021; Papapanou et al., 2023; Rahmani et al., 2019; Webster & Kaplow, 2021). Spontaneous TLS is not fully understood; one theory in solid tumors posits rapid tumor necrosis with resultant release of intracellular contents (Parsi et al., 2019). Unlike therapy-induced TLS, spontaneous TLS often presents without hyperphosphatemia, potentially due to ongoing phosphate reutilization by viable tumor cells.

Clinical Manifestations

TLS is often asymptomatic initially and typically detected through abnormal blood chemistries. Clinical manifestations caused by metabolic abnormalities may include weakness, mental changes, peripheral edema, oliguria and hematuria, flank pain, paralysis, nausea, vomiting, muscle cramps, tetany, paresthesia, fluid overload, renal failure, lethargy, seizures, cardiac arrhythmias, and sudden death occurring within one to five days of initiation of cytotoxic chemotherapy (Olsen et al., 2023). Symptoms may appear before treatment, but TLS typically develops 24–72 hours after treatment initiation, with signs and symptoms depending on the severity of metabolic abnormalities (Webster & Kaplow, 2021).

Hyperkalemia

Hyperkalemia (potassium level > 5.5 mEq/L) is life-threatening because of its effects on the heart. Elevated potassium levels can occur 6–72 hours after therapy begins. Levels above 6 mmol/L may cause the earliest electrocardiographic changes to appear, including tall, peaked T waves and a shortened QT interval. As serum potassium levels continue to rise, more severe conduction abnormalities develop, including progressive prolongation of the PR interval and widening of the QRS complex. The P wave may flatten or disappear entirely. In critical cases, the QRS complex may merge with the T wave, forming a sine wave pattern that can precede ventricular tachycardia, ventricular fibrillation, or asystole (Teymouri et al., 2022) (see Figure 10-2). Additional symptoms include ascending muscle weakness that begins with the legs and progresses to the trunk and arms, fatigue, nausea, vomiting, twitching, paresthesia, paralysis, diarrhea, lethargy, syncope, muscle cramps, and increased bowel sounds (Webster & Kaplow, 2021).

Hyperuricemia

Hyperuricemia can cause various symptoms, typically appearing 24–48 hours after therapy begins, when uric acid levels exceed 10 mg/dl (Adeyinka et al., 2024). At levels between 10–15 mg/dl, patients may experience gout, malaise, nausea, vomiting, diarrhea, lethargy, fatigue, weakness, flank pain, pruritus, and compromised renal function, including oliguria, anuria, azotemia, and acute uric acid nephropathy from uric acid crystallization (Adeyinka et al., 2024). Levels above 20 mg/dl can lead to severe complications with symptoms from progressive renal failure, such as edema, hypertension, hematuria, crystalluria, extreme lethargy, extreme somnolence, seizures, paresthesia, endocarditis, profound azotemia, and anuria, potentially resulting in acute and chronic renal failure (Adeyinka et al., 2024).

Hyperphosphatemia With Secondary Hypocalcemia

Hyperphosphatemia (serum phosphorus levels > 5 mg/dl) with secondary hypocalcemia can occur 24–48 hours after the initiation of the cancer treatment. Symptoms, often linked to renal dysfunction, include anuria, oliguria, azotemia, edema, and AKI (Adeyinka et al., 2024). Initially, the kidneys increase phosphorus excretion by increasing urinary excretion, but as the tubular transport mechanisms are overwhelmed, serum phosphorus rises. Acute renal insufficiency from uric acid or other complications can worsen hyperphosphatemia, leading to nausea, vomiting, diarrhea, lethargy, seizures, hyperreflexia, and decreased mental status. Calcium–phosphate precipitation in the renal tubules may further impair kidney function.

FIGURE 10-2. Progressive Electrocardiographic Changes in Hyperkalemia

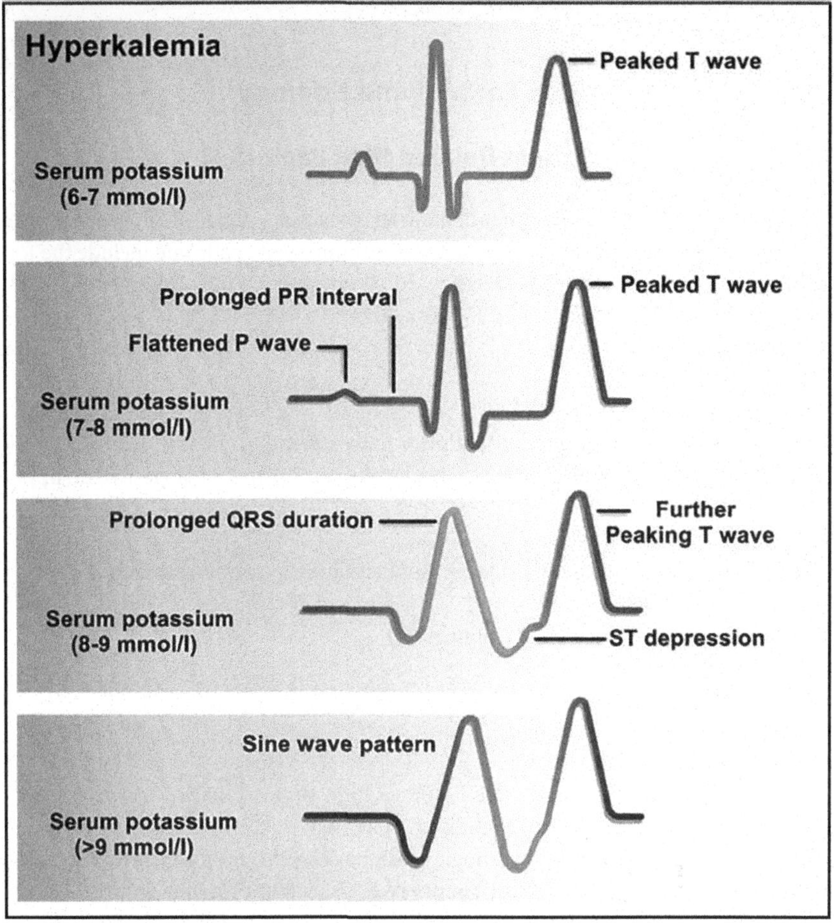

Note. Based on information from Teymouri et al., 2022.

Secondary hypocalcemia (serum calcium < 8.7 mg/dl) typically develops 24–48 hours after initiation of therapy (Adeyinka et al., 2024). It results from calcium binding to phosphorus in the systemic circulation, reducing ionized calcium. Symptoms include diarrhea, anorexia, twitching, paresthesia, muscle cramps, carpopedal spasms, anxiety, depression, confusion, hallucinations, positive Chvostek sign (facial muscle spasms following a tap on one side of the face), positive Trousseau sign (upper arm muscular spasms following pressure to the principal vessel and nerve of the limb), seizures, and laryngospasm with stridor (Webster & Kaplow, 2021).

Cardiac manifestations of TLS can include hypotension, tetany, syncope, ventricular arrhythmias, heart blocks, and, in severe cases, cardiac arrest (Rahmani et al., 2019). Hypocalcemia can lead to neurologic symptoms, such as anxiety, irritability, confusion, depression, and hallucinations (Adeyinka et al., 2024). Calcium phosphate precipitates can deposit in tissues, causing iritis, pruritus, arthritis, and gangrenous skin changes (Howard et al., 2024).

Risk Factors and Etiology

Patient-Related Risk Factors

Patient-related and pretreatment characteristics play a vital role in predisposing patients to TLS. Patient-related risk factors for tumor lysis syndrome include the following (Alqurashi et al., 2022; Delaney, 2023; Greguska, 2021; Olsen et al., 2023; Rahmani et al., 2019; Webster and Kaplow, 2021):

- Acidic urine
- Advanced age
- Bone marrow involvement
- Dehydration or poor urinary output prior to treatment
- Elevated lactate dehydrogenase (LDH) level prior to treatment (twice the upper limit of normal [ULN])
- Elevated white blood cell count (> 25,000)
- Elevated uric acid, potassium, and phosphorus levels prior to treatment
- Extensive lymphadenopathy
- High-grade tumors with rapid cell turnover
- Large tumor burden
- Liver involvement
- Lymphocytic disease
- Preexisting renal dysfunction

One of the most important predictors is high tumor burden, which refers to the overall volume or mass of malignant cells that exist in the body prior to the initiation of treatment. In hematologic malignancies, high tumor burden is often defined by notably elevated blast counts (e.g., ≥ 25,000 cells/mcl in acute leukemias), extensive bone marrow involvement, bulky lymphadenopathy (e.g., nodal mass > 10 cm), and elevated levels of LDH and uric acid (Howard et al., 2024; Olsen et al., 2023). In pediatric populations, thresholds such as a total tumor mass of greater than or equal to 500 g or greater than or equal to 300 g/m^2 of body surface area are also used to identify patients at high risk (Howard et al., 2024). In solid tumors, however, the definition is less standardized, generally including a tumor mass greater than 10 cm in diameter, multiple large metastatic lesions, or diffuse organ involvement, such as liver or bone marrow involvement (Howard et al., 2024). Although laboratory criteria guide the assessment in hematologic cancers, high tumor burden in solid tumors is primarily determined through imaging and clinical indicators, particularly when the tumor is chemosensitive and expected to respond rapidly to therapy.

Patients with preexisting dehydration, renal impairment, or renal failure are at increased risk for TLS because of reduced ability to clear the lysed tumor cells or their metabolic products during or after treatment. Patients with a lower glomerular filtration rate from advanced age are also at a higher risk (Webster & Kaplow, 2021). Furthermore, effective cytotoxic therapy can produce a large number of lysed cells, potentially overwhelming renal function.

Certain metabolic conditions may increase the risk of TLS. For example, patients with lymphocytic disease are at significant risk for TLS because the phosphorus content of lymphoblasts is three to four times greater than in healthy lymphocytes (Howard et al., 2024). Thus, cell lysis during therapy can elevate the levels of phosphorus in the circulation.

Treatment-Related Risk Factors

Chemotherapy is the most common treatment-related risk factor associated with the development of TLS. The use of a variety of chemotherapy agents may result in TLS (Durani & Hogan, 2020; Olsen et al., 2023; Rahmani et al., 2019; Webster & Kaplow, 2021) (see Table 10-1). Other therapies also pose a risk for the development

TABLE 10-1
Treatment-Related Risk Factors for Tumor Lysis Syndrome

Treatment	Agents
Biologic agents	Bispecific T-cell engagers (e.g., blinatumomab), chimeric antigen receptor T cells, BCL2 inhibitor (e.g., venetoclax), interferons, interleukins, monoclonal antibodies (e.g., alemtuzumab, brentuximab vedotin, gemtuzumab, nivolumab, obinutuzumab, pembrolizumab, rituximab), proapoptotic agents (e.g., lenalidomide), proteasome inhibitors (e.g., bortezomib, carfilzomib, oprozomib), tumor necrosis factor, tyrosine kinase inhibitors (e.g., alvocidib, dasatinib, dinaciclib, ibrutinib, imatinib, nilotinib)
Chemotherapy	Carboplatin, cisplatin, cladribine, cyclophosphamide, docetaxel, doxorubicin, etoposide, fludarabine, paclitaxel, mitoxantrone, oxaliplatin, hydroxyurea, cytosine arabinoside, intrathecal methotrexate, capecitabine
Hormone agents	Tamoxifen, corticosteroids
Miscellaneous agents	Nephrotoxic agents (e.g., amphotericin B, angiotensin-converting enzyme inhibitors, nonsteroidal anti-inflammatory drugs), agents that increase potassium (e.g., clindamycin), agents that increase uric acid (e.g., alcohol, ascorbic acid, aspirin, caffeine, cisplatin, diazoxide, thiazide diuretics, epinephrine, ethambutol, levodopa, methyldopa, nicotinic acid, pyrazinamide, phenothiazines, theophylline)
Radiation therapy	Ionizing radiation
Surgery	–

Note. Based on information from Alqurashi et al., 2022; Barbar & Jaffar Sathick, 2021; Delaney, 2023; Howard et al., 2024; Olsen et al., 2023; Salter et al., 2022; Webster & Kaplow, 2021.

of TLS, such as monoclonal antibodies, corticosteroids, hormone therapy, tyrosine kinase inhibitors, proteasome inhibitors, chimeric antigen receptor T cells, bispecific T-cell engagers, and proapoptotic agents (Barbar & Jaffer Sathick, 2021; Olsen et al., 2023; Salter et al., 2022; Webster & Kaplow, 2021). The incidence of TLS associated with these agents varies; however, the emergence of new therapies for malignancies highlights TLS as a potential risk.

Surgery and radiation therapy are also associated with TLS, although less than chemotherapy and biotherapy. TLS has been reported in patients after exposure to ionizing radiation (Kawamoto et al., 2023; Schiff et al., 2022). It can occur prior to the initiation of therapy because of autolysis of the cells or up to five days after therapy begins. Most often, it occurs a few hours to one to two days after the initiation of any treatment (Webster & Kaplow, 2021).

Specific therapies and medications may exacerbate metabolic abnormalities that can lead to TLS. Enteral and parenteral nutrition, oral potassium, and phosphorus supplements can disrupt electrolyte balance. Nephrotoxic drugs may impair renal function, leading to elevated potassium levels (Ikeda, 2024). Additionally, medications that increase uric acid levels, such as thiazide diuretics, can further disrupt electrolytes and increase TLS risk (Webster & Kaplow, 2021).

Pathophysiology and Patient Evaluation

TLS is a metabolic disturbance that is characterized by the release of intracellular components into the circulation caused by the massive lysis of malignant cells following cytotoxic therapy (Webster & Kaplow, 2021). This results in the rapid release of potassium, uric acid (from nucleic acids), and phosphorus into the bloodstream (Rahmani et al., 2019; Webster & Kaplow, 2021) (see Figure 10-3).

Hyperkalemia results directly from the intracellular release of potassium into the systemic circulation; renal failure and metabolic acidosis may further aggravate the condition. It is the most life-threatening electrolyte abnormality associated with TLS due to its cardiac effects, including arrhythmias, bradycardia, heart block, and cardiac arrest. Patients generally manifest symptoms related to hyperkalemia when the potassium level exceeds 6.5 mEq/L, which typically occurs within the first 12–24 hours after initiation of therapy (Rahmani et al., 2019).

Patients generally develop symptoms of hyperuricemia within 24–72 hours after the initiation of treatment and when uric acid levels exceed 10 mg/dl (Rahmani et al., 2019). The hyperuricemia develops when nucleic acid purines enter the circulation during massive cell lysis and are converted to hypoxanthine, then xanthine, and then to uric acid by the liver enzyme xanthine oxidase (Rieselbach et al., 1964) (see Figure 10-4). Uric acid is soluble at the healthy human body pH level (7.4); however, it can precipitate in the more acidic environment of the renal tubules (Larson & Pui, 2025; Rahmani et al., 2019). This precipitation can lead to crystallization in the collecting ducts and the ureters, causing obstructive uropathy and resulting in decreased glomerular filtration, increased hydrostatic pressure, obstructed urine flow, and potentially renal failure (Rahmani et al., 2019).

FIGURE 10-3. Metabolic Abnormalities Associated With Tumor Lysis Syndrome

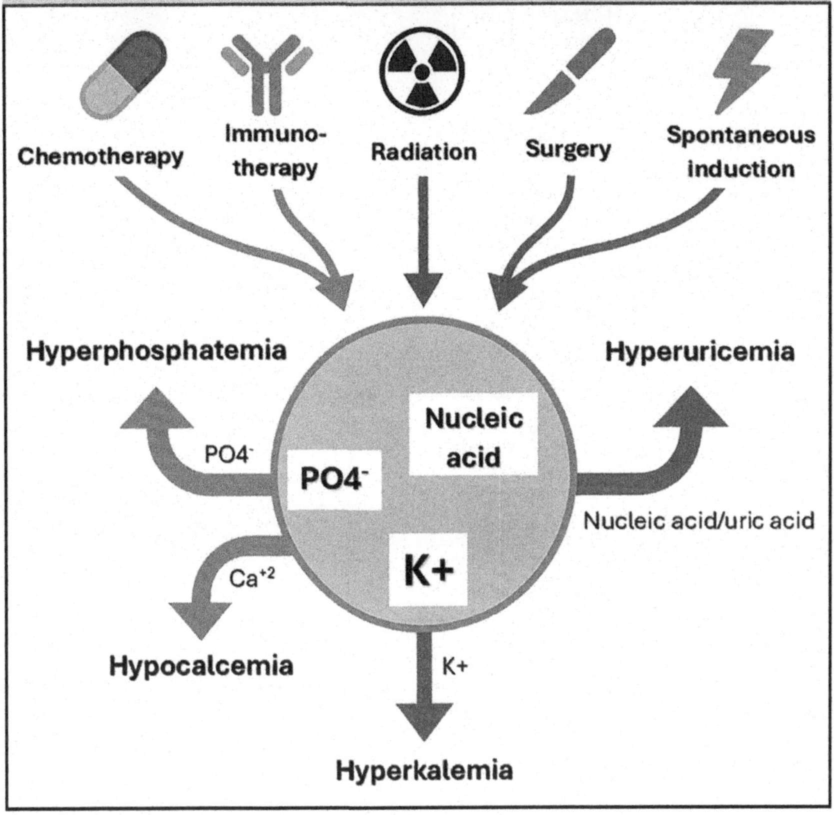

Ca^{2+}—calcium; K^{+}—potassium; $PO4^{-}$—phosphate

Note. Based on information from Barbar & Jaffer Sathick, 2021; Kawamoto et al., 2023; Rahmani et al., 2019; Webster & Kaplow, 2021.

The kidneys can excrete normal to moderate levels of uric acid; however, during TLS, excessive uric acid production can overwhelm the renal excretory capacity. AKI is a potential complication in TLS, and uric acid contributes to the development through mechanisms beyond crystal deposition, including renal vasoconstriction, inflammation, reduced renal perfusion, and impaired autoregulation (Barbar & Jaffer Sathick, 2021).

During TLS, intracellular phosphorus releases into the systemic circulation, causing hyperphosphatemia approximately 24–72 hours after initiation of therapy (Rahmani et al., 2019). Hyperphosphatemia is of particular concern in patients with lymphocytic diseases because of the high phosphorus content of lymphoblasts (Larson & Pui, 2025). Serum calcium binds with phosphorus in the circulation, leading to secondary hypocalcemia. Calcium phosphate salts may precipitate in the renal tubules and microvascular circulation, contributing to AKI. Renal

FIGURE 10-4. Purine Catabolism Pathway

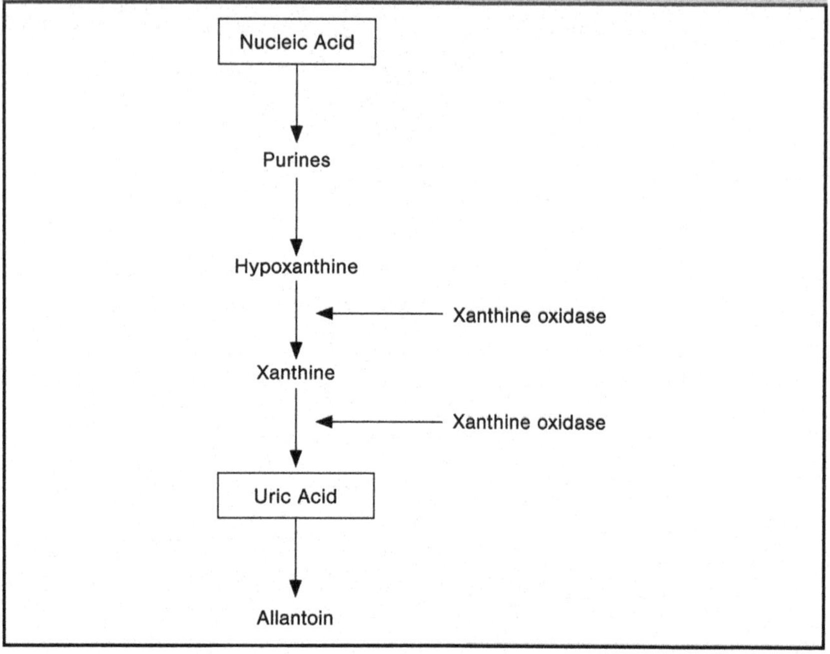

Note. Based on information from Rahmani et al., 2019; Rieselbach et al., 1964.

insufficiency exacerbates the existing hypocalcemia and hyperkalemia (Barbar & Jaffer Sathick, 2021).

Advanced Practice Considerations

TLS may develop unpredictably, sometimes within hours of treatment, so laboratory values should be closely monitored every 8–12 hours during the first 48–72 hours or more frequently if a patient's clinical status changes (Webster & Kaplow, 2021). Diagnosis is based on a combination of laboratory and clinical findings.

The Cairo-Bishop classification system, developed in 2004, remains the standard for the diagnosis of TLS. It includes specific laboratory criteria (see Figure 10-5) and a grading system for severity (on a scale from 0 to 5). This system is considered far more helpful than the National Cancer Institute Cancer Therapy Evaluation Program's *Common Terminology Criteria for Adverse Events* (2017). Laboratory diagnosis of TLS is based on changes in the serum values of uric acid, potassium, phosphorus, and calcium. An increase (e.g., potassium, phosphorus, uric acid) or decrease (e.g., calcium) of 25% from baseline laboratory values or a change above or below normal levels in two or more of these serum electrolytes within three days before or seven days after initiation of cytotoxic therapy indicates that laboratory TLS is present. Clinical TLS is defined as the presence of laboratory TLS plus one or more of the clinical TLS findings (Cairo & Bishop, 2004).

Within this system, Cairo and Bishop also developed a risk-grading classification based on the presence and severity of renal, cardiac, and neurologic clinical manifestations that can be used to help determine the need for aggressive prevention and treatment. TLS is graded along a continuum based on creatinine levels and the presence of cardiac arrhythmias and seizure activity, each of which is not considered to be caused by treatment effects (Cairo & Bishop, 2004). Grade 1 represents a laboratory creatinine level that is 1.5 times the ULN for the patient's age and gender, but without the need for interventions for cardiac arrhythmias or the presence of seizure activity. For grade 2, creatinine levels are elevated to more than 1.5–3 times the ULN.

Cardiac arrhythmias require nonurgent medical intervention, and mild seizures may be present, including a single brief generalized seizure, seizures that are well managed with anticonvulsant therapy, and focal motor seizures that occur infrequently and do not interfere with daily activities. Grade 3 is indicated by creatinine levels of more than three to six times the ULN, accompanied by cardiac arrhythmias that are symptomatic and may require a defibrillator for control. Seizure activity may result in an altered level of consciousness or be poorly controlled despite medical intervention.

In grade 4, the clinical effects of TLS are life-threatening. Creatinine is more than six times greater than the ULN. Cardiac arrhythmias may cause congestive heart failure, hypotension, and shock. Frequent and prolonged seizures may occur, leading to status epilepticus. Grade 5 is the last stage, or death, which is caused by the clinical effects of TLS (Cairo & Bishop, 2004).

A urinalysis helps to determine the urine pH and identify abnormalities, such as uric acid crystals. Patients with hyperkalemia require an electrocardiogram (ECG) to evaluate for arrhythmias or other ECG changes that may precede potentially fatal arrhythmias. The physical assessment of patients at risk should focus on those systems most affected by TLS, including the renal, cardiac, neurologic, and gastrointestinal systems. Patients' weight, vital signs, and fluid intake and output also require close monitoring. A decrease in blood pressure from baseline could be an indication that

FIGURE 10-5. Cairo-Bishop Definition of Laboratory and Clinical Tumor Lysis Syndrome

Laboratory Tumor Lysis Syndrome	Clinical Tumor Lysis Syndrome
• Potassium: > 6 mEq/L or 25% increase from baseline • Phosphorus: > 4.5 mg/dl for adults and > 6.5 mg/dl for children or 25% increase from baseline • Calcium: < 7 mg/dl or 25% decrease from baseline • Uric acid: > 8 mg/dl or 25% increase from baseline	• Creatinine: 1.5 × the upper limit of normal • Cardiac arrhythmias or sudden death • Seizures

Note. Based on information from Cairo & Bishop, 2004.

the heart is not pumping sufficient fluids into the kidneys and that renal status needs to be watched closely (McIntyre et al., 2021). Patients' weight, coupled with the intake and output, gives a good indication of their fluid and renal status, as well as the need for gentle or aggressive diuresis.

Treatment Modalities

Prevention Strategies

Prevention is the cornerstone of TLS management (see Table 10-2). Identifying at-risk patients is essential for prevention and allows for measures to be instituted 24–48 hours prior to the initiation of treatment. Prompt recognition is significant for those who have hematologic malignancies, such as acute leukemias and high-grade, aggressive lymphomas (Howard et al., 2024). In addition, LDH plays a significant role in identifying patients at high risk. It is an indicator of tissue damage, and levels of two or more times the ULN in these high-risk populations are key to identifying patients requiring more aggressive prevention approaches. Patients who fit into a high-risk profile and present with hyperuricemia and elevated LDH at baseline should be treated with aggressive volume expansion and rasburicase, rather than allopurinol, prior to treatment initiation (Adeyinka et al., 2024). Rasburicase is contraindicated in patients with a glucose-6-phosphate dehydrogenase deficiency due to the high risk of hemolytic anemia and methemoglobinemia, which can be life-threatening (Adeyinka et al., 2024). Key prevention strategies include frequent monitoring of laboratory values, aggressive hydration and diuresis prior to and during cancer treatments, and medication prophylaxis with allopurinol or rasburicase, depending on the presence of hyperuricemia at baseline.

Understanding patients' current medication regimen is essential for the prevention of TLS. Certain medications can contribute to an increase in serum potassium levels (e.g., heparin, potassium-sparing diuretics, angiotensin-converting enzyme inhibitors). Patients should avoid drugs such as aminoglycosides (e.g., gentamicin, amikacin, tobramycin, kanamycin), amphotericin B, nonsteroidal anti-inflammatory drugs, and other anti-inflammatory agents because they are known nephrotoxins and can compromise renal function (Webster & Kaplow, 2021). Radiographic dye studies should also be avoided because the dye may block tubular reabsorption of uric acid (Adeyinka et al., 2024).

Nutritional sources of potassium and phosphorus, including oral supplements and enteral or parenteral nutrition, may exacerbate hyperkalemia and hyperphosphatemia (Webster & Kaplow, 2021). Examples of foods high in potassium are oranges, bananas, tomatoes, chocolate, and orange juice. Examples of foods high in phosphorus are milk, meat, eggs, fish, nuts, cheese, bread, poultry, legumes, cereal, chocolate, and carbonated beverages. Patients should avoid these foods if their baseline potassium or phosphorus is elevated. A low purine diet can also help reduce increased uric acid levels, and patients should be educated to avoid high purine foods such as high-fat dairy products, alcohol, and fatty meats (Webster & Kaplow, 2021).

TABLE 10-2
Strategies to Prevent Tumor Lysis Syndrome

Strategy	Prevention Measures
Monitoring of laboratory values, including a complete blood count (with platelet count) and chemistries (blood urea nitrogen, creatinine, calcium, ionized calcium, phosphorus, potassium, and serum uric acid), urinalysis, and electrocardiogram	Perform at baseline and every 8–12 hours during the first 48–72 hours of treatment. Obtain urinalysis as needed to determine the presence of uric acid crystals. Obtain baseline electrocardiogram depending on patients' laboratory values or as needed to evaluate for cardiac arrhythmias.
IV hydration	Administer hydration with isotonic saline and 5% dextrose solution. Begin hydration 24–48 hours prior to initiation of therapy. Ensure urine flow of 70–100 ml/m²/hr.
Diuresis	Administer loop or osmotic diuretics to support urine flow.
Medication management	Avoid or substitute medications that contribute to an increase in serum potassium levels, such as heparin, potassium-sparing diuretics, angiotensin-converting enzyme inhibitors, and known nephrotoxins (e.g., aminoglycosides, nonsteroidal anti-inflammatory medications).
Dietary modification	Oral supplements and enteral/parenteral nutrition may exacerbate hyperkalemia and hyperphosphatemia. Depending on renal status, patients may need to avoid foods high in potassium or phosphorus. Due to increased uric acid, avoid high-purine foods such as high-fat dairy, alcohol, or fatty meats.

Note. Based on information from Adeyinka et al., 2024; Greguska, 2021; Howard et al., 2024; Olsen et al., 2023; Webster & Kaplow, 2021.

Hydration

Patients at risk for TLS should begin hydration 24–48 hours before treatment to optimize renal function and prevent TLS (Greguska, 2021; Webster & Kaplow, 2021). The type of hydration fluid should be individualized based on clinical context. Initial use of 5% dextrose and isotonic saline is commonly recommended. In regimens with high-dose steroid usage (e.g., acute lymphoblastic leukemia induction), sodium retention and hypertension could occur. In these cases, 5% dextrose with one-quarter normal (isotonic) saline is recommended (Howard et al., 2024). The goal of oral or IV hydration is to maintain a urine output between 70–100 ml/m²/hour (2 ml/kg/hour for both adults and children; 4–6 ml/kg/hour if ≤ 10 kg) (Olsen et al., 2023).

If needed, loop (e.g., furosemide) or osmotic (e.g., mannitol) diuretics may be used to support adequate diuresis and prevent renal tubular damage (Olsen et al., 2023). Effective hydration and diuresis improve glomerular filtration, inhibit calcium resorption, and promote excretion of potassium, phosphorus, and uric acid.

Medication Prophylaxis

In addition to hydration to increase urine output, prevention and management of TLS requires the use of medications, starting ideally 24 hours before cytotoxic therapy to achieve metabolic stability (Webster & Kaplow, 2021) (see Table 10-3).

Allopurinol is used to prevent TLS and works by inhibiting xanthine oxidase from converting hypoxanthine and xanthine to uric acid (see Figure 10-6). By inhibiting xanthine oxidase, allopurinol blocks the formation of uric acid, thereby preventing the development of uric acid nephropathy (Casper Pharma, 2023). It does not improve existing hyperuricemia. The oral adult dose of allopurinol is at least 300 $mg/m^2/day$ (100 mg/m^2 every eight hours), not to exceed a maximum dose of 800 mg/day (Adeyinka et al., 2024). Patients should receive allopurinol before initiation of cytotoxic therapy, during therapy, and for up to three to seven days after therapy is complete, depending on uric acid levels, tumor burden, white blood cell count (in hematologic malignancies), and other laboratory

TABLE 10-3
Medication Regimens to Prevent Tumor Lysis Syndrome

Medication	Dosing Parameters	Side Effects
Oral allopurinol	300 mg/day, max dose of 800 mg/day, to begin at least 24 hours prior to chemotherapy	Rash, diarrhea, increased liver enzymes, nausea, vomiting, hypersensitivity reactions, renal insufficiency or failure
IV allopurinol	200–400 $mg/m^2/day$ in single or divided doses, not to exceed 600 mg/day, to begin at least 24 hours prior to chemotherapy	Rash, diarrhea, increased liver enzymes, nausea, vomiting, hypersensitivity reactions, renal insufficiency or failure
Febuxostat (discontinued in the United States)	40 mg/day, to begin at least 24 hours prior to chemotherapy	Rash, nausea, dizziness, arthralgia, increased liver enzymes, cardiovascular thromboembolic events
Rasburicase	0.2 mg/kg IV once daily for 5 days, to begin 4–24 hours prior to chemotherapy	Fever, nausea, vomiting, abdominal pain, constipation, diarrhea, headache, mild to moderate hypersensitivity reactions; may cause hemolytic anemia or methemoglobinemia in patients with glucose-6-dehydrogenase deficiency (may require screening of these individuals)

Note. Based on information from Adeyinka et al., 2024; Prometheus Laboratories, 2018; Sanofi-Aventis, 2025; Takeda Pharmaceuticals, 2017; Webster & Kaplow, 2021.

FIGURE 10-6. Mechanism of Action of Allopurinol and Rasburicase

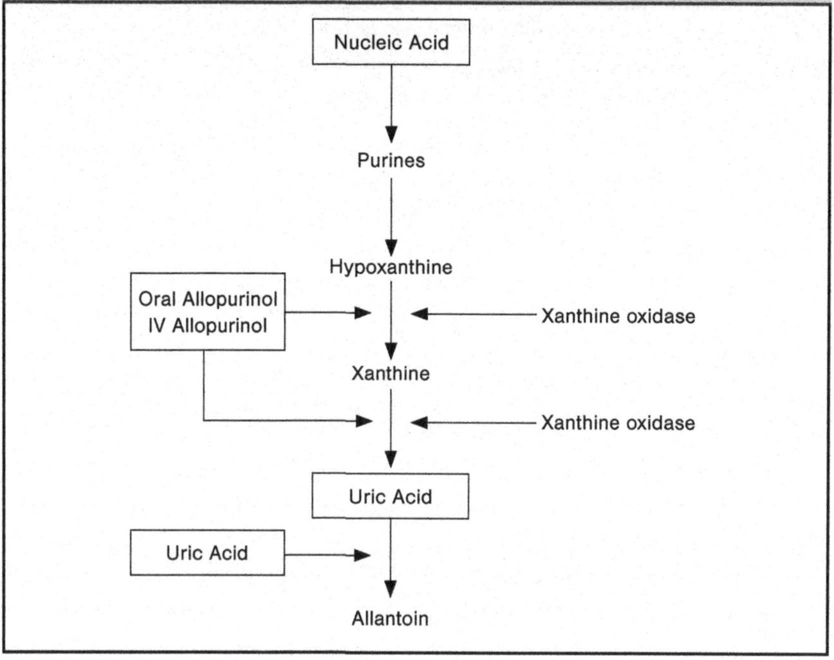

Note. Based on information from Barbar & Jaffer Sathick, 2021; Prometheus Laboratories, 2018; Sanofi-Aventis, 2025.

values. The reduction in uric acid levels occurs slowly, beginning one to three days after initiation of the drug. An IV preparation of allopurinol is available for patients unable to tolerate oral administration. The IV adult dose of allopurinol is 200–400 mg/m^2/day, in single or divided doses, not to exceed 600 mg/day, and should begin at least 24 hours before the initiation of cytotoxic therapy. The dose of allopurinol should be reduced by 50% for patients with AKI because of the risk of accumulation of the drug and its metabolites. Common side effects are nausea, diarrhea, rash, and increased liver enzymes (Prometheus Laboratories, 2018). Rare but serious side effects may include hypersensitivity reactions, such as vasculitis and Stevens-Johnson syndrome, as well as renal insufficiency or AKI (Larson & Pui, 2025; Prometheus Laboratories, 2018) (see Table 10-4). Allopurinol should be immediately discontinued if any signs of allergic reaction occur.

Allopurinol's inhibition of xanthine oxidase not only reduces uric acid formation but also impairs the catabolism of 6-mercaptopurine, 6-thioguanine, and azathioprine, resulting in increased systemic exposure and a higher risk of severe myelosuppression (Hirai et al., 2021; Turbayne & Sparrow, 2022). Because of the risk of toxicity from decreased drug clearance, it is recommended to reduce the dose of 6-mercaptopurine and azathioprine by 50%–70% when given with allopurinol (Prometheus Laboratories, 2018). This dose adjustment is essential to prevent life-threatening cytopenias.

Allopurinol may potentiate bone marrow suppression when combined with cytotoxic agents such as cyclophosphamide and may reduce the clearance of high-dose

TABLE 10-4
Treatment Recommendations for Metabolic Abnormalities Associated With Tumor Lysis Syndrome

Abnormality	Treatment
Hyperkalemia	Mild hyperkalemia (potassium < 6.5 mEq/L): sodium polystyrene sulfonate either orally or by retention enema, sodium zirconium orally Potassium > 6.5 mEq/L or with cardiac changes: IV calcium gluconate or calcium chloride (preferred if hyperkalemia is accompanied by hemodynamic instability), hypertonic glucose, and insulin accompanied by sodium polystyrene sulfonate or sodium zirconium cyclosilicate; loop diuretics, aggressive hydration
Hyperphosphatemia	Phosphate-binding agents, including calcium-containing antacids, hypertonic glucose plus insulin, aggressive hydration; loop diuretics
Hypocalcemia	Appropriate management of hyperphosphatemia, IV calcium gluconate or calcium chloride to treat arrhythmias
Hyperuricemia	Hydration, oral or IV allopurinol (best for prevention of uric acid), febuxostat, rasburicase; hemodialysis or continuous renal replacement therapy for significant renal compromise
Lactic acidosis	Volume replacement, correction of acidosis

Note. Based on information from Adeyinka et al., 2024; Barbar & Jaffer Sathick, 2021; Prometheus Laboratories, 2018; Rahmani et al., 2019; Sanofi-Aventis, 2017, 2025; Takeda Pharmaceuticals, 2017; Webster & Kaplow, 2021.

methotrexate, increasing the risk of toxicity (Coiffier et al., 2008). The risk of hypersensitivity reactions is increased when allopurinol is used with ampicillin, amoxicillin, thiazide diuretics, and bendamustine, particularly in patients with renal impairment (Conneely et al., 2020). Additionally, allopurinol can increase cyclosporine levels, requiring close monitoring for nephrotoxicity. The interaction with dicumarol may enhance anticoagulant effects, requiring periodic reassessment of coagulation parameters (Larson & Pui, 2025; Prometheus Laboratories, 2018).

Febuxostat is a nonpurine selective xanthine oxidase inhibitor used as an alternative to allopurinol for the prevention of TLS, particularly in patients intolerant to allopurinol or who have renal impairment (Takeda Pharmaceuticals, 2017). In 2025, its use in the United States was discontinued due to health concerns related to cardiovascular risks. Febuxostat effectively lowers serum uric acid levels with a safety profile comparable to allopurinol and may offer improved uric acid control while preserving kidney function, making it a viable alternative for patients who cannot tolerate allopurinol due to hypersensitivity or renal dysfunction (Barbar & Jaffer Sathick, 2021; Bellos et al., 2019). The recommended dose of febuxostat is 40 mg/day (Larson & Pui, 2025). Common side effects are rash, nausea, dizziness, arthralgia, and increased liver enzymes. Rare but serious adverse effects may include cardiovascular thromboembolic events (Takeda

Pharmaceuticals, 2017). Febuxostat should not be used in patients taking azathioprine or mercaptopurine, as these medications are metabolized by xanthine oxidase (Larson & Pui, 2025). Inhibiting this enzyme can lead to elevated levels of thiopurines in the bloodstream, increasing the risk of serious toxicity (Larson & Pui, 2025). Despite its efficacy, the higher cost of febuxostat compared to allopurinol and its noted cardiovascular risks has limited its widespread use.

Rasburicase is another medication used for both prophylaxis and management of TLS and is a recombinant urate oxidase derived from *Aspergillus.* It converts uric acid into allantoin, which is a metabolite that is 5–10 times more soluble in urine, which allows for rapid excretion (Yu et al., 2023). Rasburicase generates hydrogen peroxide, which can lead to methemoglobinemia and hemolytic anemia in individuals with glucose-6-phosphate dehydrogenase deficiency (Avidan & Quesenberry, 2023). Initially approved for pediatric TLS, rasburicase was also approved for adults with leukemia, lymphoma, and solid tumors at risk for TLS and with elevated plasma uric acid levels (Ikeda, 2024).

The recommended dosage of rasburicase is 0.2 mg/kg IV infused over 30 minutes once daily for up to five days, with chemotherapy initiation recommended 4–24 hours after the first dose (Sanofi-Aventis, 2025). Due to the high cost of this medication, alternative dosing strategies have been explored. Studies suggest that lower or single doses can be just as effective as the standard multidose regimen in reducing uric acid levels in patients at risk for or experiencing TLS (Barbar & Jaffer Sathick, 2021).

Common side effects of rasburicase are fever, nausea, vomiting, abdominal pain, mucositis, headache, constipation, and diarrhea. Other serious side effects include rash and mild to moderate hypersensitivity reactions that may result in anaphylaxis (Sanofi-Aventis, 2025). Patients should be closely monitored during infusion for signs and symptoms of infusion-related reaction, which may include hypotension, bronchospasm, urticaria, dyspnea, hypoxia, or chest tightness (Sanofi-Aventis, 2025). Rasburicase is contraindicated in patients with glucose-6-phosphate dehydrogenase deficiency due to the risk of hemolytic anemia or methemoglobinemia, particularly among those of African and Mediterranean descent (Sanofi-Aventis, 2025). To prevent degradation of uric acid, blood samples must be collected in prechilled heparinized tubes and transported in an ice bath for testing (Sanofi-Aventis, 2025).

Intervention Strategies

The metabolic abnormalities and clinical signs and symptoms associated with TLS may not appear immediately after initiating treatment but typically develop within 24–48 hours. Management should be guided by the specific symptoms that arise. Once clinical signs are present, prompt and aggressive intervention is essential.

Hyperkalemia

Hyperkalemia is often an initial sign of TLS and and represents its most common life-threatening complication. It may appear 6–72 hours after the initiation of cytotoxic therapy, and it is more dangerous when the excretory capacity of the kidney is overwhelmed due to AKI, chronic kidney disease, or concurrent acidosis that might exacerbate the hyperkalemia (Adeyinka et al., 2024; Larson & Pui, 2025). A temporary discontinuation of cytotoxic therapy may be necessary based on the degree of hyperkalemia.

Sodium polystyrene sulfonate and sodium zirconium cyclosilicate are oral treatments used for mild hyperkalemia (potassium < 6.5 mEq/L). Sodium polystyrene sulfonate can be administered orally or by retention enema and works by exchanging sodium for potassium in the digestive tract, binding potassium to reduce the total body potassium. Its onset of action is 2–12 hours orally and up to 24 hours when given rectally. Common side effects include gastrointestinal upset, and there is a rare risk of serious bowel complications (Sanofi-Aventis, 2017).

Sodium zirconium cyclosilicate also works in the digestive tract by exchanging sodium and hydrogen for potassium, which is then eliminated in the stool. It begins lowering potassium within an hour, and notable reductions are seen within two to four hours (AstraZeneca Pharmaceuticals, 2020). A common side effect is edema due to sodium content, so patients at risk for fluid overload should be closely monitored during treatment (AstraZeneca Pharmaceuticals, 2020).

IV calcium gluconate or calcium chloride can manage ECG changes. These agents help stabilize the cardiac membrane by counteracting the effects of the elevated potassium on the heart, protecting the myocardium (Webster & Kaplow, 2021). Calcium chloride contains approximately three times more elemental calcium than that found in an equal volume of calcium gluconate. Thus, if the hyperkalemia is accompanied by hemodynamic compromise, calcium chloride is the preferred medication (Rafique et al., 2021). Calcium drugs are accompanied by other therapies that work to lower the level of serum potassium. Hypertonic glucose and insulin shift the excessive extracellular potassium back into the intracellular stores, temporarily lowering serum potassium levels. The effect of these medications is not lasting; therefore, their use should be followed by medications that enhance potassium clearance, such as sodium polystyrene sulfonate. Diuresis with loop diuretics will also cause urinary potassium excretion (Russell & Kram, 2020). Patients with a serum potassium level greater than 7–7.5 mEq/L or ECG changes require continuous ECG monitoring (Rahmani et al., 2019; Russell & Kram, 2020). Frequent electrolyte monitoring is needed with these findings. Conventional hemodialysis is necessary if these measures fail to correct the hyperkalemia, immediately followed by continuous renal replacement therapy to prevent rebound hyperkalemia (Barbar & Jaffer Sathick, 2021).

Ultimately, the goal of treatment of hyperkalemia is focused on cardiac membrane stabilization, intracellular shift of potassium, and reduction in the total load of potassium.

Hyperphosphatemia and Hypocalcemia

Hyperphosphatemia usually occurs 24–48 hours after initiation of cytotoxic therapy, resulting from the rapid release of intracellular phosphate from malignant cells, which may contain up to four times more phosphate than healthy cells (Adeyinka et al., 2024). Treatment of hyperphosphatemia (serum phosphate level > 4.5 mg/dl in adults and 6.5 mg/dl in children) includes phosphate restriction and phosphate-binding agents (Webster & Kaplow, 2021). Oral calcium-based phosphate binders (e.g., calcium carbonate, calcium citrate) and non-calcium–based options (e.g., sucroferric oxyhydroxide, sevelamer, lanthanum carbonate, ferric citrate) are commonly used (Webster & Kaplow, 2021). Aluminum-based binders are generally avoided because of toxicity risks. Phosphorus levels can also be reduced by volume repletion with saline hydration and forced diuresis with a loop diuretic (e.g., furosemide, bumetanide) (Webster & Kaplow, 2021).

Once phosphorus levels normalize, secondary hypocalcemia (calcium level ≤ 7 mg/dl) often resolves without intervention. Calcium therapies should be reserved for those who are symptomatic, such as presenting with tetany, seizures, or ECG changes (Larson & Pui, 2025). Treatment of symptomatic hypocalcemia includes IV calcium gluconate and calcium chloride. IV calcium gluconate is preferred because calcium chloride must be infused through a central line, with the attendant risks of phlebitis and extravasation. Calcium infusions should be administered with continuous cardiac monitoring due to risks of arrhythmia and digitalis toxicity. Serial measurements of ionized serum calcium are recommended, and seizure precautions should be in place as appropriate (Adeyinka et al., 2024). Careful monitoring also prevents calcium–phosphorus precipitations and obstructive uropathy (Webster & Kaplow, 2021).

Hyperuricemia

The primary goals of treatment of hyperuricemia include inhibiting the formation of uric acid and enhancing renal excretion. Although the incidence of TLS has decreased with prophylactic measures, hyperuricemia remains a concern because of its potential to cause AKI. Allopurinol, a xanthine oxidase inhibitor, is commonly used for prevention. It does not affect existing uric acid, so it is less effective in rapidly lowering levels during acute TLS. Rasburicase is also an appropriate treatment for the management of hyperuricemia (Rahmani et al., 2019). It is critical to maintain aggressive hydration and diuresis (to flush out the allantoin) when administering rasburicase (Sanofi-Aventis, 2025). Patients should avoid thiazide diuretics, which decrease the renal excretion of uric acid by increasing its tubular reabsorption, potentially leading to hyperuricemia.

In patients with significant renal compromise, early intervention with hemodialysis is critical, and it is typically guided by symptoms and clinical deterioration rather than a single abnormal electrolyte level. Indications for hemodialysis include elevated uric acid level (> 10 mg/dl), uncontrolled hyperkalemia (> 7 mEq/L), symptomatic hypocalcemia, and a phosphorus level greater than 10 mg/dl. Hemodialysis is preferred over peritoneal dialysis because of its ability to rapidly and effectively correct the life-threatening electrolyte imbalances associated with TLS (Adeyinka et al., 2024). Continuous renal replacement therapy is often favored over intermittent hemodialysis to minimize the risk of rebound hyperkalemia, hyperphosphatemia, or hyperuricemia (Barbar & Jaffer Sathick, 2021).

Nursing Management

Prevention and Early Detection

Nurses play a key role in the prevention of TLS and its sequelae (see Table 10-5). The key to prevention is identifying at-risk patients, particularly those with hematologic

TABLE 10-5
Nursing Management of Patients at Risk for Tumor Lysis Syndrome

Related Event	Management
Prevention	Identify diseases that put patients at risk for tumor lysis syndrome. • Hematologic malignancies such as leukemia and high-grade non-Hodgkin lymphomas • Solid tumors, such as breast cancer, colon cancer, prostate cancer, neuroblastoma, and small cell lung cancer Identify pretreatment patient risk factors. • Dehydration or renal insufficiency • Large, bulky tumors with significant adenopathy • Hyperkalemia, hyperphosphatemia, hypocalcemia, hyperuricemia • Elevated lactate dehydrogenase level Eliminate excess sources of potassium and phosphorus. Review medications that may contribute to increased potassium and phosphorus, or those that can compromise renal function. Eliminate nutritional supplements containing potassium and phosphorus. • Oral supplements and enteral or parenteral nutrition • Foods high in potassium, such as oranges, bananas, tomatoes, chocolate, and orange juice • Foods high in phosphorus, such as milk, meat, eggs, fish, nuts, cheese, bread, poultry, legumes, cereal, chocolate, and carbonated beverages Administer prophylactic hydration and diuresis as needed to maintain urine output > 70–100 $ml/m^2/hr$. Administer prophylactic medications, including oral allopurinol, IV allopurinol, oral febuxostat, and rasburicase.
Early detection	Weigh patients daily. Adhere to strict input and output documentation requirements. Check vital signs every 4 hours or more often as needed. Monitor electrolytes at baseline and every 8–12 hours for the first 48–72 hours (or more frequently as needed). Monitor electrocardiogram as needed. Perform urinalysis as needed to observe for uric acid crystals.
Symptom management	Hyperkalemia • Check vital signs every 4 hours or more often as needed. • Monitor electrocardiogram as needed. • Restrict dietary sources of potassium. • Review the medication administration record for drugs that may contribute to the potassium level. • Administer medications as needed based on potassium level. – Sodium polystyrene sulfonate either orally or by retention enema; sodium zirconium cyclosilicate orally – IV administration of calcium gluconate or calcium chloride – Hypertonic glucose plus insulin – Loop diuretics

(Continued on next page)

TABLE 10-5
Nursing Management of Patients at Risk for Tumor Lysis Syndrome *(Continued)*

Related Event	Management
Symptom management *(Cont.)*	Hyperphosphatemia • Administer phosphate-binding agents. • Initiate forced diuresis with a loop diuretic (e.g., furosemide, bumetanide). • Restrict dietary sources of phosphorus. • Review the medication administration record for drugs that may contribute to the phosphorus level. • Perform volume repletion with saline hydration. Hypocalcemia • Administer medications for hyperphosphatemia (will likely self-correct the hypocalcemia). • Monitor the electrocardiogram as needed. • Institute seizure precautions when the calcium level is < 8 mg/dl. • Administer calcium gluconate or calcium chloride for cardiac arrhythmias. Hyperuricemia • Weigh patients daily. • Adhere to strict input and output documentation requirements. • Maintain aggressive hydration and diuresis to maintain urine output > 70–100 ml/m²/hr. • Administer rasburicase as needed. • Institute seizure precautions as necessary. • Administer allopurinol or febuxostat when uric acid is close to normal. Psychosocial support • Provide psychosocial support for patients and caregivers. • Include other healthcare team members to increase support for patients and caregivers.
Patient and caregiver education	Explain disease-, patient-, and treatment-related risk factors. Teach about the need to restrict dietary potassium and phosphorus in patients with preexisting renal impairment. Educate about treatment measures, including hydration and medication management. Provide information for patients treated at home regarding when to call their healthcare provider. Explain to patients and caregivers the potential need to hospitalize patients depending on their symptoms. Explain the potential need for a transfer of care to an intensive care setting depending on the patients' needs.

Note. Based on information from Adeyinka et al., 2024; Barbar & Jaffer Sathick, 2021; Prometheus Laboratories, 2018; Rahmani et al., 2019; Sanofi-Aventis, 2017, 2025; Takeda Pharmaceuticals, 2017; Webster & Kaplow, 2021.

malignancies, such as leukemias and aggressive lymphomas. Nurses should anticipate patient and caregiver education needs on specific prevention strategies (e.g., hydration, prophylactic medication) or implement these measures.

Understanding risk factors that contribute to the development of TLS is necessary to help prevent this syndrome. These factors include preexisting clinical conditions (e.g., dehydration, renal impairment), extent of the disease (e.g., large and bulky tumors, tumors with significant associated adenopathy), and preexisting laboratory abnormalities (e.g., hyperkalemia, hyperphosphatemia, hypocalcemia, hyperuricemia, elevated creatinine, elevated LDH that may become worse with treatment). Recognizing patients at risk for TLS allows nurses to institute preventive measures 24–48 hours prior to therapy. Dietary restrictions of potassium and phosphorus generally are indicated for patients admitted with preexisting renal impairment and metabolic abnormalities, such as hyperkalemia and hyperphosphatemia (Webster & Kaplow, 2021). Dietary consultations may help patients and caregivers understand any nutritional restrictions or necessary modifications.

Early detection of TLS is crucial for initiating prompt treatment and preventing serious complications. Regular monitoring of weight, fluid balance, and vital signs (e.g., irregular pulse) can help identify TLS-related changes (Greguska, 2021; Webster & Kaplow, 2021). Frequent monitoring of laboratory values for abnormalities is key, along with a meticulous assessment of the clinical signs and symptoms associated with the metabolic abnormalities seen in TLS (Greguska, 2021). Urine crystals suggest acidity and may indicate the need to immediately obtain the uric acid level (Adeyinka et al., 2024).

Symptom Management

The clinical course of patients at risk for TLS can change rapidly, requiring vigilant nursing care before, during, and after therapy. Monitoring should begin before therapy initiation, as spontaneous TLS may occur due to autolysis of tumor cells (Papapanou et al., 2023). Patients may experience metabolic changes within hours of treatment initiation (Webster & Kaplow, 2021). Skilled nurses need to be able to identify the clinical signs and symptoms, correlate them with laboratory results, and collaborate with the healthcare team to ensure timely and effective treatment.

For patients with hyperkalemia and cardiac changes, an ECG is appropriate for evaluation (Webster & Kaplow, 2021). Dependent on the severity, treatment may include medications, review of contributing drugs or supplements, or, in some cases, transfer to an intensive care unit setting for closer monitoring or interventions (Webster & Kaplow, 2021).

Hyperphosphatemia requires dietary restrictions and a medication review (Webster & Kaplow, 2021). Hypocalcemia may resolve with hyperphosphatemia treatment, but seizure precautions and ECG monitoring are needed for uncontrolled hypocalcemia.

If hyperuricemia is present, patients will require aggressive hydration to flush out the uric acid (Barbar & Jaffer Sathick, 2021). Allopurinol will not be able to manage existing hyperuricemia, as it inhibits the formation of uric acid but does not break it down once it is formed (Barbar & Jaffer Sathick, 2021). Patients may receive rasburicase if uric acid is elevated because this drug breaks uric acid down into allantoin, a more easily excreted metabolite (Rahmani et al., 2019).

Nurses should provide essential support to patients and caregivers during this potentially life-threatening experience, which may involve transfer to an intensive care unit and dialysis (Webster & Kaplow, 2021). Collaboration with chaplains, social workers, and other members of the interprofessional team further ensures that patients and families receive emotional, spiritual, and psychosocial support tailored to their individualized needs.

Patient and Caregiver Education

Education of patients and caregivers is essential for the prevention and management of TLS. They must be informed about risk factors, early identification, clinical manifestations, prevention and treatment (e.g., medications, hydration), dietary considerations, when to seek medical attention, and the importance of follow-up care (Webster & Kaplow, 2021). Patients at risk for TLS, often treated on an outpatient basis, need to understand the complexity of this syndrome (Webster & Kaplow, 2021). Early identification and correction of electrolyte imbalances are crucial and may reduce the need for hospitalization if clinical symptoms are recognized and treated promptly.

Nurses play a vital role in patient education and should provide written and oral instructions followed by teach-back to confirm understanding. Hospitalized patients should be informed of the potential need for escalation of care (e.g., hemodialysis, intensive care setting) depending on symptom severity. Given the diversity and complexity of symptoms and management strategies, patients and caregivers might become confused about the rationale behind specific treatments. For example, some might question the need for allopurinol if they do not have gout. This highlights the importance of clear, ongoing education to support patients' and caregivers' understanding, promote adherence, and improve outcomes (Jalali et al., 2021).

Summary

TLS is a potentially life-threatening metabolic emergency that can occur in patients with malignancies associated with large tumor burdens or rapidly proliferating cells. The symptoms of this syndrome most commonly occur because of cytotoxic therapy–induced electrolyte and metabolic disturbances. The metabolic changes may include hyperkalemia, hyperuricemia, and hyperphosphatemia with associated hypocalcemia. These electrolyte abnormalities may result in cardiac complications from the hyperkalemia; AKI caused primarily by hyperuricemia; and central nervous system complications, such as seizures from both hyperuricemia and hypocalcemia. Early identification of patients at risk and prompt treatment of the metabolic abnormalities are critical in managing this oncologic emergency. Education plays a key role in prevention and early recognition. Patients should be informed about the risks of TLS, common symptoms, and the importance of adequate hydration. They should be encouraged to report new or worsening symptoms, understand medication adherence, and follow monitoring schedules. Educating patients enhances engagement, supports early intervention, and contributes to better outcomes.

The authors would like to acknowledge Barbara Holmes Gobel, MS, RN, AOCN®, FAAN, for her contribution to this chapter that remains unchanged from the previous edition of this book.

References

Adeyinka, A., Kaur, A., & Bashir, K. (2024). Tumor lysis syndrome. In *StatPearls*. StatPearls Publishing. https://www.ncbi.nlm.nih.gov/books/NBK518985

Alqurashi, R.M., Tamim, H.H., Alsubhi, Z.D., Alzahrani, A.A., & Tashkandi, E. (2022). Tumor lysis syndrome in patients with solid tumors: A systematic review of reported cases. *Cureus, 14*(10), e30652. https://doi.org/10.7759/cureus.30652

AstraZeneca Pharmaceuticals. (2020). *Lokelma® (sodium zirconium cyclosilicate)* [Package insert]. https://www.accessdata.fda.gov/drugsatfda_docs/label/2020/207078s003lbl.pdf

Avidan, O., & Quesenberry, M. (2023). Rasburicase-induced hemolytic anemia secondary to undiagnosed G6PD deficiency. *Journal of Brown Hospital Medicine, 2*(4), 85108. https://doi.org/10.56305/001c.85108

Barbar, T., & Jaffer Sathick, I. (2021). Tumor lysis syndrome. *Advances in Chronic Kidney Disease, 28*(5), 438–446.e1. https://doi.org/10.1053/j.ackd.2021.09.007

Bellos, I., Kontzoglou, K., Psyrri, A., & Pergialiotis, V. (2019). Febuxostat administration for the prevention of tumour lysis syndrome: A meta-analysis. *Journal of Clinical Pharmacy and Therapeutics, 44*(4), 525–533. https://doi.org/10.1111/jcpt.12839

Cairo, M.S., & Bishop, M. (2004). Tumour lysis syndrome: New therapeutic strategies and classification. *British Journal of Haematology, 127*(1), 3–11. https://doi.org/10.1111/j.1365-2141.2004.05094.x

Casper Pharma. (2023). *Zyloprim (allopurinol)* [Package insert]. https://www.accessdata.fda.gov/drugsatfda_docs/label/2023/016172s065lbl.pdf

Coiffier, B., Altman, A., Pui, C.-H., Younes, A., & Cairo, M.S. (2008). Guidelines for the management of pediatric and adult tumor lysis syndrome: An evidence-based review. *Journal of Clinical Oncology, 26*(16), 2767–2778. https://doi.org/10.1200/JCO.2007.15.0177

Conneely, S.E., Cooper, S.L., & Rau, R.E. (2020). Use of allopurinol to mitigate 6-mercaptopurine associated gastrointestinal toxicity in acute lymphoblastic leukemia. *Frontiers in Oncology, 10,* 1129. https://doi.org/10.3389/fonc.2020.01129

Delaney, E. (2024). Metabolic emergencies. In J.M. Brant, D.G. Cope, & M.G. Saría (Eds.), *Core curriculum for oncology nursing* (7th ed., pp. 477–481). Elsevier.

Durani, U., & Hogan, W.J. (2020). Emergencies in haematology: Tumour lysis syndrome. *British Journal of Haematology, 188*(4), 494–500. https://doi.org/10.1111/bjh.16278

Greguska, C. (2021). Managing tumor lysis syndrome. *Journal of the American Academy of Physician Assistants, 34*(1), 10–13. https://doi.org/10.1097/01.JAA.0000723908.23506.85

Hirai, T., Shiraishi, C., Murata, T., & Iwamoto, T. (2021). Drug-drug interaction between azathioprine and allopurinol in patients with chronic kidney disease: A case series study. *BPB Reports, 4*(5), 170–174. https://doi.org/10.1248/bpbreports.4.5_170

Howard, S.C., Avagyan, A., Workeneh, B., & Pui, C.-H. (2024). Tumour lysis syndrome. *Nature Reviews Disease Primers, 10*(1), 58. https://doi.org/10.1038/s41572-024-00542-w

Ikeda, A.K. (2024, September 16). Tumor lysis syndrome treatment and management. *Medscape.* https://emedicine.medscape.com/article/282171-treatment

Jalali, R., Dalvand, S., & Tavakol, K. (2021). The effect of partnership-based education on adherence to treatment plans in patients after coronary artery bypass graft surgery. *Patient Preference and Adherence, 15,* 2977–2985.

Kawamoto, T., Karino, T., Muramoto, Y., Oshima, M., Kosugi, Y., & Shikama, N. (2023). Palliative radiotherapy induced severe tumor lysis syndrome in a patient with multiple myeloma with skin involvement: A case report and review of literature. *Cancer Diagnosis and Prognosis, 3*(2), 257–263. https://doi.org/10.21873/cdp.10210

Larson, R.A., & Pui, C.-H. (2025). Tumor lysis syndrome: Prevention and treatment. In A.G. Rosmarin (Ed.), *UpToDate*. Retrieved September 11, 2025, from http://www.uptodate.com/contents/tumor-lysis-syndrome-prevention-and-treatment

McIntyre, D., Havas, K., & Bonner, A. (2021). Monitoring for intradialytic hypotension: An audit of nursing practice. *Journal of Renal Care, 47*(1), 27–33. https://doi.org/10.1111/jorc.12343

National Cancer Institute Cancer Therapy Evaluation Program. (2017). *Common Terminology Criteria for Adverse Events* [v.5.0]. https://dctd.cancer.gov/research/ctep-trials/for-sites/adverse-events/ctcae-v5-5x7.pdf

Olsen, M., LeFebvre, K.B., Walker, S.L., & Dunphy, E.P. (Eds.). (2023). *Chemotherapy and immunotherapy guidelines and recommendations for practice* (2nd ed.). Oncology Nursing Society.

Papapanou, M., Athanasopoulos, A.E., Georgiadi, E., Maragkos, S.A., Liontos, M., Ziogas, D.C., ... Schizas, D. (2023). Spontaneous tumor lysis syndrome in patients with solid tumors: A scoping review of the literature. *Medical Oncology, 40*(8), 233. https://doi.org/10.1007/s12032-023-02108-4

Parsi, M., Rai, M., & Clay, C. (2019). You can't always blame the chemo: A rare case of spontaneous tumor lysis syndrome in a patient with invasive ductal cell carcinoma of the breast. *Cureus, 11*(11), e6186. https://doi.org/10.7759/cureus.6186

Prometheus Laboratories. (2018). *Zyloprim® (allopurinol)* [Package insert]. https://www.accessdata.fda.gov/drugsatfda_docs/label/2018/016084s044lbl.pdf

Rafique, Z., Peacock, F., Armstead, T., Bischof, J.J., Hudson, J., Weir, M.R., & Neuenschwander, J. (2021). Hyperkalemia management in the emergency department: An expert panel consensus. *Journal of the American College of Emergency Physicians Open, 2*(5), e12572. https://doi.org/10.1002/emp2.12572

Rahmani, B., Patel, S., Seyam, O., Gandhi, J., Reid, I., Smith, N., & Khan, S.A. (2019). Current understanding of tumor lysis syndrome. *Hematological Oncology, 37*(5) 537–547. https://doi.org/10.1002/hon.2668

Rieselbach, R.E., Bentzel, C.J., Cotlove, E., Frei, E., III, & Freireich, E.J. (1964). Uric acid excretion and renal function in the acute hyperuricemia of leukemia: Pathogenesis and therapy of uric acid nephropathy. *American Journal of Medicine, 37*(6), 872–884. https://doi.org/10.1016/0002-9343(64)90130-5

Russell, T.B., & Kram, D.E. (2020). Tumor lysis syndrome. *Pediatrics in Review, 41*(1), 20–26. https://doi.org/10.1542/pir.2018-0243

Salter, B., Burns, I., Fuller, K., Eshaghpour, A., Lionel, A.C., & Crowther, M. (2022). Tyrosine kinase inhibitors and tumor lysis syndrome in hematologic malignancies: A systemic review. *European Journal of Haematology, 109*(2), 166–181. https://doi.org/10.1111/ejh.13786

Sanofi-Aventis. (2017). *Kayexalate® (sodium polystyrene sulfonate) [Package insert].* https://www.accessdata.fda.gov/drugsatfda_docs/label/2017/011287s026lbl.pdf

Sanofi-Aventis. (2025). *Elitek® (rasburicase)* [Package insert]. https://products.sanofi.us/elitek/elitek.pdf

Schiff, J.P., Spraker, M.B., Duriseti, S., Shaikh, S., Murad, H.F., Mutch, D.G., ... Lin, A.J. (2022). Tumor lysis syndrome in a patient with metastatic endometrial cancer treated with lattice stereotactic body radiation therapy. *Advances in Radiation Oncology, 7*(1), 100797. https://doi.org/10.1016/j.adro.2021.100797

Takeda Pharmaceuticals. (2017). *Uloric (febuxostat)* [Package insert]. https://www.accessdata.fda.gov/drugsatfda_docs/label/2017/021856s011lbl.pdf

Teymouri, N., Mesbah, S., Navabian, S.M.H., Shekouh, D., Najafabadi, M.M., Norouzkhani, N., ... Deravi, N. (2022). ECG frequency changes in potassium disorders: A narrative review. *American Journal of Cardiovascular Disease, 12*(3), 112–124.

Turbayne, A.K., & Sparrow, M.P. (2022). Low-dose azathioprine in combination with allopurinol: The past, present and future of this useful duo. *Digestive Diseases and Sciences, 67*(12), 5382–5391. https://doi.org/10.1007/s10620-022-07719-x

Webster, J.S., & Kaplow, R. (2021). Tumor lysis syndrome: Implications for oncology nursing practice. *Seminars in Oncology Nursing, 37*(2), 151136. https://doi.org/10.1016/j.soncn.2021.151136

Yu, L., Xie, Y., Ma, J., Li, G., & Yuan, X. (2023). Rasburicase-induced falsely low measurement of uric acid in tumor lysis syndrome: A report of two cases. *Cureus, 15*(1), e34435. https://doi.org/10.7759/cureus.34435

SECTION III

HEMATOLOGIC EMERGENCIES

Diane G. Cope, PhD, APRN, BC, AOCNP®,
and Abigail Tesar, BSN, RN, OCN®, TCTCN™

CHAPTER 11

Bleeding

FAST FACTS

- **Description:** Bleeding can result from a reduction in platelets, an alteration in clotting factors, a paraneoplastic syndrome, infection, hepatic problems, or a combination of these factors.
- **Incidence:** Bleeding can occur with any cancer, but especially in patients with hematologic malignancies.
- **Clinical Manifestations:** Signs of bleeding include petechiae, ecchymoses, bruising, epistaxis, hemoptysis, hematemesis, melena, hematuria, and vaginal bleeding.
- **Risk Factors and Etiology:** Risk factors include malignancy, especially with hematologic, lung, prostate, and colorectal cancers; infection; liver disease; and coagulation disorders. Malignancy can be an etiology of bleeding and thrombosis due to local tumor invasion or adverse effects from cancer-specific therapy.
- **Pathophysiology and Patient Evaluation:** Hemostasis is regulated by a balance between clot formation (coagulation) and clot dissolution (fibrinolysis). Malignancy can lead to bleeding through alterations in platelet count and function, activation of the coagulation cascade, disruption in vascular integrity, and the effects of antineoplastic therapies.
- **Advanced Practice Considerations:** Advanced practice providers play a key role in astute assessment and execution of prompt interventions to prevent and control major bleeding episodes in patients with cancer. Tests include complete blood count, stool hemoccult, urinalysis, and coagulation tests.
- **Treatment Modalities:** Interventions for managing bleeding include transfusions, vitamin K therapy, vasopressive hormones, and mechanical measures.
- **Nursing Management:** Recognition of early signs and symptoms of bleeding or coagulation is key in the nurse's assessment. Bleeding precautions are implemented for at-risk patients.
- **Outcomes:** Patients with cancer are at high risk for bleeding, which is associated with a poor prognosis and an increased risk of morbidity and mortality. Prompt recognition and initiation of appropriate treatment are crucial to patient outcomes.

Introduction

Alterations in hemostasis, including bleeding and coagulation disorders, can have clinically significant adverse effects on patients with cancer and can greatly affect morbidity and mortality (Johnny, 2021). Several factors associated with malignancy can contribute to the etiology of bleeding and thrombosis, including local tumor invasion, tumor angiogenesis, systemic effects of the cancer, anticancer treatments, invasive diagnostic and surgical procedures, radiation therapy, central venous catheters, and anticoagulation therapy (Englisch et al., 2024; Johnstone & Rich, 2018). The risk for bleeding in patients with cancer can be tumor related or from the adverse effects of cancer-specific therapies, alterations in platelet number or function, consumption or alteration of clotting factors (e.g., disseminated intravascular coagulation [DIC]), or hyperfibrinolysis (Johnny, 2021; Wang et al., 2022). The presence of infection and liver disease can each alter the coagulation pathway, increasing the risk for bleeding (Kanikarla-Marie et al., 2021). The risk of bleeding increases in patients with cancer, and bleeding events are associated with a poor prognosis and an increased risk of death (Englisch et al., 2024).

Because bleeding poses dire consequences for patients, management plans should include bleeding prevention and patient education. To increase survival rates, rapid recognition, assessment of the precipitating factors, and knowledge of the treatment of bleeding are necessary. Ongoing bleeding can affect patients' quality of life by causing fatigue and weakness. If left untreated, bleeding may progress to a life-threatening hemorrhage. The ability to recognize early signs of bleeding and initiate interventions can dramatically improve patients' quality of life and increase their potential for survival. Oncology nurses, both in ambulatory and inpatient settings, play an important part in preventing, assessing, and managing major bleeding events and should be knowledgeable about evidence-based interventions.

Incidence

In general, bleeding can occur with any cancer, and there are no specific incidence rates for this complication. Bleeding risk is increased in patients with a history of hematologic malignancy, followed by lung, prostate, and colorectal cancers (Ajabnoor et al., 2023). Approximately 10% of all patients with advanced cancer and 30% of patients with hematologic malignancies will have at least one episode of bleeding (Johnstone & Rich, 2018).

Bleeding in individuals with hematologic cancers is associated with bone marrow alterations, often resulting in thrombocytopenia, a reduction in the number of circulating platelets. Therefore, the incidence and severity of bleeding in patients with acute leukemia are greater than in patients with solid tumors. A high percentage of blasts has been reported to increase the risk of bleeding in acute leukemia (Limijadi et al., 2021).

Clinical Manifestations

Bleeding manifests in several ways among patients with cancer. Signs of bleeding without visible hemorrhage can include petechiae, ecchymoses, bruising, tachycardia, or mental status changes. This type of bleeding may often be overlooked because it is not thought of as active bleeding and manifests as covert signs. Overt signs of bleeding include epistaxis, hemoptysis, hematemesis, melena, hematuria, vaginal bleeding, and bleeding around wounds and vascular access devices (Johnstone & Rich, 2018). In performing a patient assessment and clinical examination, nurses must evaluate the source of bleeding and the severity of bleeding that may necessitate immediate intervention. Bleeding can begin slowly and present as oozing, but it can progress to an acute hemorrhagic event. Even the smallest amount of bleeding can eventually lead to absolute anemia, defined as a reduction in the number or volume of circulating red blood cells.

Anemia is defined as a reduction in one or more of the major red blood cell measurements, including the hemoglobin concentrate, hematocrit, and red blood cell count (Turner et al., 2023). If bleeding is present in patients with cancer, anemia will most likely develop. Patients with bleeding can show symptoms of anemia, including fatigue, pallor, dizziness, irritability, weakness, chest pain, shortness of breath, decreased body temperature, and numbness in the hands and feet. Hypotension and tachycardia may be present.

Several organ systems are sensitive to the effects of bleeding and anemia (see Table 11-1). Nurses should instruct patients about the signs and symptoms of anemia and the need for immediate follow-up with their physicians.

Risk Factors and Etiology

Patients with cancer have numerous risk factors for bleeding (see Table 11-2). Bleeding can range from low-grade oozing to major episodic bleeding and can be caused by the cancer itself, with local tumor invasion, abnormal tumor vasculature, or tumor progression. It may also be related to current or prior treatments, including radiation therapy, chemotherapy, immunotherapy, an antiangiogenic agent (e.g., bevacizumab), or an anticoagulant (Johnstone & Rich, 2018). Antineoplastic therapies increase the risk for bleeding by damaging healthy tissues and altering platelet production. Radiation therapy and steroid treatment can cause blood vessels to become fragile and more prone to injury.

Tumor growth can lead to bleeding through invasion into the surrounding structures and blood vessels, as well as the bone marrow. Leukemias and lymphomas are

TABLE 11-1
Effects of Bleeding on Selected Organ Systems

Organ System	Cause	Effect
Gastrointestinal	Decreased oxygenation	Abdominal pain, tarry stools, hematemesis
Integumentary	Decreased oxygenation	Thinning and graying of hair, loss of skin elasticity, bruising, petechiae, purpura, ecchymosis, hematomas
Nervous	Myelin degeneration	Loss of nerve fibers, mental status changes
Renal	Kidneys release renin	Salt and water retention, edema, hematuria, decreased urine output

Note. Based on information from Rodriguez, 2018.

TABLE 11-2
Risk Factors Contributing to Bleeding in Patients With Cancer

Type	Risk Factors
Anatomic	Local tumor invasion Tumor involvement of vascular tissue Tumor location near major vessels Head and neck tumors
Systemic	Older age Anemia Hypoalbuminemia Hyperleukocytosis Bone marrow involvement by tumor Bone marrow suppression Concomitant disease (e.g., cirrhosis, uremia) Malnutrition Vitamin K deficiency Disseminated intravascular coagulation Infection (viral and fungal) Fever Liver failure Renal impairment Stem cell transplant Radiation therapy Medications (e.g., anticoagulants, aspirin, nonsteroidal anti-inflammatory drugs, corticosteroids, chemotherapy, immunotherapies, antiangiogenic agents, antibiotics [specifically penicillin, ceftriaxone, rifampin, and vancomycin], phenothiazines, heparin, antimalarial drugs, carbamazepine, mirtazapine, tamoxifen, methotrexate, lovastatin)

Note. Based on information from Driver et al., 2019; Escobar et al., 2022; Geng, 2024; Johnstone & Rich, 2018; Rodriguez, 2018; Yao et al., 2020.

the most common cancers associated with bone marrow invasion. In these diseases, the malignant cells crowd out the healthy cells in the marrow, leading to thrombocytopenia, anemia, and neutropenia. Tumors can also erode and enter mucous membranes and cause bleeding by local tissue disruption. Tumors that are close to large blood vessels put patients at risk for a massive hemorrhage (Englisch et al., 2024).

Platelet function can be affected by numerous drugs, especially aspirin and nonsteroidal anti-inflammatory drugs, such as ibuprofen, which can drastically reduce platelet aggregation (Driver et al., 2019). The effects of aspirin can last approximately 48 hours when platelet function starts to recover, with full recovery at 96 hours (Driver et al., 2019).

Antibiotic use can also contribute to bleeding risk, with platelet dysfunction maximized one to three days after the start of administration and continuing for several days after the antibiotic course is completed (Geng, 2024). In addition, corticosteroids affect the gastric mucosa and impair wound healing, resulting in the skin becoming thin, fragile, and at risk for gastrointestinal bleeding (Butler et al., 2019).

Infection and fever, mainly sepsis, increase the risk of bleeding in several situations. DIC, a possible complication of sepsis, can result in a fatal bleeding event (Tsantes et al., 2023). Viruses can cause myelosuppression or thrombocytopenia, and fungal infections, especially in the lungs, can lead to fatal hemorrhage (Porzionato et al., 2022; Raadsen et al., 2021).

Vitamin K is necessary for proper coagulation and is absorbed solely from the diet. Malnutrition can lead to an increased risk of bleeding because of a vitamin K deficiency, which can develop as a direct result of a dietary deficiency, biliary obstruction, malabsorption syndromes, liver disease, and anticoagulation therapy (Paulus et al., 2024).

Uremia is another risk factor for bleeding and is related to platelet dysfunction, including a reduced platelet count and increased platelet turnover. In addition, uremia can cause decreased platelet adhesion and aggregation. Uremic toxins, increased production of nitric oxide, prostacyclin, calcium, and cyclic adenosine monophosphate, along with renal anemia, cause these symptoms (Diaz et al., 2023). Bleeding in uremic patients most commonly manifests in the mucocutaneous areas and puncture sites as ecchymosis, purpura, epistaxis, gastrointestinal and genitourinary bleeding, and subdural hematomas.

Pathophysiology and Patient Evaluation

Control of bleeding (hemostasis) is maintained through a finely regulated balance between clot formation (coagulation) and clot dissolution (fibrinolysis). The presence of malignancy disrupts this essential balance. It can lead to bleeding through several different mechanisms, including alterations in platelet count and function, activation of the coagulation cascade, disruption in vascular integrity, and the effects of antineoplastic therapies. Patients with cancer often have more than one of these conditions co-occurring, putting them at increased risk for bleeding (Englisch et al., 2024).

Platelets and Thrombocytopenia

Platelets are integral to the process of hemostasis. These are not true cells but rather fragments of megakaryocytes, which are giant cells within the bone marrow integral to the production of platelets. When fragmented, a megakaryocyte can release more than 1,000 platelets. The hormone thrombopoietin regulates the platelet production process. In the event of an injury or a cut that breaks the endothelial layer of a blood vessel, platelets function as first responders to form a clot that seals the injury site and inhibits blood loss (Sang et al., 2021). Disorders of platelet function and platelet abnormalities can affect the clotting process and put an individual at risk for severe and possibly fatal bleeding.

Thrombocytopenia is the platelet abnormality most frequently associated with cancer. Several factors are linked with the development of thrombocytopenia, including reduced platelet production, a change in platelet distribution, increased platelet destruction, vascular dilution of platelets, platelet consumption as seen in DIC, and with some drug therapies, including beta-lactam antibiotics, nitrates, beta-blockers, tricyclic antidepressants, and selective serotonin reuptake inhibitors (Gauer & Whitaker, 2022; Kuter, 2022).

Decreased platelet production can occur secondary to direct invasion of the bone marrow by tumor cells or from the myelosuppressive effects of chemotherapy or radiation therapy. When a large burden of tumor cells overwhelms the normal elements of bone marrow, the resulting thrombocytopenia reflects an overall pancytopenia in which all cell lines are reduced. The occurrence and severity of treatment-associated thrombocytopenia depend on the type of chemotherapy drugs, dosage, and the time between treatments. With radiation therapy, the development of thrombocytopenia depends on the amount of bone marrow encompassed in the treatment fields. The development of thrombocytopenia may be a dose-limiting factor in delivering these treatments and can lead to a bleeding event (Kuter, 2022).

Thrombocytopenia may arise indirectly in patients with cancer whose spleens have enlarged because of infection, inflammation, autoimmune disorder, or neoplasm within the spleen. Splenic pooling of platelets has been identified as a cause of thrombocytopenia. Splenic enlargement may occur with metastasis to the spleen. The spleen is involved in approximately 1% of all metastases with common primary malignant tumors involving breast, lung, ovarian, and colorectal cancers, as well as melanomas and gastric carcinomas (Kang et al., 2023).

Thrombocytopenia may develop when platelet destruction increases, a feature of idiopathic thrombocytopenic purpura, an autoimmune disorder in which autoantibodies are formed against the individual's own platelets. Immature platelets accumulate in the bone marrow as the number of circulating mature platelets diminishes. Individuals with idiopathic thrombocytopenic purpura have an increased risk of hematologic malignancies, such as Hodgkin and non-Hodgkin lymphoma and myeloproliferative neoplasms (Ekstrand et al., 2020).

Thrombocytopenia may occur within four days after an operation; however, this can be viewed as a normal process resulting from hemodilution and the stress response from surgery (Skeith et al., 2020). Pathologic etiologies of thrombocytopenia postoperatively may include DIC, idiopathic thrombocytopenic purpura, bacterial infection, or heparin-induced thrombocytopenia associated with thrombosis and heparin exposure (Skeith et al., 2020).

Platelet Refractoriness

Platelet refractoriness is defined as a platelet level that does not increase to the desired level following a platelet transfusion (Cohn, 2020; Youk et al., 2022). Platelet refractoriness has been reported in 30%–70% of patients who receive platelet transfusions (Hagino et al., 2021). Two categories of platelet refractoriness exist: nonimmune and immune.

Nonimmune

Causes of nonimmune refractoriness include DIC, sepsis, fever, bleeding, splenomegaly, hematopoietic stem cell transplantation, graft-versus-host disease, vaso-occlusive diseases, drug-induced thrombocytopenia, and hemorrhage (Cohn, 2020;

Hagino et al., 2021; Youk et al., 2022). DIC leads to an increased rate of platelet consumption, which can result in refractoriness. Splenomegaly is a well-established cause of poor response to platelet transfusion. Typically, approximately one-third of a person's platelets are sequestered in the spleen, which is in equilibrium with the circulating platelet pool.

Immune

Refractoriness to platelet transfusion caused by an immune response is known as alloimmunization and has the greatest potential for prevention and management. Some platelet antigens, such as human leukocyte antigens (HLAs), are shared by other blood cells and tissues, with HLA-A and HLA-B antigens most likely responsible for alloimmunization. To counteract this effect, transfusions of leukoreduced platelets, in which the white blood cells (leukocytes) have been removed from the blood product, can be used to decrease the potential for alloimmunization. Another type of antigen, the human platelet antigen, is specific to platelets only. It can cause changes in platelet membranes that can stimulate the production of antibodies once exposed to foreign platelets with different human platelet antigens through platelet transfusions (Chen et al., 2024).

Clotting Factor Deficiencies

Clotting factors are the blood components responsible for the conversion of fibrinogen to fibrin, which is needed to form a clot. Deficiencies can contribute to bleeding risk and may occur with certain cancers. Patients with hematologic cancers, myeloproliferative disorders, macroglobulinemia, lymphoproliferative disorders, and, to a lesser extent, solid tumors may acquire von Willebrand disease, in which factor VIII and von Willebrand factor procoagulant activity is diminished or absent (Colonne et al., 2022).

Clotting factors I, II, V, VII, IX, X, and XIII are synthesized in the liver; therefore, conditions that compromise liver function, such as infection, chemotherapy treatment, tumor invasion, and surgery, can contribute to prolonged bleeding times and alter normal coagulation. The liver also clears fibrin degradation products and activated clotting factors from circulation. Deficiency of clotting factor XIII may exist with acute leukemias and myelodysplastic syndrome and is associated with impaired procoagulant activities and abnormal platelet function because of alterations in platelet size, shape, and aggregation responses (Lv & Li, 2023).

Patient Assessment

Patient assessment should include a thorough history and physical examination. Nurses must identify patients at risk of bleeding or with active bleeding and be aware of symptoms that require immediate identification and intervention to prevent massive hemorrhage. A complete bleeding history should be obtained, including signs of bleeding such as easy bruising, nosebleeds, bloody sputum, gingival bleeding, excessive bleeding with invasive procedures, unusually heavy menstrual bleeding, petechiae, and changes in the color of stools or urine. Nurses should question patients about the presence of symptoms associated with anemia, such as fatigue, headache, and weakness, and whether they have a history of heavy menstrual bleeding, bloody stools, bloody sputum, or prior anemia. A complete medication history should occur and focus on medications that may put patients at risk for bleeding, including antibiotics; nonsteroidal anti-inflammatory drugs; chemotherapy, biologics, and supportive agents; and all over-the-counter medications and supplements. The patient history should also include transfusions, immunologic disorders (e.g., idiopathic thrombocytopenic purpura), and family history of bleeding abnormalities. Patients' nutritional status needs to be assessed to possibly identify any vitamin deficiencies, such as vitamin B_{12}, folic acid, or iron deficiencies (Williams et al., 2023).

A systematic physical examination to assess for signs of bleeding follows the patient history. Bleeding within the central nervous system can manifest as mental status changes, headache, lethargy, restlessness, altered level of consciousness, seizures, or coma, as well as changes in neurologic signs (e.g., pupil size, reactivity), motor strength and coordination, and speech. Examination of the eyes and ears may reveal partial visual field loss, increased redness in the eyes, periorbital edema, and subconjunctival hemorrhage. Patients may report blurred vision and eye or ear pain. Examination of the nose, mouth, and throat may reveal petechiae on the nasal or oral mucosa, ulceration, gingivitis, mucous membrane bleeding, or epistaxis. Signs of bleeding manifested by the cardiovascular system include changes in vital signs, changes in the color and temperature of all extremities, changes in the peripheral pulses, tachycardia, or hypotension. During examination of the pulmonary system, it is important to note changes in the respiratory rate and depth, dyspnea, tachypnea, shortness of breath, crackles, wheezing, orthopnea, hemoptysis, or cyanosis. Examination of the gastrointestinal system could reveal increased or vague abdominal pain, blood around the rectum, tarry stools, and occult blood in the stool or hematemesis. Indications of bleeding in the genitourinary system present as blood in the urine, dysuria, burning and frequency with urination, decreased urine output, and a change in the character or amount of menses. Bleeding in the musculoskeletal system could manifest as warm, tender, and swollen joints with diminished mobility. Indications of bleeding in the integumentary system include signs of bruising, petechiae, purpura, ecchymoses, hematomas, pallor or jaundice, and oozing from injection sites, biopsy sites, central lines, catheters, or nasogastric tubes (Chi & Green, 2021).

Advanced Practice Considerations

Many diagnostic tests are used to determine if bleeding is present. Hemoccult tests can identify blood in stool, and a urine dipstick is typically used to test for microscopic hematuria. Imaging scans can also be used to assess for internal bleeding. Laboratory values are the most commonly used tools to determine bleeding and coagulation status and include tests to evaluate platelet counts, bleeding times, D-dimer levels, and levels of specific coagulation factors. Hemoglobin and hematocrit values are measured to monitor blood loss (Bannow & Konkle, 2023). Patients with cancer may present with existing anemia and have reduced hemoglobin and hematocrit levels. Sudden drops in these levels could indicate an acute blood loss and should be treated immediately.

A bone marrow aspiration may be performed if no other causes are identified for thrombocytopenia. It can assess whether the number of megakaryocytes in the marrow is normal or altered. If the number is reduced, the cause relates to primary thrombocytopenia or a decreased production of platelets. When the number is normal or elevated, thrombocytopenia is a result of increased uptake or peripheral destruction of platelets (Thiagarajan, 2025).

The platelet count, which quantifies the number of platelets in the blood volume, is the best gauge of possible bleeding in patients with cancer. The *Common Terminology Criteria for Adverse Events* grades a decreased platelet count from 1 to 5 (National Cancer Institute Cancer Therapy Evaluation Program, 2017). Nurses should always reference the version of this documentation used by their institutions or protocols. Table 11-3 presents the grading system for decreased platelet count.

After a patient receives a platelet transfusion for thrombocytopenia, the response to the transfusion must be evaluated. The corrected count increment (CCI) is a formula based on a platelet count obtained 10 minutes to 1 hour after transfusion. If the CCI is less than 5,000 cells/mcl on at least two sequential occasions, the patient is determined to be refractory to platelets (Arabi et al., 2021; Cohn, 2020). Often, CCI is not the most practical means of assessing response because the formula for calculating it uses the number of platelets transfused, which often is unavailable. Therefore, a more common definition for CCI uses measurements of platelet recovery and platelet response to indicate refractoriness. Platelet recovery is defined as the increment in platelet count measured 10 minutes to 1 hour following transfusion. Platelet survival is evaluated by a platelet count obtained 18–24 hours after transfusion. When assessing both platelet recovery and survival, platelet refractoriness is present if the absolute platelet count rises less than 10,000 cells/mcl after administration of a unit of platelets or if it rapidly returns to pretransfusion levels (Arabi et al., 2021; Cohn, 2020).

Besides laboratory tests, certain radiographic studies can be used to determine whether any bleeding is present, such as computed tomography scans, magnetic resonance imaging, or ultrasound. Endoscopic examinations can be used to assess for bleeding in the upper or lower gastrointestinal tract; however, an invasive procedure could also put patients at an increased risk for bleeding and should be performed with caution (Guglielmo et al., 2021).

TABLE 11-3
Grading of Decreased Platelet Count

Grade	Platelet Levels
1	< LLN–75,000 cells/mcl; < LLN–75 × 10^9/L
2	< 75,000–50,000 cells/mcl; < 75–50 × 10^9/L
3	< 50,000–25,000 cells/mcl; < 50–25 × 10^9/L
4	< 25,000 cells/mcl; < 25 × 10^9/L
5	Death

LLN—lower limit of normal

Note. From *Common Terminology Criteria for Adverse Events* [v.5.0], by National Cancer Institute Cancer Therapy Evaluation Program, 2017 (https://dctd.cancer.gov/research/ctep-trials/for-sites/adverse-events/ctcae-v55x7.pdf). In the public domain.

Treatment Modalities

Prophylaxis

Transfusions of red blood cells, platelets, and plasma have been used effectively in patients with thrombocytopenia to prevent bleeding. The decision for red blood cell transfusions can vary per patient-specific factors. According to the Association for the Advancement of Blood and Biotherapies guideline, red blood cell transfusion is recommended on an individualized basis, dependent on signs, symptoms, comorbidities, and patient values and preferences (Carson et al., 2023). For most adult patients who are hospitalized and hemodynamically stable, a transfusion should be considered when the hemoglobin concentration is less than 7 g/dl. Transfusion should be considered for a hemoglobin of 7.5 g/dl for patients undergoing cardiac surgery and 8 g/dl for patients undergoing orthopedic surgery or those with preexisting cardiovascular disease. For adult patients who are hospitalized with hematologic and oncologic disorders, a transfusion is recommended when hemoglobin concentration is less than 7 g/dl (Carson et al., 2023).

The transfusion of platelets plays an important role in bleeding prevention and management (Yuan & Otrock, 2021). Usually, one unit of platelets can increase platelet count by 6,000–10,000 cells/mcl, but each individual is unique and may not have the same results. Patients with acute leukemia or solid tumors and those undergoing stem cell transplantation should maintain a platelet threshold of 10,000 cells/mcl to prevent spontaneous bleeding. Patients undergoing any invasive procedure will need a prior evaluation for adequate platelet counts. Those with major or severe bleeding, including trauma and DIC, should have a threshold for platelet transfusion of less than 50,000 cells/mcl (Yuan & Otrock, 2021). Patients with multiple trauma, central nervous system, or ocular bleeding should maintain a platelet count of greater than 100,000 cells/mcl (Yuan & Otrock, 2021).

Several factors can influence the effectiveness of platelet transfusions, including fever, sepsis, and hypersplenism. Another important factor in the efficacy of platelet transfusions is the proper storage of platelets to maintain freshness and metabolic activity. Platelets can be stored for up to five days at room temperature with constant agitation to prevent clumping (American Red Cross, 2025). After the platelets are obtained, they should be transfused at a rate of 2–5 ml/min, with completion of the transfusion within one hour (Garraud et al., 2023).

Treatment Interventions

A variety of interventions can be used to manage bleeding in patients with cancer. A specific plan designed to treat bleeding should be individualized for each patient and depends on many factors, including the underlying causes, likelihood of reversing or controlling the bleeding etiology, disease status, goals of therapy, presence of comorbidities, and whether the treatment benefits outweigh the risks. If a benefit is expected, specific measures are put in place to control the bleeding. The mainstay of treatment for bleeding is the transfusion of blood products. Treatments used to control bleeding include vitamin K therapy and mechanical measures (Johnstone & Rich, 2018).

Platelet transfusions reduce morbidity and mortality from thrombocytopenia and are likely to prevent and manage bleeding in patients with cancer who are actively bleeding (Yuan & Otrock, 2021). The traditional management of patients with HLA antibodies is to provide platelets from HLA-matched donors. Unfortunately, for many patients, HLA-matched donors are unavailable. In this case, platelets from partially mismatched donors may provide adequate responses. Patients generally respond well to HLA-matched donor platelets if alloimmunization alone is responsible for platelet refractoriness. These platelets should be irradiated to prevent transfusion-associated graft-versus-host disease (Cohn, 2020).

In patients with cancer, decreased red blood cell production typically is caused by the disease process or myelosuppressive therapy. Transfusion of packed red blood cells is used most often because it can provide more than 70% of the hematocrit of whole blood and one-third of the plasma, thus minimizing fluid overload issues (Cywinski, 2025).

Human plasma, which is derived from whole blood products or plasmapheresis, is used to correct coagulopathy. Fresh frozen plasma is commonly given when a patient's international normalized ratio level is greater than two times baseline with an abnormal partial thromboplastin time level. Plasma can be used in patients who present with shock, severe bleeding, and bleeding associated with an infection, as well as in the management of acute DIC. Typically, plasma is infused quickly so that the maximum plasma level is reached before any metabolic changes occur (Cywinski, 2025). Another agent, cryoprecipitate, is used most commonly for replacement of fibrinogen in patients who are bleeding or at increased risk of bleeding, as well as in patients with a consumptive coagulopathy (e.g., DIC). Cryoprecipitate is prepared by slowly thawing fresh frozen plasma to form an insoluble precipitate. Factor VIII, fibrinogen, and factor XIII are its major components. Other proteins in the concentrate include vitronectin and fibronectin (Stanford et al., 2023).

The indirect plasmin inhibitors, tranexamic acid and aminocaproic acid, have also been used to decrease bleeding by reducing fibrinolysis. These agents have been shown to decrease blood loss and subsequent transfusions with no increased risk of venous thromboembolism. These drugs do not help the body to form a clot; instead, they stop the body's enzymes and plasmin from breaking down a clot. Aminocaproic acid and tranexamic acid may be taken orally or intravenously (Kaseer & Sanghavi, 2023; Ockerman et al., 2021).

Thrombopoietin receptor agonists have been used for chemotherapy-induced thrombocytopenia to prevent delay and dose reduction of chemotherapy (Al-Samkari et al., 2021). Romiplostim dosing strategies include weekly dosing beginning at 2–4 mcg/kg, increased no more than 1–2 mcg/kg/week to a target platelet count of 100,000–150,000 cells/mcl. The maximum dose is 10 mcg/kg/week. Thrombopoietin receptor agonists for chemotherapy-induced thrombocytopenia may increase the risk of venous thromboembolism in patients with cancer and should be given with caution (Al-Samkari et al., 2021).

Vitamin K is necessary for the hepatic production of several clotting factors, including factors II, VII, IX, and X. Patients who have small bowel disease or resection or biliary obstruction are prone to deficiencies of these clotting factors. Vitamin K therapy is effective if a deficiency of these factors or excessive warfarin therapy is implicated in bleeding in patients with advanced cancer. The preferred route to administer vitamin K is oral, which reduces the potential for additional bleeding or infection in patients who are already compromised (Imbrescia & Moszczynski, 2023).

Mechanical measures can be used to manage active bleeding, including applying direct steady pressure to the site of bleeding or, if the bleeding site is not directly exposed, inserting a balloon catheter or nasal packing, especially when dealing with epistaxis. Extreme care must be taken when removing or replacing packing to avoid disturbing the clot that has formed (Rodriguez, 2018). If the bleeding is from peripheral phlebotomy sites or central venous catheter sites, direct pressure and hemostatic bioabsorbable dressings can be applied (Rodriguez, 2018). Other usable topical agents include absorbable gelatin, collagen, and fibrin sealants (Johnstone & Rich, 2018; Zhong et al., 2021).

Nursing Management

Nurses are fundamental to the prevention, recognition, and management of bleeding in patients with cancer. They must be able to recognize the early signs and symptoms of bleeding through astute observation and physical assessment. Table 11-4 provides an overview of the clinical assessments and nursing interventions in the care of patients who have active bleeding or are at risk for bleeding.

Vital signs, hemodynamic status, oxygenation, and fluid status are closely monitored in patients at risk for bleeding. All unnecessary procedures should be avoided, including intramuscular injections, subcutaneous injections, rectal temperatures, and suppositories. Injection sites could put patients at risk for hematomas and lead to infection. If an injection must be given, the smallest gauge needle should be used and direct pressure applied for several minutes. This is followed by application of a pressure dressing to avoid a hematoma. Cold compresses can also be used to induce vasoconstriction (Rodriguez, 2018).

Because bleeding is a very common and potentially fatal event in patients with cancer, nurses must instruct patients and caregivers on strategies to help prevent bleeding and what to do if it occurs. Nurses should also advise patients to do an environmental check at home to identify fall risks, such as throw rugs, and to remove clutter from rooms and pathways. They also must ensure that patients wear shoes or slippers at all times to minimize the potential for injury. To maintain good skin integrity, nurses should teach patients to use lotion that prevents dryness and breaks in skin and to avoid the use of adhesive tape, which causes skin trauma; only paper tape should be used. The mouth and gums of patients with thrombocytopenia are susceptible to injury; therefore, patients should apply a nonpetroleum lubricant to the lips and gums to keep them moist and use a soft-bristle toothbrush to avoid trauma. Patients should avoid substances that can irritate the tissues of the mouth and gums, including hot and spicy foods, alcoholic beverages, and mouthwashes that contain alcohol. To prevent bleeding from the nose, patients should be taught to clean the nostrils with a soft

TABLE 11-4
Nursing Management of Patients With Actual or Potential Bleeding

System	Clinical Assessment	Nursing Management
Central nervous	Mental status changes, including confusion, lethargy, restlessness, changes in cognition, alteration in level of consciousness, obtundation, seizures, and coma Changes in neurologic signs, including widening pulse pressure, pupil size, and reactivity; motor strength and coordination; speech and paralysis; and complaints of headache	Review the head CT scan for an accurate diagnosis of intracranial bleeding. Monitor vital signs. Administer blood product transfusion as ordered to maintain platelet level above 20,000 cells/mcl Administer corticosteroids or mannitol as ordered to decrease intracranial pressure. Instruct patients to avoid the Valsalva maneuver. Administer pain medication as ordered for severe headache. Administer cough suppressant as ordered to prevent further spontaneous bleeding caused by forceful coughing.
Eyes and ears	Visual disturbances, including diplopia, blurred vision, and partial field loss Increased injection on the sclera Periorbital edema Subconjunctival hemorrhage (homogenous red color that is sharply outlined on the sclera) Eye or ear pain	Administer blood product transfusion as ordered. Instruct patients to use artificial tears to provide lubrication and relieve burning or itching from eye irritation.
Nose, mouth, and throat	Petechiae on the nasal/oral mucosa Ulcerations Gingivitis or mucous membrane bleeding Epistaxis	Ensure that patients maintain good oral hygiene. Apply topical thrombin/hemostatic agents to bleeding and lesions. Instruct patients to avoid forceful blowing of the nose. Manage epistaxis. • Place patients in high Fowler position. • Apply direct pressure on the nares. • Apply a cold compress for vasoconstriction. • Apply topical epinephrine or silver nitrate.

(Continued on next page)

TABLE 11-4
Nursing Management of Patients With Actual or Potential Bleeding *(Continued)*

System	Clinical Assessment	Nursing Management
Nose, mouth, and throat *(Cont.)*		• Use nasal packing with aminocaproic, acid–saturated dressing as ordered. • Apply direct pressure with balloon catheters (i.e., Foley).
Cardiovascular	Changes in vital signs Changes in color and temperature of all extremities Changes in peripheral pulses Tachycardia Hypotension	Monitor vital signs. Administer blood product transfusion as ordered. Provide hemodynamic support with fluids or vasopressors.
Pulmonary	Respiratory rate and depth, dyspnea, tachypnea, and shortness of breath Crackles, wheezing, and stridor Orthopnea Hemoptysis (usually bright red in color and frothier than hematemesis) Cyanosis	Support patients during thoracentesis for pleural effusions. Assist with the sclerosis of the bleeding site. Administer as ordered: • Codeine or hydrocodone to control coughing • Glucocorticoids to control bleeding • Oxygen therapy for shortness of breath • Antianxiety medication Place patients in high Fowler position to relieve dyspnea. Intubate for severe bleeding.
Abdominal	Pain (location, occurrence, duration, quality) • Right upper quadrant pain and abdominal distension may indicate hepatomegaly. • Left flank or shoulder pain may indicate splenomegaly. • Vague abdominal pain may indicate retroperitoneal bleeding. Palpable spleen Blood around the rectum Tarry stools Frank or occult blood in stool Hematemesis	Administer as ordered: • Antiemetics • Antacids • H_2 blockers • IV desmopressin acetate for massive esophageal varices bleeding • Antibiotics • Sucralfate to coat the mucosal lining • Stool softeners Avoid rectal manipulation (rectal thermometer, suppositories, and rectal tubes). Anticipate possible surgery for a ruptured spleen.

(Continued on next page)

TABLE 11-4
Nursing Management of Patients With Actual or Potential Bleeding *(Continued)*

System	Clinical Assessment	Nursing Management
Genitourinary	Blood in urine (measure for frequency and size of clots) Dysuria, burning, and frequency of urination Decreased urine output Character and amount of menses	Administer cytoprotectants as ordered, such as mesna, prior to high-dose chemotherapy. Perform continuous bladder irrigation. Instruct patients to void frequently if without an indwelling Foley catheter. Administer as ordered: • Phenazopyridine hydrochloride for pain and burning • Oxybutynin chloride to relieve spasms Perform bladder sclerosis with formalin, silver nitrate, or prostaglandin for uncontrolled bladder hemorrhage. Monitor menstrual bleeding (number of saturated sanitary pads used). Administer hormone therapy as ordered for uncontrolled heavy menses. Administer blood product transfusion as ordered.
Musculoskeletal	Warm, tender, swollen joints with diminished mobility for active and passive range of motion, indicating bleeding into the joints	Correct coagulation deficits by vitamin K administration and plasma product transfusion as ordered. Administer pain medication as needed for joint pain as ordered.
Integumentary	Bruising, petechiae, purpura, ecchymoses, hematomas Acrocyanosis (irregularly shaped cyanotic patches on the periphery of the arms and legs associated with bleeding from DIC) Pallor and jaundice Oozing from venipuncture or injection sites, biopsy sites, central lines, catheters, or nasogastric tubes	Apply direct pressure to the site of bleeding. Apply a cold compress to promote vasoconstriction. Apply topical absorbable hemostats: collagen, fibrins. Provide wound care using • Nonadherent dressings • Gentle dressing removal • Moist wound products

CT—computed tomography; DIC—disseminated intravascular coagulation

Note. From "Bleeding" (pp. 863–865), by A.L. Rodriguez in C.H. Yarbro, D. Wujcik, and B.H. Gobel (Eds.), *Cancer Nursing: Principles and Practice* (8th ed.), 2018, Jones and Bartlett Learning, www.jblearning.com. Copyright 2018 by Jones and Bartlett Learning. Adapted with permission.

tissue and to avoid vigorous nose blowing. The use of saline nose drops and sprays, as well as a small amount of moisturizing ointment (e.g., petroleum jelly) inside the nostrils, will help to prevent nosebleeds (Tunkel et al., 2020).

Bleeding events can be very distressing for patients and caregivers, so excellent communication should be maintained with the care team, and a plan should be developed in the case of an acute bleeding episode. Patients and caregivers should be prepared for the distress of visualizing a massive bleeding episode. To lessen the visual shock of bleeding, patients should be encouraged to use dark sheets, towels, blankets, and clothing (Johnstone & Rich, 2018). If a massive bleed occurs, patients should be placed in the lateral decubitus position to avoid suffocation (Sood et al., 2019).

Summary

Bleeding in patients with cancer can be caused by a variety of underlying factors, including the disease process and cancer therapies, which can reduce the quantity and functional quality of platelets and alter clotting factors. The initial step in managing bleeding is the identification of underlying causes, with the type and origin of bleeding directing treatment. The patient's status, goals of treatment, and comorbidities must be considered before deciding on a care plan.

The authors would like to acknowledge Colleen M. O'Leary, MSN, RN, AOCNS®, for her contribution to this chapter that remains unchanged from the previous edition of this book.

References

Ajabnoor, A.M., Parisi, R., Zghebi, S.S., Ashcroft, D.M., Faivre-Finn, C., Morris, C., ... Kontopantelis, E. (2023). Common cancer types and risk of stroke and bleeding in patients with nonvalvular atrial fibrillation: A population-based study in England. *Journal of the American Heart Association, 12*(19). https://doi.org/10.1161/JAHA.123.029423

Al-Samkari, H., Parnes, A.D., Goodarzi, K., Weitzman, J.I., Connors, J.M., & Kuter, D.J. (2021). A multicenter study of romiplostim for chemotherapy-induced thrombocytopenia in solid tumors and hematologic malignancies. *Haematologica, 106*(4), 1148–1157. https://doi.org/10.3324/haematol.2020.251900

American Red Cross. (2025). *Blood components.* https://www.redcrossblood.org/donate-blood/how-to-donate/types-of-blood-donations/blood-components.html

Arabi, S., Almahayni, A.O., Alomair, A.A., Masuadi, E.M., Damlaj, M., & Al-Dorzi, H.M. (2021). Prevalence, risk factors, and outcomes of platelet transfusion refractoriness in critically ill patients: A retrospective cohort study. *Critical Care Research and Practice, 2021*(1), 5589768. https://doi.org/10.1155/2021/5589768

Bannow, B.S., & Konkle, B.A. (2023). How I approach bleeding in hospitalized patients. *Blood, 142*(9), 761–768. https://doi.org/10.1182/blood.2021014766

Butler, E., Møller, M.H., Cook, O., Granholm, A., Penketh, J., Rygård, S.L., ... Perner, A. (2019). The effect of systemic corticosteroids on the incidence of gastrointestinal bleeding in critically ill adults: A systematic review with meta-analysis. *Intensive Care Medicine, 45*(11), 1540–1549. https://doi.org/10.1007/s00134-019-05754-3

Carson, J.L., Stanworth, S.J., Guyatt, G., Valentine, S., Dennis, J., Bakhtary, S., ... Pagano, M.B. (2023). Red blood cell transfusion: 2023 AABB International Guidelines. *JAMA, 330*(19), 1892–1902. https://doi.org/10.1001/jama.2023.12914

Chen, X., Zhao, Y., Lv, Y., & Xie, J. (2024). Immunological platelet transfusion refractoriness: Current insights from mechanisms to therapeutics. *Platelets, 35*(1). https://doi.org/10.1080/09537104.2024.2306983

Chi, M., & Green, J.R. (2021). Assessing bleeding disorders: Keys for hem/onc fellows. *Onclive, 13*(4). https://www.onclive.com/view/assessing-bleeding-disorders-keys-for-hem-onc-fellows

Cohn, C.S. (2020). Platelet transfusion refractoriness: How do I diagnose and manage? *Hematology American Society of Hematology Education Program, 2020*(1), 527–532. https://doi.org/10.1182/hematology.2020000137

Colonne, C.K., Favaloro, E.J., & Pasalic, L. (2022). The intriguing connections between von Willebrand Factor, ADAMTS13 and cancer. *Healthcare, 10*(3), 557. https://doi.org/10.3390/healthcare10030557

Cywinski, J.B. (2025). Blood products transfusion. In E. Farag, M. Argalious, J.E. Tetzlaff, & D. Sharma (Eds.), *Basic sciences in anesthesia* (pp. 465–481). Springer. https://doi.org/10.1007/978-3-319-62067-1_27

Diaz, C., Quintero, J.A., Zarama, V., & Bustamante-Cristancho, L.A. (2023). Bleeding complications in uremic patients after ultrasound-guided central venous catheter placement. *Open Access Emergency Medicine, 15*, 21–28. https://doi.org/10.2147/OAEM.S384081

Driver, B., Marks, D.C., & van der Wal, D.E. (2019). Not all (N)SAID and done: Effects of nonsteroidal anti-inflammatory drugs and paracetamol intake on platelets. *Research and Practice in Thrombosis and Haemostasis, 4*(1), 36–45. https://doi.org/10.1002/rth2.12283

Ekstrand, C., Bahmanyar, S., Cherif, H., Kieler, H., & Linder, M. (2020). Cancer risk in patients with primary immune thrombocytopenia–A Swedish nationwide register study. *Cancer Epidemiology, 69*, 101806. https://doi.org/10.1016/j.canep.2020.101806

Englisch, C., Moik, F., Steiner, D., Starzer, A.M., Berghoff, A.S., Preusser, M., ... Ay, C. (2024). Bleeding events in patients with cancer: Incidence, risk factors, and impact on prognosis in a prospective cohort study. *Blood, 144*(22), 2349–2359. https://doi.org/10.1182/blood.2024025362

Escobar, A., Salem, A.M., Dickson, K., Johnson, T.N., Burk, K.J., Bashoura, L., & Faiz, S.A. (2022). Anticoagulation and bleeding in the cancer patient. *Supportive Care in Cancer, 30*(10), 8547–8557. https://doi.org/10.1007/s00520-022-07136-w

Garraud, O., Hamzeh-Cognasse, H., Chalayer, E., Duchez, A.C., Tardy, B., Oriol, P., ... Cognasse, F. (2023). Platelet transfusion in adults: An update. *Transfusion Clinique et Biologique, 30*(1), 147–165. https://doi.org/10.1016/j.tracli.2022.08.147

Gauer, R.L., & Whitaker, D.J. (2022). Thrombocytopenia: Evaluation and management. *American Family Physician, 106*(3), 288–298.

Geng, C. (2024). Drug-induced thrombocytopenia. In M. Armstrong (Ed.), *Medical News Today*. https://www.medicalnewstoday.com/articles/drug-induced-thrombocytopenia

Guglielmo, F.F., Wells, M.L., Bruining, D.H., Strate, L.L., Huete, A., Gupta, A., ... Fidler, J.L. (2021). Gastrointestinal bleeding at CT angiography and CT enterography: Imaging atlas and glossary of terms. *RadioGraphics, 41*(6), 1632–1656. https://doi.org/10.1148/rg.2021210043

Hagino, T., Sato, T., Tsuno, N.H., & Tasaki, T. (2021). Incidence and management of nonimmune platelet transfusion refractoriness: A narrative review. *Annals of Blood, 6*. https://aob.amegroups.org/article/view/6483

Imbrescia, K., & Moszczynski, Z. (2023). Vitamin K. In *StatPearls*. StatPearls Publishing. https://www.ncbi.nlm.nih.gov/books/NBK551578

Johnny, J.D. (2021). Hemostatic disorders: Physiology, diagnostics, and management. *Clinical Journal of Oncology Nursing, 25*(4), 379–382. https://doi.org/10.1188/21.CJON.379-382

Johnstone, C., & Rich, S. (2018). Bleeding in cancer patients and its treatment: A review. *Annals of Palliative Medicine, 7*(2), 265–273. https://doi.org/10.21037/apm.2017.11.01

Kang, D., Zhao, D., Jiang, X., & Li, D. (2023). Isolated splenic metastasis from primary fallopian tube carcinoma and the application of laparoscopic splenectomy: A case report and literature review. *Frontiers in Oncology, 13*, 1079044. https://doi.org/10.3389/fonc.2023.1079044

Kanikarla-Marie, P., Fowlkes, N.W., Afshar-Kharghan, V., Martch, S.L., Sorokin, A., Shen, J.P., ... Menter, D.G. (2021). The provocative roles of platelets in liver disease and cancer. *Frontiers in Oncology, 11,* 643815. https://doi.org/10.3389/fonc.2021.643815

Kaseer, H., & Sanghavi, D.K. (2023). Aminocaproic acid. In *StatPearls.* StatPearls Publishing. https://www.ncbi.nlm.nih.gov/books/NBK554475

Kuter, D.J. (2022). Treatment of chemotherapy-induced thrombocytopenia in patients with non-hematologic malignancies. *Haematologica, 107*(6). https://doi.org/10.3324/haematol.2021.279512

Limijadi, E.K.S., Cantika, Q.C., Retnoningrum, D., Devi, W.R., & Riansari, A. (2021). Blast cells count influences bleeding incidence in acute leukemia: Preliminary study in South Kalimantan, Indonesia. *Macedonian Journal of Medical Sciences, 9*(B), 900–902. https://doi.org/10.3889/oamjms.2021.6860

Lv, X.Y., & Li, Z.J. (2023). Reduced plasma coagulation factor XIII in patients with acute leukemia in remission during consolidation chemotherapy cycles. *Annals of Hematology, 102*(7), 1739–1744. https://doi.org/10.1007/s00277-023-05261-y

National Cancer Institute Cancer Therapy Evaluation Program. (2017). *Common Terminology Criteria for Adverse Events* [v.5.0]. https://ctep.cancer.gov/protocoldevelopment/electronic_applications/docs/CTCAE_v5_Quick_Reference_5x7.pdf

Ockerman, A., Vanassche, T., Garip, M., Vandenbriele, C., Engelen, M.M., Martens, J., ... Verhamme, P. (2021). Tranexamic acid for the prevention and treatment of bleeding in surgery, trauma and bleeding disorders: A narrative review. *Thrombosis Journal, 19*(1), 54. https://doi.org/10.1186/s12959-021-00303-9

Paulus, M.C., Drent, M., Kouw, I.W.K., Balvers, M.G.J., Bast, A., & van Zanten, A.R.H. (2024). Vitamin K: A potential missing link in critical illness–A scoping review. *Critical Care, 28*(1), 212. https://doi.org/10.1186/s13054-024-05001-2

Porzionato, A., Stocco, E., Emmi, A., Macchi, V., & De Caro, R. (2022). Case report: Sudden fatal hemorrhage in ulcerative fungal laryngotracheitis—A pediatric case report. *Frontiers in Pediatrics, 9,* 764027. https://doi.org/10.3389/fped.2021.764027

Raadsen, M., Du Toit, J., Langerak, T., van Bussel, B., van Gorp, E., & Goeijenbier, M. (2021). Thrombocytopenia in virus infections. *Journal of Clinical Medicine, 10*(4), 877. https://doi.org/10.3390/jcm10040877

Rodriguez, A.L. (2018). Bleeding. In C.H. Yarbro, D. Wujcik, & B.H. Gobel (Eds.), *Cancer nursing: Principles and practice* (8th ed., pp. 851–881). Jones and Bartlett Learning.

Sang, Y., Roest, M., de Laat, B., de Groot, P.G., & Huskens, D. (2021). Interplay between platelets and coagulation. *Blood Reviews, 46,* 100733. https://doi.org/10.1016/j.blre.2020.100733

Skeith, L., Baumann Kreuziger, L., Crowther, M.A., & Warkentin, T.E. (2020). A practical approach to evaluating postoperative thrombocytopenia. *Blood Advances, 4*(4), 776–783. https://doi.org/10.1182/bloodadvances.2019001414

Sood, R., Mancinetti, M., Betticher, D., Cantin, B., & Ebneter, A. (2019). Management of bleeding in palliative care patients in the general internal medicine ward: A systematic review. *Annals of Medicine and Surgery, 50,* 14–23. https://doi.org/10.1016/j.amsu.2019.12.002

Stanford, S., Roy, A., Cecil, T., Hegener, O., Schulz, P., Turaj, A., ... Arbuthnot, E. (2023). Differences in coagulation-relevant parameters: Comparing cryoprecipitate and a human fibrinogen concentrate. *PLOS ONE, 18*(8), e0290571. https://doi.org/10.1371/journal.pone.0290571

Thiagarajan, P. (2025, April 17). Platelet disorders overview of platelet disorders. *Medscape.* https://emedicine.medscape.com/article/201722-overview

Tsantes, A.G., Parastatidou, S., Tsantes, E.A., Bonova, E., Tsante, K.A., Mantzios, P.G., ... Sokou, R. (2023). Sepsis-induced coagulopathy: An update on pathophysiology, biomarkers, and current guidelines. *Life, 13*(2), 350. https://doi.org/10.3390/life13020350

Tunkel, D.E., Anne, S., Payne, S.C., Ishman, S.L., Rosenfeld, R.M., Abramson, P.J., ... Monjur, T.M. (2020). Clinical practice guideline: Nosebleed (epistaxis). *Otolaryngology–Head and Neck Surgery, 162*(1, Suppl.), S1–S38. https://doi.org/10.1177/0194599819890327

Turner, J., Parsi, M., & Badireddy, M. (2023). Anemia. In *StatPearls.* StatPearls Publishing. https://www.ncbi.nlm.nih.gov/books/NBK499994

Wang, T.-F., Leader, A., & Sanfilippo, K.M. (2022). Thrombosis and bleeding in hematological malignancy. *Best Practice and Research Clinical Haematology, 35*(1), 101353. https://doi.org/10.1016/j.beha.2022.101353

Williams, A.M., Brown, K.H., Allen, L.H., Dary, O., Moorthy, D., & Suchdev, P.S. (2023). Improving anemia assessment in clinical and public health settings. *Journal of Nutrition, 153*(1, Suppl.), S29–S41. https://doi.org/10.1016/j.tjnut.2023.05.032

Yao, T.-C., Huang, Y.-W., Chang, S.-M., Tsai, S.-Y., Wu, A.C., & Tsai, H.-J. (2020). Association between oral corticosteroid bursts and severe adverse events: A nationwide population-based cohort study. *Annals of Internal Medicine, 173*(5), 325–330. https://doi.org/10.7326/M20-0432

Youk, H.-J., Hwang, S.-H., Oh, H.-B., & Ko, D.-H. (2022). Evaluation and management of platelet transfusion refractoriness. *Blood Research, 57*(Suppl. 1), S6–S10. https://doi.org/10.5045/br.2022.2021229

Yuan, S., & Otrock, Z.K. (2021). Platelet transfusion: An update on indications and guidelines. *Clinics in Laboratory Medicine, 41*(4), 621–634. https://doi.org/10.1016/j.cll.2021.07.005

Zhong, Y., Hu, H., Min, N., Wei, Y., Li, X., & Li, X. (2021). Application and outlook of topical hemostatic materials: A narrative review. *Annals of Translational Medicine, 9*(7), 577. https://doi.org/10.21037/atm-20-7160

Diane G. Cope, PhD, APRN, BC, AOCNP®,
and Abigail Tesar, BSN, RN, OCN®, TCTCN™

CHAPTER 12

Venous Thromboembolism

FAST FACTS

- **Description:** Patients with cancer are at increased risk for developing blood clots (thromboemboli), particularly in the venous circulation. Venous thromboembolism includes both deep vein thrombosis and pulmonary embolism.
- **Incidence:** The annual incidence of venous thromboembolism is five times greater in patients with cancer than in the general population. Certain chemotherapy agents and targeted agents are associated with higher rates of venous thromboembolism.
- **Clinical Manifestations:** Deep vein thrombosis presents as unilateral swelling of the extremity, edema, warmth, localized pain, vein dilation, limb color changes, and pyrexia. Pulmonary embolism presents as dyspnea, pleuritic pain, tachypnea, apprehension, and tachycardia.
- **Risk Factors and Etiology:** Risk factors for venous thromboembolism include malignancy and can be related to patient-, disease-, or treatment-related factors.
- **Pathophysiology and Patient Evaluation:** Changes in blood flow, vessel integrity, cellular components, and malignancy can predispose individuals to the development of venous thromboembolism.
- **Advanced Practice Considerations:** Deep vein thrombosis can be diagnosed with venous duplex ultrasound and computed tomography scans. Pulmonary embolism can be diagnosed using computed tomography scans, pulmonary angiograms, and ventilation or perfusion scans. Advanced practice providers should be knowledgeable about risk factors for venous thromboembolism and apply appropriate treatment strategies to decrease associated patient complications.
- **Treatment Modalities:** Prophylaxis includes low-molecular-weight heparin, unfractionated heparin, factor Xa inhibitors, and mechanical prophylaxis for at-risk nonambulatory hospitalized patients. Therapy with low-molecular-weight heparin or vitamin K antagonists may continue indefinitely for patients with active cancer.
- **Nursing Management:** Nursing measures are instituted to prevent venous thromboembolism in hospitalized patients and those at risk. The disease is the most preventable cause of death in hospitalized patients.
- **Outcomes:** Patients with cancer are at high risk for venous thromboembolism. Early recognition and initiation of appropriate treatment are crucial to patient outcomes. Those at risk are considered for pharmacologic prophylaxis, balancing the risk of venous thromboembolism with the increased risk of bleeding.

Introduction

Risk of venous thromboembolism (VTE), which includes deep vein thrombosis (DVT) and pulmonary embolism (PE), is strongly associated with hospitalization during cancer treatment and up to three months after discharge (Centers for Disease Control and Prevention [CDC], 2025; Jordan Bruno et al., 2022). An estimated 900,000 people in the United States (1–2 per 1,000) will experience VTE, with approximately 60,000–100,000 deaths each year (CDC, 2025). Sudden death is the first symptom in about 25% of individuals who have a PE (CDC, 2025). VTE is a leading cause of preventable hospital death in the United States (CDC, 2025).

Patients with cancer are at increased risk of developing a new VTE or having DVT recur compared to patients who do not have cancer (Lyman et al., 2021). The risks of VTE, bleeding, and early mortality among patients receiving systemic cancer therapy vary by cancer type and treatment, as well as patient-specific factors.

VTE has been shown to adversely affect quality of life (Arteaga et al., 2024). Marin-Barrera et al. (2020) conducted a multicenter, prospective, case-control study that found that acute symptomatic VTE adversely affected the quality of life of patients with malignancies.

Incidence

VTE develops in 5%–20% of patients with cancer, with an estimated 20% of all VTE cases occurring in this population (Lyman et al., 2021). In addition to the overall increased risk for VTE among patients with cancer, VTE risk is exceptionally high among certain cancer subgroups, hospitalized patients, those undergoing active antineoplastic therapy, and those receiving certain supportive care measures. The first few months following a cancer diagnosis pose the highest risk for DVT recurrence, but the risk persists for many years after the initial DVT (Gervaso et al., 2021). Often, these incidental VTEs are discovered during initial or restaging computed tomography (CT) scans. VTE rates in patients with cancer are four to seven times higher than in healthy individuals and are increasing (Gervaso et al., 2021; Lyman et al., 2021). The reasons for this increased incidence of VTE in patients with cancer are multifactorial, including the use of thrombogenic cancer treatments (e.g., antiangiogenic agents, anti–epidermal growth factor receptor antibodies, cyclin-dependent kinase inhibitors, tyrosine kinase inhibitors, lenalidomide-based regimens, thalidomide, platinum-based therapies, monoclonal antibodies, antihormone therapies), extensive use of central catheters, and increasing awareness (Dave & Khorana, 2024; Grover et al., 2021). VTE is associated with a high risk of morbidity and mortality in patients with cancer and necessitates early recognition and treatment.

Clinical Manifestations

Although VTE has classic clinical manifestations, 50% of the cases of DVT and up to 40% of cases of PE have no initial observable symptoms (Lin, 2024). PE should be considered in patients who present with the four most frequent signs: dyspnea, pleuritic chest pain, hypoxia, and tachypnea. Less frequent signs are cough, hemoptysis, fever, syncope, diaphoresis, nonpleuritic chest pain, apprehension, rales, wheezing, hypotension, tachycardia, cyanosis, or pleural rub. Massive PE can present with hemodynamic instability or shock (Sandy, 2022). Recent unilateral swelling and pain above or below the knee without explanatory bone or joint trauma suggests DVT (Faiman & Wilks, 2022). Other signs of DVT include edema, warmth, localized pain, dilation of veins, color changes of the limb, and pyrexia. Edema may be caused by decreased venous return resulting from the embolism or capillary damage, producing leakage of intravascular fluid into the surrounding tissue, distal to the thrombosis site. When the affected limb is warm, it is most likely because of localized venous congestion and accumulation of tissue metabolites. Patients can experience pain in the calf muscle during dorsiflexion of the foot, known as Homans' sign. However, it is not a very specific finding for VTE and is positive in less than 50% of cases with a high incidence of false positives (Faiman & Wilks, 2022). Initially, pallor of the skin might be the only indicator of DVT. In other cases, erythema occurs immediately over the DVT site because of superficial thrombophlebitis. Pyrexia, a systemic increase in body temperature, can be caused by the accumulation of tissue metabolites at the site of the thrombosis.

Upper extremity DVT has become an increasingly recognized source of morbidity and mortality and represents less than 10% of all cases (Patel et al., 2020). It is often associated with central venous catheters and can occur in the subclavian, axillary, or brachial veins, with clinical symptoms consisting of edema, arm pain or discoloration, or the development of collateral veins involving the affected arm, neck, or chest wall.

Risk Factors and Etiology

Thrombophilia is the general term for a condition where the blood has an increased tendency to form clots. Two distinct types of thrombosis exist: venous and arterial, with VTE occurring more often than arterial thromboembolism (Ashorobi et al., 2024). The presence of cancer is a well-established independent risk factor for the development of VTE. In addition to the independent variable of cancer, risk for VTE development can be divided into patient-, disease-, and treatment-related factors. Several studies have indicated that both erythropoiesis-stimulating agents and blood transfusions can increase the risk of venous thrombosis in patients with cancer. Lee et al. (2023) conducted a case-crossover study that explored the association between the use of erythropoiesis-stimulating agents, blood transfusions, and the risk of venous thrombosis in patients with cancer using the National Health Insurance Database of Korea. Results indicated that there was an increased risk of thrombosis associated with red blood cell transfusions; however, the use of erythropoiesis-stimulating agents did not show a significant association with thrombotic events. See Figure 12-1 for a list of factors associated with increased VTE risk.

Pathophysiology and Patient Evaluation

Coagulation or clotting is the process whereby blood changes from a liquid form to a gel, creating a clot that potentially will stop bleeding. Many factors contribute to the

FIGURE 12-1. Risk Factors for Venous Thromboembolism

Patient Related	Cancer Related	Treatment Related
• Advanced age • African American race • Male gender • Obesity • Smoking • Pregnancy • Central venous catheters • Elevated white and red blood cell counts • First 6 months after cancer diagnosis and after progression • Factor V Leiden variant • Diabetes • Infection • Prothrombin G20210A variant • Prior venous thromboembolism • Pulmonary disease • Renal insufficiency	• Acute leukemia • Bladder • Brain • Central nervous system lymphoma • Colon/rectum • Kidney • Lung • Multiple myeloma • Myeloproliferative neoplasms • Non-Hodgkin lymphoma, especially aggressive lymphoma • Ovary • Pancreas • Stomach	• Antiangiogenesis agents • Bevacizumab • Biotherapy • Chemotherapy • Cisplatin • 5-Fluorouracil • L-Asparaginase • Lenalidomide • Surgery, especially vascular, orthopedic, and neurologic procedures • Red blood cell transfusion • Thalidomide

Note. Based on information from Falanga et al., 2023; Gervaso et al., 2021; Gong et al., 2021; Halsema & McMahon, 2023; Jordan Bruno et al., 2022; Khorana et al., 2022; Lee et al., 2023; Meknas et al., 2023; Moik & Ay, 2022; Pastori et al., 2023; Sanfilippo, 2022.

general prothrombotic state present in patients with cancer. In 1856, German physician Rudolf Virchow described three mechanisms integral to thrombosis formation, commonly referred to as the Virchow triad: aberrant blood flow, vascular integrity, and blood components (Wolberg et al., 2012). Figure 12-2 depicts the Virchow triad. French internist Armand Trousseau further elaborated on the cellular components within blood and was the first to discuss the relationship between malignancy and coagulation (Wolberg et al., 2012).

Blood Flow

The first mechanism involved in coagulation is blood flow. The normal fluidity, or viscosity, of blood depends on a balance between the plasma fluid in the blood and the cellular components. Changes in one or both elements may occur in patients with cancer, resulting in atypical blood flow and an increased prothrombotic risk. Under normal physiologic conditions, whole blood viscosity is a function of plasma viscosity, hematocrit, and red cell aggregation. When plasma viscosity increases, as may happen with high levels of plasma proteins or high fibrinogen levels, hyperviscosity of whole blood occurs, contributing to thrombotic risk. The brain, myocardium, lungs, and kidneys are especially vulnerable to the development of microthrombi, which most often manifest as headache, visual changes, chest pain, and dyspnea (Saffarieh et al., 2024).

Immunoglobulins, which are plasma proteins, also affect viscosity and blood flow. They can cause red cell dysplasia, in which healthy red blood cells have reduced ability to change their shape to flow through small spaces, especially in the microvasculature, and red cell aggregation can result. In the presence of high levels of plasma proteins, red cells begin to stack together or create long chains that can be seen in peripheral blood smears, or a rouleaux formation (Rosenthal & Freed, 2025). Plasma viscosity increases proportionately to the quantity and size of the plasma protein. Hyperviscosity is linked to increased levels of the proteins immunoglobulin M and immunoglobulin A (Alcantara & Klemisch, 2025b).

The cellular components of blood also influence the blood's ability to flow freely. High hematocrit and hemoglobin have been found to be associated with increased long-term risk of VTE, predominantly provoked VTE (Folsom et al., 2020). The consequences of high hematocrit levels have been studied with conflicting results. In earlier studies, it was believed that a high hematocrit was a thrombotic risk factor, which led to the recommendation of maintaining a hematocrit level less than 45% (Fox et al., 2021). Elevated platelet levels have also been identified in the pathogenesis of VTE.

Hyperleukocytosis, a high white blood cell count, is a common finding in acute and chronic leukemias, leading to leukostasis, an oncologic emergency in which white blood cell plugs develop within the microcirculation of the central nervous and respiratory systems. This is most commonly found in acute myeloid leukemia and acute

FIGURE 12-2. Virchow Triad

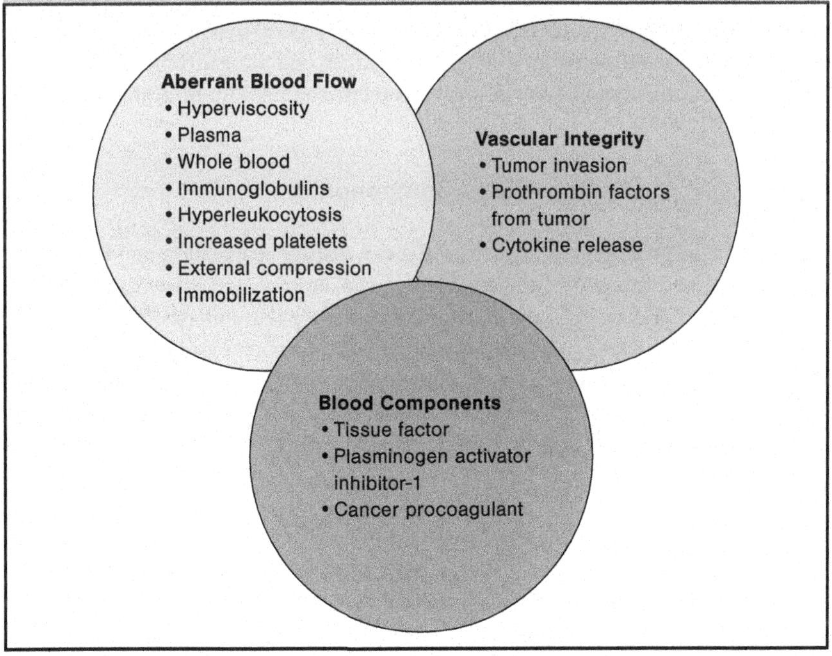

Note. Based on information from Wolberg et al., 2012.

promyelocytic leukemia because the myeloblasts are larger and less able to change shape than normal neutrophils (Alcantara & Klemisch, 2025a). Leukostasis occurs less in lymphoid leukemias because the cells are smaller, more deformable, and have lower adherence to the vasculature.

External compression resulting from tumor growth can impede blood flow. Intrinsic thrombus formation can also be secondary to the presence of vascular access devices (Azizi et al., 2020).

Immobilization associated with surgery or hospitalization can result in decreased and impaired blood flow. Patients who undergo oncologic surgery have twice the risk of thrombosis because of the underlying cancer and the resulting immobility (Pastori et al., 2023). A cohort study indicated an increased rate of VTE with the risk persisting for about two to four months postoperatively (Björklund et al., 2024).

Vessel Integrity

Vascular integrity is breached when the tumor directly invades or extends into the endothelial cell wall. Tumor cells produce prothrombotic factors that can be a significant constituent of the resulting clot, especially when the breached vessel is adjacent to the primary tumor (Gi et al., 2023).

Cytokines produced by tumor cells are key in the formation of thrombi and compromise of vascular integrity. The proximity of tumor cells, endothelial cells, and stromal cells provides the opportunity for cytokine-mediated interactions. Tumor cells produce proinflammatory cytokines, including interleukin-1, interleukin-6, and tumor necrosis factor-beta. Once released, these cytokines stimulate tissue factor (TF) expression on monocytes, thereby causing the monocyte to bind to the platelet. At the same time, they downregulate anticoagulant factors, including thrombomodulin and plasminogen activator inhibitor-1, creating an environment for thrombus formation (Pastori et al., 2023).

Blood Components

Tumor cells produce several factors that can disrupt coagulation and fibrinolytic systems and lead to a prothrombotic state in cancer, such as TF and cancer procoagulant. TF is a transmembrane glycoprotein receptor that initiates the coagulation cascade. When activated, it assembles several complexes that lead to thrombin production. TF can also be induced by proinflammatory cytokines or by vascular trauma. Elevated levels of plasma TF antigen and leukocyte TF have been found in patients with DVT (Pastori et al., 2023).

Patient History

A complete thrombosis history is important, including the age of onset and the location and results of diagnostic examinations for patients and their families. A history of VTE in one or more first-degree relatives is particularly notable because it suggests a hereditary defect or increased susceptibility to VTE disease (Faiman & Wilks, 2022).

Assessing for risk of VTE is important because half of the patients with VTE are asymptomatic. Nurses should discuss information with patients regarding conditions that could increase risk, such as recent surgery, trauma, heart failure, and immobility. Discussion of a female's use of oral contraceptive medications should take place. A complete cancer history, including any previous incidence of VTE, is also necessary because recurrent thrombosis, despite therapeutic anticoagulation, is more common in patients with cancer (Faiman & Wilks, 2022). In a general physical examination, special attention should be directed to the vascular and pulmonary systems and extremities. Because many clinical manifestations and examination findings can be nonspecific, further diagnostic testing is required to confirm or exclude the diagnosis of VTE.

Advanced Practice Considerations

The American Society of Hematology and the American Academy of Family Physicians recommend the use of prediction rules to establish the pretest probability of VTE (Lim et al., 2018; Randel, 2019). The Wells Clinical Prediction Rule is a clinical decision-making tool used to determine the probability of VTE prior to performing additional diagnostic tests. In the Wells test for DVT, patient assessment and symptoms determine the number of points given (Randel, 2019). One point each is scored if the patient has active cancer; paralysis, paresis, or plaster immobilization; previous DVT; or is recently bedridden. In addition, one point each is scored if the patient has localized tenderness, entire leg swelling, calf swelling, pitting edema in the affected leg, or collateral superficial veins. Two points are deducted if an alternative diagnosis is just as likely as DVT. A low probability of DVT is defined as a score of 0 or less, intermediate probability as a score of 1–2, and high probability as 3 or greater. In patients with symptoms in both legs, the more symptomatic leg is used for scoring.

There is also a prediction rule for PE. In this probability test, a score of 0–1 indicates low probability of PE; a score of 2–6 indicates intermediate probability; and a score of 7 or greater indicates high probability (Lo, 2020).

Historically, when a patient has been shown to have a low pretest probability of VTE, a D-dimer test is the next step. The D-dimer has a high sensitivity for the presence of an acute thrombosis. It can be used to exclude VTE with a high sensitivity for negative probability. In other words, patients with low pretest predictability and a negative D-dimer are considered to have DVT ruled out, and no further testing is needed (Lim et al., 2018). However, studies confirming the use of D-dimer as predictive of VTE have not included large numbers of patients with cancer.

For PE, a chest radiograph, arterial blood gases, and an electrocardiogram should be performed to rule out other disorders. Chest x-rays may reveal atelectasis, pleural-based infiltrates, or effusions. Arterial blood gases can show hypoxemia and hypocapnia. An electrocardiogram can show supraventricular arrhythmia, right axis deviation, or cor pulmonale. If the D-dimer is positive, further testing should be completed, including duplex ultrasound for both VTE and PE and chest CT angiography for PE (Lim et al., 2018; Lo, 2020).

Patients with an intermediate to high pretest predictability for VTE should have a venous duplex ultrasound performed as the first test when DVT is suspected (Lim et al., 2018; Lo, 2020). D-dimer can be used in addition after a negative ultrasound to determine whether further testing is needed (Lo, 2020). When DVT is suspected and D-dimer is positive despite a negative ultrasound, serial ultrasonography, CT venography, or contrast venography can be performed.

When PE is suspected in the presence of an intermediate to high pretest predictability, noninvasive pulmonary vascular imaging, including a CT pulmonary angiography and ventilation/perfusion scan, is recommended as initial radiologic evaluation (Lim et al., 2018; Lo, 2020). Both CT pulmonary angiography and ventilation/perfusion scans have a high degree of sensitivity to diagnose PE; therefore, the choice of imaging modality depends on the availability of the test, the resolution of images obtained, underlying conditions (including renal status), and the experience of the radiologist. Extra care should be taken when using dye in patients with renal insufficiency. In some areas, CT pulmonary angiography has become easier to obtain than ventilation/perfusion scans. In addition, it is more useful in patients with underlying cardiac disease and chronic obstructive pulmonary disease.

Treatment Modalities

Prophylaxis

Three professional groups issuing medical guidelines—the American College of Chest Physicians (ACCP), the American Society of Clinical Oncology (ASCO), and the National Comprehensive Cancer Network (NCCN)—recommend routine thromboprophylaxis with low-molecular-weight heparin (LMWH) or unfractionated heparin (UFH) for patients with cancer who do not have contraindications to anticoagulation and are undergoing surgical procedures or confined to bed with an acute illness (Key et al., 2023; NCCN, 2024; Stevens et al., 2021). Contraindications to anticoagulation are those conditions that put patients at an increased risk for bleeding, including clinically significant active or chronic bleeding, thrombocytopenia or platelet dysfunction, a high risk for falls, lumbar puncture, interventional spine and pain procedures, and clotting factor abnormalities that lead to prolonged prothrombin time or activated partial thromboplastin time (NCCN, 2025). Frequent reevaluation of these contraindications is recommended because they can be temporary in many patients. A risk–benefit analysis is critical when determining whether to administer thromboprophylaxis to patients.

Extended duration thromboprophylaxis should also be considered for all high-risk patients with cancer undergoing major abdominopelvic surgery. In a Cochrane review investigating extended duration thromboprophylaxis using LMWH following major abdominopelvic surgery, findings suggested a significant decrease in VTE with no difference in the incidence of bleeding complications or mortality between the control and LMWH group (Felder et al., 2019). Based on these findings, the National Institute for Health and Care Excellence, the American Society of Colon and Rectal

Surgeons, the American Society of Hematology, ASCO, and ACCP suggested the use of extended-duration thromboprophylaxis up to four weeks post-discharge for all high-risk patients undergoing major abdominopelvic surgery (Fleming et al., 2018; Gould et al., 2012; Key et al., 2023; Lyman et al., 2021; National Institute for Health Care Excellence, 2018).

For those with contraindications who are undergoing a major surgical procedure, mechanical prophylaxis with the use of venous compression devices, including graduated compression stockings and intermittent pneumatic compression, should be considered (Anderson et al., 2019). Mechanical prophylaxis should not be used alone except in the presence of contraindications to pharmacologic prophylaxis. The advantage of venous compression devices is that they can be used in patients with an increased risk of bleeding. Anticoagulation should be resumed as soon as the clinical picture allows.

Guidance for Treatment

Guidelines for the treatment of VTE from ACCP, ASCO, and NCCN are based on the findings of three major studies and differ slightly among each organization (Key et al., 2023; NCCN, 2025; Stevens et al., 2021). ACCP guidelines recommend an oral Xa inhibitor (e.g., apixaban, edoxaban, rivaroxaban) instead of LMWH for the initiation and treatment phases of therapy (Stevens et al., 2021). ASCO guidelines state that LMWH is preferred for the first 5–10 days of anticoagulation (Key et al., 2023). For long-term anticoagulation, LMWH, edoxaban, rivaroxaban, or apixaban for at least six months are preferred instead of vitamin K antagonists. NCCN guidelines recommend that direct oral anticoagulants and LMWH are preferable to warfarin in patients with cancer (NCCN, 2025). Duration of anticoagulation should be at least three months or as long as there is active cancer or cancer therapy. For patients with non–catheter-associated DVT or PE, indefinite anticoagulation is recommended while cancer is active, under treatment, or if risk for recurrence persists.

Heparin-Induced Thrombocytopenia

Both UFH and LMWH are associated with heparin-induced thrombocytopenia (HIT), which is an immune-mediated reaction to the presence of heparin. HIT occurs in 0.5%–1% of patients exposed to unfractionated heparin (Arepally & Padmanabhan, 2020). The incidence of HIT is lower (0.1%–0.5%) in patients receiving LMWH (Arepally & Padmanabhan, 2020). Patients with HIT have an increased risk for developing VTE for up to 100 days following diagnosis. Patients with a history of HIT should not be treated with UFH or LMWH. HIT should be suspected in patients who develop skin lesions at the injection site, have a systemic reaction to a bolus administration of heparin, or experience a greater than 50% decrease in platelet count from baseline laboratory values while receiving heparin (May et al., 2023). Another form, delayed-onset HIT, typically presents as thromboembolic complications at least five days after the final dose of LMWH or UFH (Naji et al., 2022). These patients usually have mild or moderate thrombocytopenia. If HIT is not suspected, patients are typically rechallenged with heparin. If HIT is suspected, heparin therapy should be stopped while antibody testing is completed. In the interim, patients can be effectively treated with non-heparin anticoagulant agents, such as direct thrombin inhibitors (Naji et al., 2022).

Nursing Management

Preventive measures for VTE for all hospitalized patients are a crucial part of the nurse's role (Yang et al., 2023). Positioning is an important aspect of prevention. Ensuring that patients avoid prolonged sitting and elevating the legs when in bed helps to promote venous return. Daily assessment of extremities for pain, erythema, and size discrepancy is vital. Proper use of compression devices, incentive spirometry, adequate hydration, and early ambulation are encouraged to prevent VTE. Nurses must vigilantly monitor patients who are immobilized or have had their activity restricted for unexplained tachypnea, tachycardia, and restlessness. These signs should not be attributed to anxiety unless a physical reason has been ruled out. Although patients are on anticoagulation therapy, nurses should pay attention to identify bleeding complications. If nurses observe a change in mental status or new focal neurologic deficits in patients receiving thrombolytics, intracranial hemorrhage must be evaluated as a possible cause. Nursing interventions related to VTE include (Yang et al., 2023):

- Instruct patients to do the following:
  - Avoid prolonged sitting.
  - Elevate legs when in bed.
  - Use an incentive spirometer.
  - Ambulate early.
  - Avoid medications that interfere with coagulation (e.g., aspirin, nonsteroidal anti-inflammatory drugs).
- Assess extremities for pain, erythema, and size discrepancy daily.
- Apply mechanical compression devices as ordered.
- Ensure adequate hydration.

Education regarding VTE should include information on the clinical condition itself, as well as treatments implemented and potential lifestyle changes that could reduce patient risk. Treatments that require teaching include early and frequent ambulation and proper and timely use of compression devices. When anticoagulation therapy is initiated, education regarding the administration and side effects of each medication is required. Patients or caregivers may need to learn to give subcutaneous injections if LMWH is to be continued after discharge. They should also learn the signs and symptoms of bleeding, including bleeding precautions, as well as the signs of subsequent or recurrent VTE. Education provided to patients and caregivers is essential for patients to maintain adherence to ongoing anticoagulation therapy. Patients continuing warfarin therapy will need to be instructed to maintain a consistent dietary intake of vitamin K–containing foods, such as dark green vegetables and apricots, to prevent decreased warfarin action (Card et al., 2020). Patients should be taught that their blood counts will need to be monitored to keep their international normalized ratio between 2 and 3 when on warfarin therapy (Garcia & Vazquez, 2025). Because patients with a history of VTE are at greater risk for subsequent VTE, they should be instructed to keep well hydrated and stretch every hour during confined travel (Key et al., 2023).

Thorough education for patients and caregivers can help them recognize potential problems and also reduce the risk of bleeding and recurrent VTE. Good communication, including possible interventions, needs to be in place to keep patients and caregivers calm and focused should bleeding or VTE occur.

Summary

Patients with cancer have an increased risk of developing VTE, which is associated with considerable morbidity and mortality. Hospitalized medical and surgical patients with cancer are at increased risk for VTE and should be considered for pharmacologic prophylaxis if no contraindications are present. When considering prophylactic anticoagulation in these patients, the risk of VTE must be carefully balanced with the increased risk of bleeding. Proper patient and family education regarding the risk of bleeding, as well as the signs and symptoms of both bleeding and VTE recurrence, is paramount in the care of patients with cancer.

The authors would like to acknowledge Colleen M. O'Leary, MSN, RN, AOCNS®, for her contribution to this chapter that remains unchanged from the previous edition of this book.

References

Alcantara, R., & Klemisch, R. (2025a). Hyperleukocytosis and leukostasis. *ACEP Critical Care Medicine.* https://www.acep.org/criticalcare/newsroom/newsroom-articles/january-2025/hyperleukocytosis -and-leukostasis

Alcantara, R., & Klemisch, R. (2025b). Hyperviscosity syndrome. *ACEP Critical Care Medicine.* https://www.acep.org/criticalcare/newsroom/newsroom-articles/january-2025/hyperviscosity-syndrome

Anderson, D.R., Morgano, G.P., Bennett, C., Dentali, F., Francis, C.W., Garcia, D.A., ... Dahm, P. (2019). American Society of Hematology 2019 guidelines for management of venous thromboembolism: Prevention of venous thromboembolism in surgical hospitalized patients. *Blood Advances, 3*(23), 3898–3944. https://doi.org/10.1182/bloodadvances.2019000975

Arepally, G.M., & Padmanabhan, A. (2020). Heparin-induced thrombocytopenia: A focus on thrombosis. *Arteriosclerosis, Thrombosis, and Vascular Biology, 41*(1), 141–152. https://doi.org/10.1161/ATVBAHA.120.315445

Arteaga, A.J.M., Font, C., & Rojas Hernandez, C.M. (2024). Quality of life in oncological patients with venous thromboembolic disease. *Research and Practice in Thrombosis and Haemostasis, 8*(5), 102510. https://doi.org/10.1016/j.rpth.2024.102510

Ashorobi, D., Ameer, M.A., & Fernandez, R. (2024). Thrombosis. In *StatPearls.* StatPearls Publishing. https://www.ncbi.nlm.nih.gov/books/NBK538430

Azizi, A.H., Shafi, I., Shah, N., Rosenfield, K., Schainfeld, R., Sista, A., & Bashir, R. (2020). Superior vena cava syndrome. *Journal of the American College of Cardiology: Cardiovascular Intervention, 13*(24), 2896–2910. https://doi.org/10.1016/j.jcin.2020.08.038

Björklund, J., Rautiola, J., Zelic, R., Edgren, G., Bottai, M., Nilsson, M., ... Akre, O. (2024). Risk of venous thromboembolic events after surgery for cancer. *JAMA Network Open, 7*(2), e2354352. https://doi.org/10.1001/jamanetworkopen.2023.54352

Card, D.J., Hall, A., Watson, H.G., Kitchen, D.P., & Harrington, D.J. (2020). Portion-controlled spinach for improved vitamin K antagonist anticoagulant control. *British Journal of Haematology, 189*(3), e71–e73. https://doi.org/10.1111/bjh.16481

Centers for Disease Control and Prevention. (2025). *Venous thromboembolism (blood clots): Data and statistics on venous thromboembolism.* https://www.cdc.gov/blood-clots/data-research/facts-stats/index.html

Dave, H.M., & Khorana, A.A. (2024). Management of venous thromboembolism in patients with active cancer. *Cleveland Clinic Journal of Medicine, 91*(2), 109–117. https://doi.org/10.3949/ccjm.91a.23017

Faiman, B., & Wilks, M. (2022). Deep vein thrombosis. In D. Camp-Sorrell, R. Hawkins, & D. Cope (Eds.), *Clinical manual for the oncology advanced practice nurse* (4th ed., pp. 313–322). Oncology Nursing Society.

Falanga, A., Ay, C., Di Nisio, M., Gerotziafas, G., Jara-Palomares, L., Langer, F., ... Jordan, K. (2023). Venous thromboembolism in cancer patients: ESMO Clinical Practice Guideline. *Annals of Oncology, 34*(5), 452–467. https://doi.org/10.1016/j.annonc.2022.12.014

Felder, S., Rasmussen, M.S., King, R., Sklow, B., Kwaan, M., Madoff, R., & Jensen, C. (2019). Prolonged thromboprophylaxis with low molecular weight heparin for abdominal or pelvic surgery. *Cochrane Database of Systematic Reviews, 3*(3), CD004318. https://doi.org/10.1002/14651858.CD004318.pub5

Fleming, F., Gaertner, W., Ternent, C.A., Finlayson, E., Herzig, D., Paquette, I.M., ... Steele, S.R. (2018). The American Society of Colon and Rectal Surgeons clinical practice guideline for the prevention of venous thromboembolic disease in colorectal surgery. *Diseases of the Colon and Rectum, 61*(1), 14–20. https://doi.org/10.1097/DCR.0000000000000982

Folsom, A.R., Wang, W., Parikh, R., Lutsey, P.L., Beckman, J.D., & Cushman, M. (2020). Hematocrit and incidence of venous thromboembolism. *Research and Practice in Thrombosis and Haemostasis, 4*(3), 422–428. https://doi.org/10.1002/rth2.12325

Fox, S., Griffin, L., & Harris, D.R. (2021). Polycythemia vera: Rapid evidence review. *American Family Physician, 103*(11), 680–687. https://www.aafp.org/pubs/afp/issues/2021/0601/p680.html

Garcia, D.A., & Vazquez, S.R. (2025). Patient education: Warfarin (beyond the basics). In J.S. Tirnauer (Ed.), *UpToDate.* Retrieved September 16, 2025, from https://www.uptodate.com/contents/warfarin-beyond-the-basics#H15

Gervaso, L., Dave, H., & Khorana, A.A. (2021). Venous and arterial thromboembolism in patients with cancer: JACC: CardioOncology state-of-the-art review. *JACC: CardioOncology, 3*(2), 173–190. https://doi.org/10.1016/j.jaccao.2021.03.001

Gi, T., Kuwahara, A., Yamashita, A., Matsuda, S., Maekawa, K., Moriguchi-Goto, S., ... Asada, Y. (2023). Histopathological features of cancer-associated venous thromboembolism: Presence of intrathrombus cancer cells and prothrombotic factors. *Arteriosclerosis, Thrombosis, and Vascular Biology, 43*(1), 146–159. https://doi.org/10.1161/ATVBAHA.122.318463

Gong, J., Drobni, Z.D., Alvi, R.M., Murphy, S.P., Sullivan, R.J., Hartmann, S.E., ... Neilan, T.G. (2021). Immune checkpoint inhibitors for cancer and venous thromboembolic events. *European Journal of Cancer, 158*, 99–110. https://doi.org/10.1016/j.ejca.2021.09.010

Gould, M.K., Garcia, D.A., Wren, S.M., Karanicolas, P.J., Arcelus, J.I., Heit, J.A., & Samama, C.M. (2012). Prevention of VTE in nonorthopedic surgical patients: Antithrombotic Therapy and Prevention of Thrombosis, 9th ed: American College of Chest Physicians Evidence-Based Clinical Practice Guidelines. *Chest, 141*(2, Suppl.), e227S–e277S. https://doi.org/10.1378/chest.11-2297

Grover, S.P., Hisada, Y.M., Kasthuri, R.S., Reeves, B.N., & Mackman, N. (2021). Cancer therapy–associated thrombosis. *Arteriosclerosis, Thrombosis, and Vascular Biology, 41*(4), 101063. https://doi.org/10.1161/ATVBAHA.120.314378

Halsema, K., & McMahon, B. (2023). Cancer-associated thrombosis: Risk assessment, prevention, and treatment. *Journal of the Advanced Practitioner in Oncology, 14*(3), 213–217. https://doi.org/10.6004/jadpro.2023.14.3.6

Jordan Bruno, X., Koh, I., Lutsey, P.L., Walker, R.F., Roetker, N.S., Wilkinson, K., ... Zakai, N.A. (2022). Venous thrombosis risk during and after medical and surgical hospitalizations: The medical inpatient thrombosis and hemostasis (MITH) study. *Journal of Thrombosis and Haemostasis, 20*(7), 1645–1652. https://doi.org/10.1111/jth.15729

Key, N.S., Khorana, A.A., Kuderer, N.M., Bohlke, K., Lee, A.Y.Y., Arcelus, J.I., ... Falanga, A. (2023). Venous thromboembolism prophylaxis and treatment in patients with cancer: ASCO guideline update. *Journal of Clinical Oncology, 41*(16), 3063–3074. https://doi.org/10.1200/JCO.23.00294

Khorana, A.A., Mackman, N., Falanga, A., Pabinger, I., Noble, S., Ageno, W., ... Lee, A.Y.Y. (2022). Cancer-associated venous thromboembolism. *Nature Reviews Disease Primers, 8*(1), 11. https://doi.org/10.1038/s41572-022-00336-y

Lee, T.C., Almeida, N., Pelletier, P., & McDonald, E.G. (2023). Comparison of blood transfusion rates before and after implementation of a quality improvement initiative for transfusion safety and appropriateness. *JAMA Network Open, 6*(1), e2252253. https://doi.org/10.1001/jamanetworkopen.2022.52253

Lim, W., Le Gal, G., Bates, S.M., Righini, M., Haramati, L.B., Lang, E., ... Mustafa, A. (2018). American Society of Hematology 2018 guidelines for management of venous thromboembolism: Diagnosis of venous thromboembolism. *Blood Advances, 2*(22), 3226–3256. https://doi.org/10.1182/bloodadvances.2018024828

Lin, J.L. (2024, November 14). Deep venous thrombosis (DVT). *Medscape.* https://emedicine.medscape.com/article/1911303-overview

Lo, B.M. (2020, October 30). Deep venous thrombosis risk stratification. *Medscape.* https://emedicine.medscape.com/article/1918446-overview

Lyman, G.H., Carrier, M., Ay, C., Di Nisio, M., Hicks, L.K., Khorana, A.A., ... Alonso-Coello, P. (2021). American Society of Hematology 2021 guidelines for management of venous thromboembolism: Prevention and treatment in patients with cancer. *Blood Advances, 5*(4), 927–974. https://doi.org/10.1182/bloodadvances.2020003442

Marin-Barrera, L., Muñoz-Martin, A.J., Rios-Herranz, E., Garcia-Escobar, I., Beato, C., Font, C., ... Jara-Palomares, L. (2020). A case-control analysis of the impact of venous thromboembolic disease on quality of life of patients with cancer: Quality of Life in Cancer (Qca) study. *Cancers, 12*(1), 75. https://doi.org/10.3390/cancers12010075

May, J., Westbrook, B., & Cuker, A. (2023). Heparin-induced thrombocytopenia: An illustrated review. *Research and Practice in Thrombosis and Haemostasis, 7*(5), 100283. https://doi.org/10.1016/j.rpth.2023.100283

Meknas, D., Brækkan, S.K., Hansen, J.-B., & Morelli, V.M. (2023). Surgery as a trigger for incident venous thromboembolism: Results from a population-based case-crossover study. *TH Open, 7*(3), e244–e250. https://doi.org/10.1055/a-2159-9957

Moik, F., & Ay, C. (2022). Venous and arterial thromboembolism in patients with cancer treated with targeted anti-cancer therapies. *Thrombosis Research, 213*(1, Suppl.), S58–S65. https://doi.org/10.1016/j.thromres.2022.01.004

Naji, F.S., Shafie, M., Issaiy, M., Jalalabadi, N.Z., & Parsa, S. (2022). Delayed-onset heparin-induced thrombocytopenia complicated with saddle embolus. *Clinical Case Reports, 10*(7), e6085. https://doi.org/10.1002/ccr3.6085

National Comprehensive Cancer Network. (2025). *NCCN Clinical Practice Guidelines in Oncology (NCCN Guidelines®): Cancer-associated venous thromboembolic disease* [v.3.2025]. https://www.nccn.org

National Institute for Health Care Excellence. (2018). *NICE guideline [NG89]: Interventions for people having abdominal, thoracic or head and neck surgery.* https://www.nice.org.uk/guidance/ng89/chapter/Recommendations#interventions-for-people-having-abdominal-thoracic-or-head-and-neck-surgery

Pastori, D., Cormaci, V.M., Marucci, S., Franchino, G., Del Sole, F., Capozza, A., ... Pignatelli, P. (2023). A comprehensive review of risk factors for venous thromboembolism: From epidemiology to pathophysiology. *International Journal of Molecular Sciences, 24*(4), 3169. https://doi.org/10.3390/ijms24043169

Patel, P., Braun, C., Patel, P., Bhatt, M., Begum, H., Wiercioch, W., ... Mustafa, R.A. (2020). Diagnosis of deep vein thrombosis of the upper extremity: A systematic review and meta-analysis of test accuracy. *Blood Advances, 4*(11), 2516–2522. https://doi.org/10.1182/bloodadvances.2019001409

Randel, A. (2019). Diagnosing VTE: Guidelines from the American Society of Hematology. *American Family Physician, 100*(11), 716–717. https://www.aafp.org/pubs/afp/issues/2019/1201/p716.html

Rosenthal, D.S., & Freed, J. (2025). Evaluation of the peripheral blood smear. In J.S. Tirnauer (Ed.), *UpToDate.* Retrieved September 16, 2025, from https://www.uptodate.com/contents/evaluation-of-the-peripheral-blood-smear

Saffarieh, E., Nokhostin, F., Yousefnezhad, A., & Yousefi Sharemi, S.R. (2024). Cancer-associated thrombotic microangiopathy: A review article. *Journal of Renal Injury Prevention, 13*(2), e32248. https://doi.org/10.34172/jrip.2023.32248

Sandy, B. (2022). Pulmonary embolism. In D. Camp-Sorrell, R. Hawkins, & D. Cope (Eds.), *Clinical manual for the oncology advanced practice nurse* (4th ed., pp. 229–236). Oncology Nursing Society.

Sanfilippo, K.M. (2022). Venous thromboembolism and risk stratification in hematological malignancies. *Thrombosis Research, 213*(1, Suppl.), S16–S21. https://doi.org/10.1016/j.thromres.2022.01.008

Stevens, S.M., Woller, S.C., Kreuziger, L.B., Bounameaux, H., Doerschug, K., Geersing, G.-J., ... Moores, L.K. (2021). Antithrombotic therapy for VTE disease: Second update of the CHEST Guideline and Expert Panel Report. *Chest, 160*(6), 2247–2259. https://doi.org/10.1016/j.chest.2021.07.056

Wolberg, A.S., Aleman, M.M., Leiderman, K., & Machlus, K.R. (2012). Procoagulant activity in hemostasis and thrombosis: Virchow's triad revisited. *Anesthesia and Analgesia, 114*(2), 275–285. https://doi.org/10.1213/ANE.0b013e31823a088c

Yang, B., Liu, C., Lin, Z., Geng, C., & Zhang, Z. (2023). Nursing management of treatment-related venous thromboembolism in patients with multiple myeloma. *Frontiers in Medicine, 10,* 1153694. https://doi.org/10.3389/fmed.2023.1153694

Diane G. Cope, PhD, APRN, BC, AOCNP®,
and Abigail Tesar, BSN, RN, OCN®, TCTCN™

CHAPTER 13

Disseminated Intravascular Coagulation

FAST FACTS

- **Description:** Disseminated intravascular coagulation is characterized by simultaneous bleeding and thrombosis. Platelet and coagulation factor consumption lead to hemorrhage, whereas thrombus formation leads to organ damage or failure.
- **Incidence:** This condition is primarily associated with severe sepsis, trauma, obstetric conditions, and malignancy, especially acute promyelocytic leukemia and mucin-secreting adenocarcinomas of the prostate, lung, and breast.
- **Clinical Manifestations:** Disseminated intravascular coagulation presents with clinical signs and symptoms of both bleeding and thrombosis. This condition can go undetected or result in an abrupt, life-threatening event.
- **Risk Factors and Etiology:** A wide range of malignancies may trigger disseminated intravascular coagulation related to tumor-driven procoagulant activity, endothelial disruption, and immune-mediated mechanisms.
- **Pathophysiology and Patient Evaluation:** Disseminated intravascular coagulation develops through activation of both intrinsic and extrinsic coagulation pathways. No one test can diagnose this condition. Diagnostic findings include evidence of a clinical condition known to be associated with disseminated intravascular coagulation and assessment of results of characteristic sequential laboratory findings that include low or rapidly decreasing platelet counts, prolonged coagulation tests, low plasma levels of coagulation factors and inhibitors, and increased markers of fibrin formation and degradation (i.e., fibrin degradation products, including D-dimer).
- **Advanced Practice Considerations:** Healthcare providers should assess bleeding and clotting history, review medications, and conduct a thorough physical examination of all organ systems.
- **Treatment Modalities:** Effective treatment of the underlying disorder is key. Supportive therapies include blood component replacement therapy to control bleeding, restoration of anticoagulation, and inhibition of fibrinolysis. Treatment is individualized based on clinical presentation, laboratory studies, and initiating pathology.
- **Nursing Management:** Nurses must conduct careful physical assessment to recognize subtle signs and symptoms of bleeding or thrombosis. They should also closely monitor vital signs, hemodynamic status, oxygenation, fluid status, and laboratory results. Blood products may be administered. Patient education is essential and should include prevention, recognition, and reporting of bleeding and symptoms of thrombosis.
- **Outcomes:** Early recognition and treatment initiation may improve patient outcomes. Supportive care measures aimed at breaking the cycle of thrombosis and hemorrhage

may provide time for antineoplastic therapies to control the precipitating malignancy and ablate the mechanisms leading to disseminated intravascular coagulation. However, it is associated with a poor prognosis and death, usually related to the underlying pathology.

Introduction

Disseminated intravascular coagulation (DIC) is a potentially fatal oncologic emergency. It is characterized by the systemic activation of intravascular coagulation, depletion of clotting factors and platelets, inadequate fibrin removal, and widespread deposition of fibrin in the microvasculature of small and midsize vessels, leading to thrombotic occlusion, tissue ischemia, and multiorgan failure. The excessive activation of platelets and coagulation factors, which are subsequently consumed, coincides with thrombi formation, inducing severe bleeding (Popescu et al., 2022; Smith, 2021). Thus, DIC is both a bleeding and a thrombotic disorder.

Underlying malignancy accounts for more than 25% of DIC cases in patients who are critically ill, and mortality can range anywhere from 31%–86% (Popescu et al., 2022). The presence of simultaneous thrombosis and bleeding can lead to devastating sequelae and presents complex treatment challenges. Oncology nurses should be knowledgeable about DIC, as recognizing signs and symptoms early may allow for prompt diagnosis and intervention. Early recognition and emergent treatment are crucial to help minimize the morbidity and mortality associated with DIC.

DIC can develop in acute and chronic forms. Acute DIC is a severe systemic disorder that occurs when the blood is suddenly exposed to procoagulants, activating intravascular coagulation. Compensatory hemostatic mechanisms are quickly overwhelmed with the ongoing activation of coagulation, and, as a result, a severe state of consumptive coagulopathy occurs, leading to profuse bleeding from multiple sites. According to Adelborg et al. (2021), clinically significant bleeding may occur in up to 50% of patients with cancer-related DIC. The simultaneous development of widespread thrombosis within the microvasculature compromises blood supply, causes ischemia, and leads to multiorgan failure. Microthrombus formation is typically more pronounced in sepsis-related DIC and frequently leads to renal or hepatic dysfunction.

In contrast, chronic DIC reflects a compensated state that develops when blood is continuously or intermittently exposed to small amounts of procoagulant. Compensatory mechanisms in the liver and bone marrow can sufficiently maintain stability, and there may be little obvious clinical or laboratory indication of the presence of DIC. However, chronic DIC is a risk factor for venous thromboembolism (VTE) and is associated with increased mortality (Adelborg et al., 2021). Chronic DIC is more likely to be seen in patients with an underlying malignancy or aortic disorder (Okamoto et al., 2024).

Incidence

DIC occurs secondary to an underlying pathologic condition, such as sepsis, trauma, malignancy, hematologic disorders, or obstetric disorders. DIC is associated mainly with sepsis, occurring in approximately 29%–61% of cases, and with trauma and systemic inflammatory response syndrome, occurring in approximately 36%–41% of cases (Adelborg et al., 2021). DIC associated with malignancy is most frequently seen in patients with a diagnosis of acute promyelocytic leukemia (APL) or advanced malignancy. Patel et al. (2024) found that approximately 19% of hospitalized patients with APL exhibited DIC. According to Sohal et al. (2020), 15% of patients with cancer develop DIC. It is estimated to occur in approximately 7% of patients with solid tumor malignancies, increasing up to 21% for patients with advanced malignancies.

Clinical Manifestations

DIC is characterized by widespread coagulation activation leading to microvascular thrombosis and bleeding due to the consumption of clotting factors and platelets, with a highly variable presentation. Acute DIC is characterized by generalized bleeding, which may occur at any site and range from oozing to uncontrolled hemorrhage. Most frequently occurring in sepsis, acute leukemia, and tumor lysis syndrome, acute DIC can progress rapidly from an asymptomatic presentation to diffuse bleeding from multiple sites as the underlying etiology progresses (Adelborg et al., 2021). Common sites of bleeding include the mucous membranes, the gingiva, the gastrointestinal system, surgical sites, venipuncture sites, drain sites, and wound sites. Signs of bleeding may include epistaxis, petechiae, ecchymoses, hematomas, wound bleeding, and blood oozing at a venipuncture or catheter site. Blood may be evident in the urine, stool, or emesis. Mental status changes, including headache, papilledema, confusion, disorientation, and irritability, may reflect intracerebral bleeding.

Chronic (clinically non-overt or occult) DIC is usually a mild, clinically insignificant condition that occurs when blood is exposed to small amounts of tissue factor (TF). Compensatory mechanisms in the liver and bone marrow usually can sufficiently control the condition, and there is a gradual systemic activation of the coagulation system (Adelborg et al., 2021). Chronic DIC is more frequently observed in patients with solid tumors or large aortic aneurysms (Okamoto et al., 2024).

Patients with DIC secondary to an underlying cancer usually present with chronic DIC. They are commonly asymptomatic with no clinical evidence of bleeding or thrombosis and have only laboratory evidence of DIC. In contrast to DIC associated with sepsis and trauma, which may have a fulminant presentation, DIC in patients with cancer may proceed gradually and silently until platelets and coagulation factors are depleted and bleeding occurs, usually at the tumor site (Popescu et al., 2022).

Signs and symptoms associated with thrombosis at any organ site develop as a result of hypoperfusion, ischemia, infarction, necrosis, and organ failure. Thrombi occurring in superficial and small veins may be clinically undetectable. Widespread thrombosis may manifest as focal ischemia with tender, red, indurated areas over organ sites; peripheral acrocyanosis (blue fingers, toes, earlobes, and nose tip); and gastrointestinal ulcers, including stress ulcers that may cause obvious bleeding (Adelborg et al., 2021). Dyspnea, hemoptysis, and cough may indicate the presence of pulmonary emboli. Thrombosis in the central nervous system may present as neurologic symptoms, such as paresthesias, obtunded mental status, convulsions, delirium, and coma (Smith, 2021). Early recognition and prompt treatment are crucial; if unrecognized, DIC can be fatal from severe hemorrhage.

Risk Factors and Etiology

A wide variety of clinical conditions are associated with the risk of DIC development, including sepsis, severe trauma, injury, malignancy, infections, environmental factors, obstetric disorders, surgical complications, shock, malignancy, and cardiovascular, pancreatic, hepatic, and connective tissue disorders (Ahuja & Conran, 2025). In most situations, the risk of extensive coagulation depends on the severity of the associated systemic inflammatory response in combination with underlying pathologic conditions, such as liver dysfunction (Iba et al., 2023).

Acute DIC occurs frequently in patients with severe trauma and tissue injury, particularly following brain injuries (Iba et al., 2023). Chronic DIC may occur in patients with rheumatoid arthritis, Raynaud disease, ulcerative colitis, Crohn disease, and sarcoidosis (Levi, 2022). Although acute DIC can be seen in patients with cancer, it tends to be more often chronic, with mild abnormalities in laboratory values (Ahuja & Conran, 2025). Disorders that mimic the clinical picture of DIC include the microangiopathic hemolytic anemias, such as thrombocytopenic thrombotic purpura, hemolytic uremic syndrome, and chemotherapy-induced microangiopathic hemolytic anemia. These syndromes may lead to organ failure (Levi, 2022). Most of the conditions associated with DIC share common features, including the expression of TF by mononuclear or cancer cells and the release of TF-bearing cells following tissue injury that initiates the coagulation cascade (Levi, 2022).

Malignancy

DIC is the most common coagulopathy in malignancy and can present in three different forms: procoagulant, hyperfibrinolytic, and subclinical (Sohal et al., 2020). In the procoagulant form, thrombotic features in the microvasculature are observed due to the production of excess thrombin. In contrast, the hyperfibrinolytic form manifests clinically with bleeding due to activation of the fibrinolytic system. The subclinical form presents in some patients who lack overt thrombosis or bleeding but do have laboratory markers indicating activation of coagulation or fibrinolysis.

DIC may complicate solid and hematologic cancers. Among solid cancers, mucin-secreting adenocarcinoma is predominantly associated with DIC, with tumors involving the gastrointestinal tract, pancreas, lung, breast, or prostate, and occasionally glioblastomas or other brain tumors (Sohal et al., 2020). Additionally, in patients with cancer, tumor cells that generate TF or increase tumor factor generation on the surface of monocytes or macrophages initiate the pathophysiologic process in DIC. TF then binds to factor VII and activates factors IX and X. Endothelial cells also express TF and are involved in the regulation of blood coagulation because of the role of the endothelium in protein C activation and the expression of TF pathway inhibitor and thrombomodulin. Furthermore, some tumors generate a cysteine protease, which directly activates factor X. Proinflammatory cytokines and tumor necrosis factor (TNF) may further trigger procoagulant pathways and may be aggravated by chemotherapy (Smith, 2021). Other pathologic changes arising from the malignant process are also associated with the development of coagulation disorders in patients with cancer, including derangements in the endothelial linings of new blood vessels stimulated by angiogenesis, bone marrow dysfunction, hypoproteinemia, and impairment of organs involved with metastatic deposits.

DIC associated with solid tumors is usually subclinical in nature and characterized by an absence of clinical evidence of clotting or bleeding (Sohal et al., 2020). However, metastatic prostate cancer may be associated with a hyperfibrinolytic form of DIC. In prostate cancer–related DIC, interactions between the TF–secreting cancer cells and the aggregates formed between the patient's monocytes and platelets lead to upregulation of TF (Hell et al., 2021).

In APL, malignant cells produce the procoagulants TF, cysteine proteinase procoagulant, and procoagulant microparticles. TF forms a complex with factor VII to activate factor X, generating thrombin. Cysteine proteinase procoagulant directly activates factor X and generates thrombin in the absence of factor VII. APL cells also release procoagulant microparticles involved in hypercoagulability, as seen in the more aggressive, microgranular form of the disease that is associated with a higher risk of hemorrhagic death (Ten Cate & Leader, 2021).

Patients with APL also develop severe hyperfibrinolysis, a characteristic feature of DIC associated with the presence of annexin II, a cell surface phospholipid-binding protein in patients with APL (Ten Cate & Leader, 2021). Annexin II is expressed on endothelial cells and macrophages and acts as a cell surface receptor for plasmin and tissue plasminogen activator (tPA). APL cells express higher levels of annexin II that facilitate tPA-mediated conversion of plasminogen to plasmin. Another substance that may be related to the hemorrhagic process in APL is thrombin activatable fibrinolysis inhibitor. Thrombin, bound to thrombomodulin, protects fibrin clots from plasmin-mediated fibrinolysis. Thrombomodulin activates thrombin-activatable fibrinolysis inhibitor, hampering fibrinolysis by removing lysine residues on fibrin, which act to bind plasminogen and tPA and generate plasmin. Fibrinolysis is also increased by granulocytic proteases produced by APL cells, which act to separate fibrinogen and degrade fibrinolytic inhibitors (Ten Cate & Leader, 2021).

Pathophysiology and Patient Evaluation

The Normal Coagulation Process

The normal hemostasis process that controls bleeding following vascular or tissue injury results from an intricate balance between blood clot formation (coagulation) and blood clot dissolution (fibrinolysis). In general, all the substances necessary for clotting to occur circulate within the bloodstream in a soluble, inactive form. A stimulus, such as injury to small blood vessels or endothelial tissue, triggers a series of events called the coagulation cascade, in which each clotting factor is activated sequentially and acts to convert soluble fibrinogen into fibrin and form a stable, insoluble fibrin clot. When a stimulus triggers the coagulation cascade, opposing fibrinolytic pathways are activated to defend against excessive clot formation and ultimately lyse the clots and restore normal blood flow. In the process of fibrinolysis, plasmin digests fibrinogen and fibrin into fragments—fibrin degradation products (FDPs) or fibrin split products. FDPs impart an anticoagulant effect and prevent further clotting. See Table 13-1 for a list of normal coagulation factors and Figure 13-1 for a diagram of the coagulation cascade and fibrinolysis.

The coagulation cascade is initiated via two pathways: the TF pathway (extrinsic pathway) and the contact activation pathway (intrinsic pathway), which merge into the common pathway of coagulation with the activation of factor X (Park & Park, 2024). Both pathways are required for normal hemostasis, and positive feedback loops exist between the two pathways that amplify reactions to produce enough fibrin to form a lifesaving plug. Deficiencies or abnormalities in any single factor can slow the overall process, increasing the risk of hemorrhage. The TF pathway is considered the first step in coagulation. A transmembrane glycoprotein present on several cell types, including monocytes, vascular endothelial cells, cancer cells, and TF, is released into

TABLE 13-1
Plasma Coagulation Factors

Factor	Common Names	Actions
I	Fibrinogen	Cleaved by thrombin to form a fibrin clot
II	Prothrombin	Activated on the surface of activated platelets Active form activates factors I, V, VII, VIII, X, XI, and XIII, as well as protein C and platelets
III	Tissue factor (TF) Tissue thromboplastin	A subendothelial cell-surface glycoprotein that binds phospholipids; complexes with activated factor VIIaa (TF–VIIa) to initiate the extrinsic pathway
IV	Calcium ion (Ca^{2+})	Required in every step of the clotting process, other than the initial two steps for clotting factors to bind to phospholipid
V	Labile factor Proaccelerin Ac-globulin	Complexes with factor Xa to convert prothrombin to thrombin
VI—obsolete term (same as Va)	Accelerin	Same as factor V
VII	Stable factor Proconvertin	Complexes with tissue factor (TF–VIIa) to activate factor X and factor IX in the presence of Ca^{2+}

(Continued on next page)

TABLE 13-1
Plasma Coagulation Factors *(Continued)*

Factor	Common Names	Actions
VIII	Antihemophilic factor A Antihemophilic globulin	Cofactor of factor IX in the intrinsic pathway to form the tenase complex
IX	Plasma thromboplastin component Christmas factor Antihemophilic factor B	Activates factor X in the intrinsic pathway to form tenase complex with factor VIII
X	Stuart-Prower factor Stuart factor	Activated on the surface of activated platelets and by TF–VIIa complex in the presence of Ca^{2+} Activated when intrinsic and extrinsic pathways converge, forming the prothrombinase complex with factor V
XI	Plasma thromboplastin antecedent Antihemophilic factor C	Involved in the intrinsic pathway activation to activate factor IX
XII	Hageman factor Contact factor Antihemophilic factor D	Involved in the first step of the intrinsic pathway activation to activate factors XI, VII, and prekallikrein
XIII	Fibrin stabilizing factor Plasma transglutaminase	Synthesized by platelets; stabilizes the fibrin clot by cross-linkage of fibrin
Antithrombin	Antithrombin III	Natural inhibitor of factors Xa, IXa, XIa, XIIa, thrombin, and TF–VIIa complex
Plasminogen	–	Converts to plasmin to lyse fibrin and other proteins
Protein C	–	Inactivates factors Va and VIIIa
Protein S	–	Cofactor for activated protein C
Thrombomodulin	–	Protein on the surface of the endothelial cell binds to thrombin and activates protein C

[a]Indicates the clotting factor has been activated

Note. Based on information from National Bleeding Disorders Foundation, 2025.

FIGURE 13-1. Coagulation Cascade and Fibrinolysis

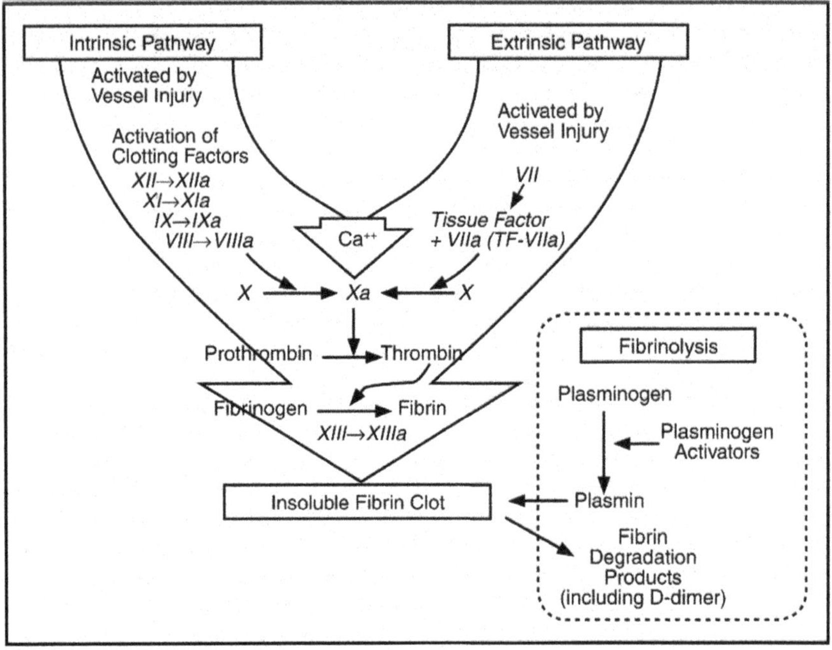

The letter "a" indicates the clotting factor has been activated.

Note. Image courtesy of Marcelle Kaplan. Used with permission.

the circulation following damage to capillary endothelial cells and tissue injury (e.g., severe trauma, sepsis, cancer), exposure to endotoxin, expression of inflammatory cytokines, or expression of procoagulant molecules (e.g., TF) by tumor cells (Iba et al., 2023). Once released, TF binds with activated clotting factor VII (denoted as VIIa) and calcium to form the TF–VIIa complex, which acts to initiate the coagulation cascade via the TF pathway. The formation of the TF–VIIa complex, in turn, activates factor IX and factor X, leading to the generation of thrombin, the end point in the coagulation cascade. The contact activation pathway, initiated by events that take place within the lumen of blood vessels, is a parallel pathway for thrombin formation. The pathway begins with factor XII and factor XI, which results in the activation of factor XI. Activated factor XI further activates factor IX, which then acts with its cofactor, factor VIII, to form a tenase complex on a phospholipid surface to activate factor X, resulting in thrombin formation (Unar et al., 2023).

Pathogenesis

The pathogenesis of DIC is based on a hemostatic activation process that involves both the contact activation (intrinsic) pathway and TF (extrinsic) pathway, and regulates the coagulation cascade. Four simultaneous pathologic mechanisms have primary roles in promoting a procoagulant state in DIC, including TF–mediated thrombin generation, suppression of anticoagulant mechanisms, inhibition and impairment of the fibrinolytic system, and activation of proinflammatory cytokines, mainly interleukin-6 and TNF-α (Iba et al., 2023). Although many different clinical conditions can trigger DIC, once coagulation is activated, the pathologic processes are similar for all disorders.

The physiologic effects of excessive thrombin production in DIC are initiated by TF, which is present on the surface of many cell types and functions as a receptor and activator of factor VII, leading to its activation (Unar et al., 2023). Vascular damage, which may be caused by endothelial disruption, inflammation, or tumor cell expression of procoagulant molecules, leads to the release of TF into the circulation. Table 13-2 lists the effects of excess thrombin generation on coagulation.

Normally, opposing reactions that prevent coagulation balance mechanisms that promote thrombin formation. However, in DIC, the anticoagulant pathways that tightly regulate thrombin are suppressed. Antithrombin, the protein C system, and TF pathway inhibitor are all impaired. Thrombomodulin, a protein found on the surfaces

TABLE 13-2
Effects of Excess Thrombin Generation on Coagulation

Action of Thrombin	Outcome
Converts fibrinogen to fibrin	Widespread microvasculature fibrin deposition; depletion of fibrinogen
Activates platelet activity	Increased platelet aggregation; platelet consumption leading to thrombocytopenia
Activates clotting factors V, VIII, XI, and XIII	Increased thrombin generation and thrombosis; consumption of clotting factors
Activates opposing anticoagulant reactions by antithrombin and activated protein C	Degraded clotting factors (V, VIII, XI, XIII); promotion of fibrinolysis; consumption of antithrombin; decreased protein C levels Thrombosis and bleeding caused by depletion of all the prothrombotic clotting factors and antithrombin
Activates fibrinolysis	Increased circulating fibrinogen leading to increased formation and lysis of fibrin clots; increased circulating fibrin split products have anticoagulant effects (inhibit platelet aggregation); fibrinogen depleted; hemorrhage promoted
Activates endothelial cells, especially in the skin	Coagulation initiated by tissue factor expression from damaged endothelium; downregulation of thrombomodulin; protein C activation inhibited; activated protein C levels reduced
Enhances activation of proinflammatory factors	Promotion of inflammatory effects of white blood cells; release of cytokines

Note. Based on information from Iba et al., 2023; Unar et al., 2023.

of a variety of cells, acts to inhibit thrombin formation by binding to thrombin and activating protein C. Inflammatory cytokines released by endothelial cells, including interleukin-1, interleukin-6, and TNF, downregulate thrombomodulin, leading to impaired production of activated protein C. Levels of protein C are further reduced by consumption, capillary leakage, and decreased protein synthesis in the liver, which results in limited inactivation of coagulation factors Va and VIIIa (Unar et al., 2023). TF pathway inhibitor inhibits early phases of the procoagulant response. It is localized on the endothelium surface, where it is a potent inhibitor of TF–VIIa complexes that initiate blood coagulation. In DIC, TF pathway inhibitor activity is suppressed and unable to counterbalance the increase in TF-induced activation of coagulation (Iba et al., 2023).

Fibrinolysis becomes hyperactive in response to widespread intravascular fibrin deposition. The increase in plasminogen activator inhibitor-1 level causes fibrinolytic suppression and is an important predictor of multiorgan dysfunction and poor prognosis (Adelborg et al., 2021). Eventually, the magnitude of increased fibrin formation overwhelms the process of fibrinolysis, resulting in further fibrin deposition in the vasculature, occlusion of blood flow, and development of peripheral ischemia and end-organ damage. Ongoing intravascular coagulation leads to the consumption of clotting factors, platelets, and anticoagulant substances, and thus bleeding occurs.

Excessive circulating thrombin stimulates the increased conversion of plasminogen to plasmin, a protein that cleaves fibrinogen and releases FDPs, such as D-dimer. FDPs act as circulating anticoagulants, inhibiting the activity of platelets and leading to hemorrhage. The presence of plasmin and TNF in circulation activates the complement pathway and induces lysis of red blood cells and platelets, causing thrombocytopenia and releasing more procoagulant material (Unar et al., 2023). Activation of factor XII leads to the conversion of kininogen into circulating kinins. Clinically, activation of the complement system and kinin system in DIC causes increased vascular permeability, hypotension, and shock.

Another important mechanism in the pathogenesis of DIC is the interaction between the inflammatory cascade and the coagulation pathways. Inflammation activates the clotting cascade, and the subsequent coagulation stimulates increased inflammatory activity. Factor Xa, thrombin, and the TF–VIIa complex have been found to stimulate endothelial cell release of proinflammatory cytokines. In contrast, suppression of activated protein C and antithrombin enhances a proinflammatory state (Iba et al., 2023). Interactions between inflammatory and coagulation pathways in DIC create a vicious circle of bleeding, clotting, and fibrinolysis.

The pathophysiology of DIC is complex and centers primarily on enhanced thrombin generation triggered by vascular endothelium damage and the subsequent dysregulated systemic coagulation following initiation of the TF pathway (Popescu et al., 2022). Inappropriate activation of thrombin-mediated systems leads to widespread fibrin deposition in the microvasculature, impaired fibrinolysis, and consumption coagulopathy. Figure 13-2 presents a schema of the processes involved in DIC. The clinical picture is one of bleeding, intravascular thrombosis, and multiorgan damage and failure. As nurses gain a complete understanding of the pathophysiology of DIC,

FIGURE 13-2. Processes in Disseminated Intravascular Coagulation

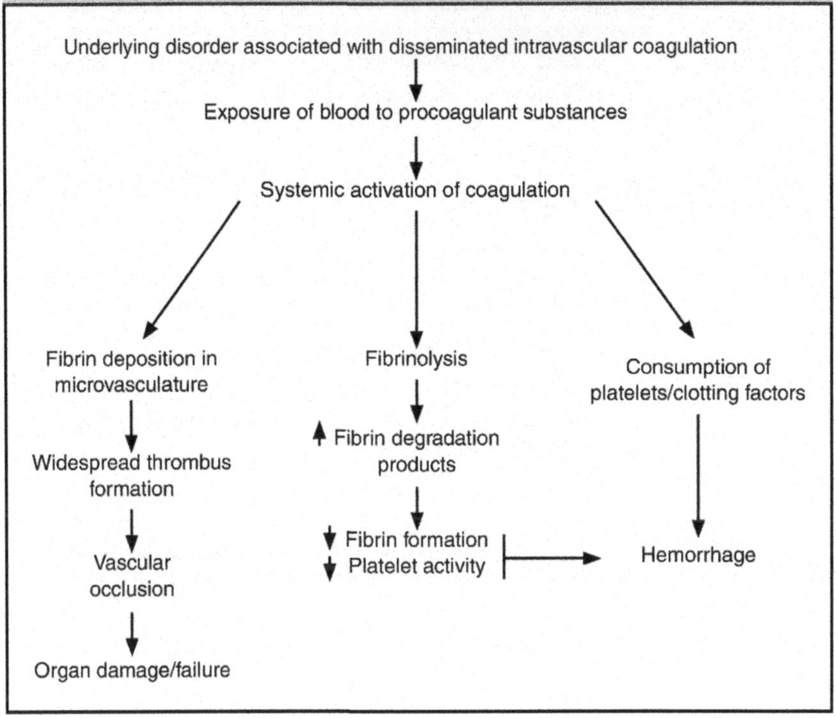

they will be able to more readily identify and monitor the underlying pathologic conditions that predispose patients to developing this complication.

Patient Assessment

History

DIC may be fulminant or low grade depending on the disease triggering the syndrome. Because DIC is not a specific disease entity but a manifestation of an underlying disorder, a thorough history includes a search for the presence of a clinical condition that may increase the risk of DIC. Nurses should question patients about previous bleeding or clotting events, such as gastrointestinal bleeding or deep vein thrombosis, transfusion history, nutritional status to evaluate for vitamin K deficiency, and medications, including over-the-counter drugs (Sohal et al., 2020).

Physical Examination

Assessment of patients at risk for developing DIC includes evaluation of clinical manifestations that may occur because of bleeding or thrombosis. Nurses should conduct a thorough assessment of each organ system when evaluating patients for risk or presence of bleeding (Smith, 2021) (see Table 13-3).

TABLE 13-3
Physical Assessment for Patients at Risk for Bleeding or Thrombosis

Site/System	Assessment
Central nervous system (symptoms dependent on site and size of bleeding or clot)	Headache, nausea, vomiting, retching, mental status changes (restlessness, confusion, lethargy, obtundation, coma), vertigo, seizures, changes in pupil size and reactivity, eye deviations, sensory or motor strength alterations, speech alterations, paralysis
Eyes	Visual disturbances: blurring, diplopia, absent or altered fields of vision, nystagmus, increased injections in the sclera, conjunctival hemorrhage, periorbital edema; note if sclerae are icteric
Nose	Petechiae, blood-tinged drainage, epistaxis
Mouth	Petechiae of the oral mucosa, pain, dysphagia, hematemesis, bleeding gums/mucosa, blood-tinged secretions, ulcerations with frank bleeding
Upper gastrointestinal (esophagus/stomach)	Dysphagia, hematemesis, blood-tinged secretions, substernal burning and pain, epigastric discomfort (burning, tenderness, or cramping), coffee-ground emesis, nausea, vomiting, fever, weakness, anorexia, melena, hyperactive bowel sounds
Lower gastrointestinal (duodenum/anus)	Pain (location, occurrence, duration, quality), nausea, vomiting, tarry stools, diarrhea, bowel sounds (hyperactive or hypoactive), cramping, occult blood in stools, frank blood in stools (rectum or lower), blood around anus, frequency and quantity of stools, pain with bowel movements (hemorrhoids)
Lungs	Tachypnea, dyspnea, air hunger, respiration rate, depth, exertion, crackles, rubs, wheezing, diminished breath sounds, hemoptysis (frothy bright red blood in sputum—major airway bleeding), stridor, tickling in throat or chest with desire to cough
Cardiovascular	Tachycardia and hypotension (characteristic of anemia and acute blood loss) Changes in vital signs, color and temperature of extremities, peripheral pulses (present, quality), changes in peripheral perfusion Pericardial effusions: dyspnea, cough, pain, orthopnea, venous distension, tamponade (muted heart sounds, hypotension, pulsus paradoxus, angina, palpitations)

Advanced Practice Considerations

DIC is a highly dynamic condition, and no single laboratory test can definitively establish a diagnosis. Patient history, clinical evidence, and a multitude of associated laboratory tests are necessary to confirm a diagnosis. Table 13-4 describes common laboratory abnormalities associated with DIC. In clinical practice, the diagnosis of DIC is based on the clinical impression and the abnormal results of a combination of

TABLE 13-4
Laboratory Data in Disseminated Intravascular Coagulation

Laboratory Test	Result	Comments
Activated partial thromboplastin time	Prolonged	Prolonged, shortened, or normal Decreased quantity of coagulation factors Nonspecific in DIC; may be caused by heparin therapy, increased fibrin degradation products, and consumption of clotting factors
Alpha-2 antiplasmin	Decreased	Hyperfibrinolysis
Antithrombin	Decreased	Anticoagulant activity inhibited Accelerated coagulation
D-dimer	Elevated	Indicates hyperfibrinolysis Common in DIC, trauma, recent surgery, inflammation, and venous thromboembolism
Fibrin degradation products	Elevated	Indicates breakdown of fibrin and fibrinogen Elevated levels possible with surgery, obstetric complications, inflammation, and venous thromboembolism
Fibrinogen	Decreased	Plasma concentration of fibrinogen decreases; seen only in severe cases of DIC Nonspecific in DIC; may be low because of congenital or acquired hypofibrinogenemia, fibrinolysis, severe liver disease, malignant disease, or obstetric trauma
Fibrinopeptide A	Elevated	Indicates an accelerated rate of fibrin formation and coagulation
International normalized ratio	Prolonged	Prolonged, shortened, or normal Nonspecific in DIC Evaluates overall coagulation
Peripheral smear	Schistocytes (red cell fragments) present	Nonspecific finding in DIC
Plasminogen	Decreased	Hyperfibrinolysis
Platelet count	Decreased	A frequent finding, but nonspecific in DIC Decreasing trend in serial platelet counts; may show a steep drop Absolute platelet count < 100,000 cells/mcl
Protein C	Decreased	Anticoagulant activity inhibited Accelerated coagulation

(Continued on next page)

TABLE 13-4
Laboratory Data in Disseminated Intravascular Coagulation *(Continued)*

Laboratory Test	Result	Comments
Prothrombin time	Prolonged	Prolonged, shortened, or normal Nonspecific in DIC; may be prolonged because of liver disease, vitamin K deficiency, obstructive biliary disease, or warfarin therapy
Thrombin time	Elevated	Estimate of plasma fibrinogen Prolonged with heparin, streptokinase, or urokinase therapy Prolonged in DIC, liver disease, or fibrinogen deficiency
Thrombin–antithrombin complex	Elevated	Indicates an accelerated rate of fibrin formation and coagulation

DIC—disseminated intravascular coagulation

Note. Based on information from Adelborg et al., 2021; Cope, 2016; Levi, 2022.

tests that include platelet count, global clotting times (e.g., activated partial thromboplastin time, prothrombin time, thrombin time), clotting factors (e.g., protein C, protein S), antithrombin, and FDPs (Adelborg et al., 2021; Smith, 2021). These values may change markedly as the clinical situation evolves and need to be tested serially.

Interpretation of laboratory data is difficult because tests are not specific to DIC. Serial coagulation tests are more helpful than a single laboratory result in diagnosing DIC. They can reveal a sudden shift from an initially mild abnormality to severe DIC. The classic laboratory findings for DIC are prolonged prothrombin time, activated partial thromboplastin time, and thrombin time; increased levels of FDPs and D-dimer; low platelet count; low fibrinogen levels; and low plasma levels of coagulation factor, antithrombin, and protein C (Adelborg et al., 2021; Iba et al., 2023). A low initial platelet count (< 100,000 cells/mcl) or a rapid platelet decline over serial measurements can indicate DIC. A peripheral blood smear that reveals schistocytes (fragmented red blood cells) may help confirm a diagnosis of DIC (Sohal et al., 2020). Prolonged clotting times may indicate consumption of various coagulation factors, including factors V and VII, but can be caused by chronic liver disease or vitamin K deficiency (Adelborg et al., 2021). Although fibrinolysis is an important component of DIC, plasma fibrinogen levels have a low sensitivity for diagnosing DIC because fibrinogen has a half-life of four days. Thus, low plasma levels are detected only in severe cases of DIC. In addition, evidence of fibrin breakdown, such as elevated D-dimer and FDPs, is not specific for DIC because levels may be elevated in patients with trauma, inflammation, or recent surgery.

Professional organizations have developed guidelines to assist in the diagnosis of DIC. The International Society on Thrombosis and Haemostasis scoring system is the most frequently used in clinical practice and considered the global standard (Iba et al., 2023; Kiya et al., 2025). It is designed to provide an objective measurement of DIC and to serve as the reference standard for diagnostic and therapeutic purposes (Larsen et al., 2021). The scoring system takes into account international normalized ratio, D-dimer, platelet count, and fibrinogen laboratory values, assigning a higher score for increasingly abnormal values. In this algorithm, after DIC risk is determined, the presence of overt DIC is indicated by a cumulative score of 5 or greater. A score of less than 5 is suggestive of subclinical DIC or a DIC-negative case. Scoring is performed daily until the condition resolves. Initial validation studies have demonstrated the feasibility and prognostic relevance of this system, with the DIC score found to have a 91% sensitivity and 97% specificity (Larsen et al., 2021).

Besides the global coagulation tests, other molecular markers have been proposed for diagnosing DIC. However, many of the more sensitive and sophisticated tests are not routinely available in general hematology laboratories, so specialized testing may be limited to clinical trials or specialized settings. Markers of thrombin generation are one area that has future potential for improving DIC diagnoses, as excess thrombin formation is a central component of DIC (Adelborg et al., 2021). Viscoelastic tests to assess clot formation capacity could also help guide diagnosis and treatment decisions in the future for patients with DIC who have acute bleeding.

Diagnostic studies to determine the presence of bleeding are also helpful in evaluating the severity of DIC. Bedside hemoccult testing of stools, emesis, nasogastric output, and urinalysis or urine dipstick are important to determine the presence of bleeding. Radiologic studies are useful only to detect an underlying cause or to assess for the presence of internal bleeding or thrombosis. Endoscopic examinations may be performed to determine the presence of bleeding in the upper or lower gastrointestinal tract. Angiography may be ordered to determine the presence of bleeding or thrombosis. Invasive procedures are performed with caution because of the potential for bleeding and should be preceded by repletion of clotting factors and platelets (Sohal et al., 2020).

Treatment Modalities

The cornerstone of DIC management is early recognition and correction of the underlying disorder. Controlling the precipitating malignancy may be sufficient to resolve DIC in patients with cancer. Antineoplastic treatment can lead to complete remission of DIC in patients with APL and should be treated as a medical oncologic emergency (Ten Cate & Leader, 2021). However, additional supportive care measures aimed at breaking the cycle of thrombosis and hemorrhage are required until treatment of the underlying condition becomes effective.

Therapy for DIC is individualized based on the initiating pathology, the clinical presentation (e.g., bleeding, clotting, neither), and the severity of laboratory abnormalities. DIC management may include replacement of depleted coagulation factors and coagulation inhibitors, use of anticoagulants, restoration of anticoagulant pathways, inhibition of the fibrinolytic system, and use of other pharmacologic agents (Smith, 2021; Ten Cate & Leader, 2021). Practice guidelines are available from both the International Society on Thrombosis and Haemostasis and the Japanese Society on Thrombosis and Hemostasis (Asakura, 2025; Wang et al., 2020).

Replacement Therapy

The goal of blood component replacement is to prevent bleeding or arrest active bleeding by replenishing the substances consumed in the DIC process. This may include platelet or red blood cell transfusions, coagulation factors, and coagulation inhibitors (Adelborg et al., 2021).

Platelet transfusions may be administered to patients who have active bleeding or are at high risk for bleeding. In general, the bleeding status of patients determines the transfusion threshold. A platelet count of less than 50,000 cells/mcl is associated with significantly increased bleeding risk in patients who are critically ill and is the threshold for platelet transfusion in patients who are actively bleeding or are at high risk for bleeding. In patients with platelet counts less than 20,000 cells/mcl, the threshold to transfer is much lower, regardless of the presence or absence of bleeding (Adelborg et al., 2021; Wang et al., 2020).

Red blood cell transfusions may be considered for patients who are bleeding. Transfusion of packed red blood cells can provide more than 70% of the hematocrit of whole blood and one-third of the plasma, minimizing fluid overload issues (Cywinski, 2025). Stored blood cells lack factors V and VIII, so repletion with fresh frozen plasma (FFP) is recommended (Horstman & Tormey, 2022).

FFP and cryoprecipitate are transfused with a prolonged prothrombin time, activated partial thromboplastin time, or fibrinogen less than 50 mg/dl (Smith, 2021). FFP contains all of the necessary coagulation factors and inhibitors and is used to replace depleted factors during active bleeding. No evidence has shown that infusion of plasma stimulates the ongoing activation of coagulation. FFP is administered intravenously in a starting dose of 15–30 ml/kg and is indicated in patients with significant DIC-associated bleeding and a fibrinogen level below 150 mg/dl (Adelborg et al., 2021).

Cryoprecipitate, enriched with fibrinogen, factor VIII, von Willebrand factor, factor XIII, and fibronectin, may be administered to patients with significant bleeding and is dispensed with less volume than FFP. Transfusion of 10 units of cryoprecipitate (1 U/10 kg body weight) is expected to maintain the plasma fibrinogen level above 100–150 mg/dl (Horstman & Tormey, 2022). A dose of 3 g would raise plasma fibrinogen by around 1 g/L. It can be given as approximately 4 units of FFP, 2 cryoprecipitate pools (10 donor units), or 3 g of fibrinogen concentrate, with the aim of bringing prothrombin time and activated partial thromboplastin time to less than 1.5 times the upper limit of normal. Response to blood component therapy should be monitored frequently by repeating platelet counts and coagulation tests to determine that repletion was adequate and to promptly identify the appearance of new coagulation defects.

Anticoagulant Therapy

Heparin acts as an anticoagulant by activating antithrombin. It cannot lyse clots that have already formed, but it inhibits further thrombus formation by preventing the conversion of fibrinogen to fibrin. Patients who are critically ill are at high risk for VTE because of risk factors such as a history of VTE, older age, recent surgery, immobilization, and indwelling vascular catheters. VTE prophylaxis using either unfractionated or low-molecular-weight heparin has become standard care in patients who are not bleeding but with DIC (Levi, 2022). Additionally, decreased mortality has been noted in pre-DIC or early DIC in patients who are started on anticoagulation with heparin (Omidkhoda et al., 2022). Therapeutic doses of heparin are commonly used in cases of chronic DIC where thrombosis predominates (e.g., solid tumors, hemangiomas, purpura fulminans, dead fetus syndrome). Because of the potential for bleeding, close patient monitoring is mandatory during heparin therapy. Monitoring the partial thromboplastin time is critical, along with close observation for clinical signs of bleeding.

Restoration of Anticoagulant Pathways

Antithrombin is the most abundant anticoagulant circulating in the plasma and the primary inhibitor of circulating thrombin. Reduced levels of antithrombin in DIC are caused by several circumstances, including ongoing activation of coagulation, production of elastase by activated neutrophils that degrades antithrombin, capillary leakage of antithrombin, and impaired production secondary to liver damage from underperfusion and microvascular thrombi. Low antithrombin levels in DIC are associated with increased mortality, particularly in patients with sepsis. Antithrombin III may be administered when levels are significantly reduced in patients with severe DIC. Chung et al. (2023) investigated the effects of antithrombin III administration on the prognosis of severe trauma patients with DIC. Results indicated that it significantly improved sequential organ failure assessment score and aided in multiorgan dysfunction recovery. The drug is usually administered in a loading dose of 100 U/kg over three hours and then as a continuous maintenance infusion of 100 U/kg/day for three days. Patients must be closely monitored for bleeding, hypotension, shock, thrombi, and hematoma during administration (Harper, 2024).

Inhibition of Fibrinolysis

Activation of coagulation in DIC is accompanied by suppression of the fibrinolytic system caused by a sustained increase in plasma levels of plasminogen activator inhibitor-1, the principal inhibitor of the fibrinolytic system. The existing fibrinolytic activity is not sufficient to counteract the systemic deposition of fibrin. Because of possible thrombotic complications, such as myocardial infarction or renal artery thrombosis with systemic clotting, antifibrinolytic agents should be avoided in DIC (Levi, 2022). It has been suggested that antifibrinolytic agents may be used for local intravascular coagulation or for patients with trauma and massive blood loss (Levi, 2022).

Recombinant Factor VII Activated

Recombinant factor VII activated (rFVIIa) has been used as a final option to increase thrombin production to control ongoing intractable hemorrhage in patients with DIC who have been resistant to all other therapies (Navarro et al., 2024). The U.S. Food and Drug Administration has approved its use for hemophilia treatment. The rFVIIa agent is a potent and synthetic hemostatic that controls bleeding via two different mechanisms of action. One way is by binding to TF and initiating the coagulation pathway by activating factor X and factor IX. The second way is through binding to the surface of activated platelets, leading to the activation of factor X and the generation of thrombin.

Recombinant Human Soluble Thrombomodulin

Recombinant human soluble thrombomodulin (rhTM) is an agent that has been investigated to inhibit thrombus formation. Although rhTM is widely used in clinical settings throughout Japan and recommended for the treatment of sepsis-induced DIC by the *Japanese Clinical Practice Guidelines for Management of Sepsis and Septic Shock 2024* (Shime et al., 2025), it is not approved for DIC treatment in other countries. The rhTM agent binds to thrombin to form a thrombin–rhTM complex, which supports activation of protein C and the subsequent inhibition of thrombin generation. Because of the downregulation of thrombomodulin, the activated protein C system (an important anticoagulant pathway) is impaired in DIC. Activation of protein C diminishes when thrombomodulin levels are reduced.

Thrombin Inhibitors

Other agents investigated for efficacy in treating DIC are gabexate mesylate, hirudin, and nafamostat. Gabexate mesylate is a synthetic inhibitor of serine proteases (e.g., thrombin) and has demonstrated anticoagulant activity in the absence of antithrombin. In limited studies, it was found to be more effective than heparin alone in treating patients with low antithrombin levels. No randomized clinical trials of gabexate mesylate in patients with DIC have been conducted; however, one case report described the successful management of the enhanced-fibrinolytic type of DIC in a patient when treated with gabexate mesylate and tranexamic acid (Okamoto et al., 2024). A direct inhibitor of thrombin and a natural anticoagulant occurring in leeches, hirudin has been investigated in animal studies. Recombinant hirudin appeared to be effective in treating DIC but is associated with a high risk of bleeding. Nafamostat is especially effective in enhanced fibrinolytic-type DIC, yet hyperkalemia is a potential adverse effect that requires careful consideration (Asakura, 2025).

Nursing Management

Nurses must be able to identify patients at increased risk for developing DIC and remain alert to its signs and symptoms. Careful physical assessment of patients at risk for DIC, including a thorough neurologic assessment, is essential to recognize the subtle signs and symptoms of bleeding or thrombosis (Levi, 2022; Patel et al., 2024). Early recognition leads to the prompt initiation of treatment and the potential for improved patient outcomes.

During the clinical course of DIC, nurses must assess and document the extent of hemorrhage and thrombosis and for the administration of anticoagulant therapy and other medications, blood products, and IV fluids (Levi, 2022). Monitoring of coagulation studies during heparin therapy is important to titrate infusion rates and maintain a therapeutic range. Blood component therapy may include transfusion of red blood cells, platelets, FFP, and cryoprecipitate as indicated (Adelborg et al., 2021).

Nurses also play a significant role in providing patient education regarding the risks of bleeding and thrombosis, as well as the management of DIC. Collaboration among healthcare team members is imperative to determine treatment effectiveness and minimize the risk of clinical sequelae of DIC. Nurses should provide instructions to patients and caregivers regarding strategies to help prevent bleeding, what to do if it occurs, and VTE.

Patients and caregivers will require support from social, spiritual, and psychological services during this critical time. Discussion regarding code status and end-of-life decisions with patients and caregivers should take place before a decline occurs in patients' clinical status. Advance directives should be discussed to identify patients' wishes and should include a power of attorney for health care and a living will that specifies what medical treatment is desired.

Summary

DIC is a complex syndrome characterized by inappropriate activation of the coagulation system precipitated by an underlying pathologic disorder. Widespread intravascular thrombosis leads to multiorgan damage and failure. Overwhelming consumption of coagulation factors and platelets results in hemorrhage. Many clinical conditions are associated with acute DIC, especially sepsis, trauma, and cancer, and diagnosis is often complex and challenging.

Definitive treatment of DIC involves treating the underlying disorder and providing supportive care to maintain hemodynamic status and control bleeding and thrombus development. Nurses are vital in preventing and recognizing the subtle manifestations of bleeding or clotting so that early treatment can be initiated and potentially improve the patient's outcome.

References

Adelborg, K., Larsen, J.B., & Hvas, A.-M. (2021). Disseminated intravascular coagulation: Epidemiology, biomarkers, and management. *British Journal of Haematology, 192*(5), 803–818. https://doi.org/10.1111/bjh.17172

Ahuja, K., & Conran, R.M. (2025). Educational case: Disseminated intravascular coagulation in a patient with cancer. *Academic Pathology, 12*(1), 100162. https://doi.org/10.1016/j.acpath.2025.100162

Asakura, H. (2025). Clinical practice guidelines for management of disseminated intravascular coagulation in Japan 2024: Significance of guidelines developed for each underlying disease. *International Journal of Hematology, 121*(5), 586–591. https://doi.org/10.1007/s12185-025-03928-y

Chung, J.S., Kim, M.J., Choi, Y.U., Kim, J.G., & Bae, K.S. (2023). Effect of antithrombin III administration on the prognosis of severe trauma patients with disseminated intravascular coagulation. *Healthcare, 11*(10), 1476. https://doi.org/10.3390/healthcare11101476

Cope, D.G. (2016). Metabolic emergencies. In B.H. Gobel, S. Triest-Robertson, & W.H. Vogel (Eds.), *Advanced oncology nursing certification review and resource manual* (2nd ed., pp. 643–692). Oncology Nursing Society.

Cywinski, J.B. (2025). Blood products transfusion. In E. Farag, M. Argalious, J.E. Tetzlaff, & D. Sharma (Eds.), *Basic sciences in anesthesia* (pp. 465–481). Springer. https://doi.org/10.1007/978-3-319-62067-1_27

Harper, J.L. (2024, March 21). Antithrombin III deficiency follow-up. *Medscape.* https://emedicine.medscape.com/article/954688-followup

Hell, L., Däullary, T., Burghart, V., Mauracher, L.M., Grilz, E., Moser, B., ... Thaler, J. (2021). Extracellular vesicle-associated tissue factor activity in prostate cancer patients with disseminated intravascular coagulation. *Cancers, 13*(7), 1487. https://doi.org/10.3390/cancers13071487

Horstman, E.E., & Tormey, C.A. (2022). Plasma products for transfusion: An overview. *Annals of Blood, 7,* 4. https://doi.org/10.21037/aob-22-7

Iba, T., Helms, J., Neal, M.D., & Levy, J.H. (2023). Mechanisms and management of the coagulopathy of trauma and sepsis: Trauma-induced coagulopathy, sepsis-induced coagulopathy, and disseminated intravascular coagulation. *Journal of Thrombosis and Haemostasis, 21*(12), 3360–3370. https://doi.org/10.1016/j.jtha.2023.05.028

Kiya, G.T., Abebe, G., Mekonnen, Z., Tadasa, E., Milkias, G., & Asefa, E.T. (2025). A comparison of disseminated intravascular coagulation scoring systems and their performance to predict mortality in sepsis patients: A systematic review and meta-analysis. *PLOS ONE, 20*(1), e0315797. https://doi.org/10.1371/journal.pone.0315797

Larsen, J.B., Aggerbeck, M.A., Granfeldt, A., Schmidt, M., Hvas, A.-M., & Adelborg, K. (2021). Disseminated intravascular coagulation diagnosis: Positive predictive value of the ISTH score in a Danish population. *Research and Practice in Thrombosis and Haemostasis, 5*(8), e12636. https://doi.org/10.1002/rth2.12636

Levi, M.M. (2022, August 23). Disseminated intravascular coagulation. *Medscape.* https://emedicine.medscape.com/article/199627-overview

National Bleeding Disorders Foundation. (2025, January 1). *The clotting cascade.* https://www.bleeding.org/educational-programs/education/online-education/the-clotting-cascade

Navarro, R., Bojic, S., Fatima, R., El-Tahan, M., & El-Diasty, M. (2024). Recombinant activated factor VII (rFVIIa) for bleeding after thoracic aortic surgery: A scoping review of current literature. *Journal of Cardiothoracic and Vascular Anesthesia, 38*(1), 275–284. https://doi.org/10.1053/j.jvca.2023.09.041

Okamoto, H., Ozawa, T., Suzuki, T., & Nakagawa, Y. (2024). The two therapeutic strategies of surgical intervention and medical management in a patient with enhanced-fibrinolytic type of disseminated intravascular coagulation after aortic replacement for Stanford type A aortic dissection with chronic heart and renal failure. *BMC Cardiovascular Disorders, 24*(1), 78. https://doi.org/10.1186/s12872-024-03750-0

Omidkhoda, N., Abedi, F., Ghavami, V., Rahimi, H., Samadi, S., Arasteh, O., & Mohammadpour, A.H. (2022). The effect of heparin and its preparations on disseminated intravascular coagulation mortality and hospitalization: A systematic review. *International Journal of Clinical Practice, 2022*(1), 2226761. https://doi.org/10.1155/2022/2226761

Park, S., & Park, J.K. (2024). Back to basics: The coagulation pathway. *Blood Research, 59*(1), 35. https://doi.org/10.1007/s44313-024-00040-8

Patel, R., Patel, D., Patel, M., Ohemeng-Dapaah, J., Onyechi, A., Patel, Z., ... Shaikh, S. (2024). Disseminated intravascular coagulation in acute promyelocytic leukemia patients: A retrospective analysis of outcomes and healthcare burden in US hospitals. *Turkish Journal of Hematology, 41*(1), 1–8. https://doi.org/10.4274/tjh.galenos.2024.2023.0479

Popescu, N.I., Lupu, C., & Lupu, F. (2022). Disseminated intravascular coagulation and its immune mechanisms. *Blood, 139*(13), 1973–1986. https://doi.org/10.1182/blood.2020007208

Shime, N., Nakada, T.-A., Yatabe, T., Yamakawa, K., Aoki, Y., Inoue, S., ... Matsumoto, T. (2025). The Japanese Clinical Practice Guidelines for Management of Sepsis and Septic Shock 2024. *Acute Medicine and Surgery, 12*(1), e70037. https://doi.org/10.1002/ams2.70037

Smith, L. (2021). Disseminated intravascular coagulation. *Seminars in Oncology Nursing, 37*(2), 151135. https://doi.org/10.1016/j.soncn.2021.151135

Sohal, S., Thakur, A., Zia, A., Sous, M., & Trelles, D. (2020). Disseminated intravascular coagulation and malignancy: A case report and literature review. *Case Reports in Oncological Medicine, 2020,* 9147105. https://doi.org/10.1155/2020/9147105

Ten Cate, H., & Leader, A. (2021). Management of disseminated intravascular coagulation in acute leukemias. *Hämostaseologie, 41*(2), 120–126. https://doi.org/10.1055/a-1393-8302

Unar, A., Bertolino, L., Patauner, F., Gallo, R., & Durante-Mangoni, E. (2023). Pathophysiology of disseminated intravascular coagulation in sepsis: A clinically focused overview. *Cells, 12*(17), 2120. https://doi.org/10.3390/cells12172120

Wang, T.-F., Makar, R.S., Antic, D., Levy, J.H., Douketis, J.D., Connors, J.M., ... Zwicker, J.I. (2020). Management of hemostatic complications in acute leukemia: Guidance from the SSC of the ISTH. *Journal of Thrombosis and Haemostasis, 18*(12), 3174–3183. https://doi.org/10.1111/jth.15074

Mary Elizabeth Davis, DNP, RN, CHPN®, AOCNS®,
and Michelle K. Maiers, MSN, RN, AGPCNP-BC, OCN®

CHAPTER 14

Febrile Neutropenia

FAST FACTS

- **Description:** Febrile neutropenia, characterized by a fever and low neutrophil count, is one of the most common emergencies in patients with malignancy.
- **Incidence:** Approximately 50% of patients with solid tumors receiving chemotherapy develop febrile neutropenia; this number rises to more than 80% for those with hematologic disease receiving chemotherapy or transplants.
- **Clinical Manifestations:** Fever is often the only sign or symptom of infection in patients who are neutropenic; this is due to their decreased ability to mount an inflammatory response.
- **Risk Factors and Etiology:** Patient-, disease-, and treatment-related factors can be predictive for the development of a neutropenic fever.
- **Pathophysiology and Patient Evaluation:** Contributing factors to the pathogenesis of febrile neutropenia are multifactorial.
- **Advanced Practice Considerations:** Clinicians need to differentiate between low- and high-risk patients with fever and neutropenia, as this information may be helpful in diagnosing and determining the approach to treatment.
- **Treatment Modalities:** IV antibiotics should be administered within one hour of the determination of febrile neutropenia and preferably after cultures have been obtained.
- **Nursing Management:** Nurses should know the myelosuppressive capability of different chemotherapy, biotherapy, and radiation therapy regimens and the expected time frame of the nadir.
- **Outcomes:** Febrile neutropenia is a common oncologic emergency that presents a significant burden on patients with cancer regarding morbidity, mortality, financial cost, and quality of life. Clinicians working in the oncology specialty need to be knowledgeable of factors that may increase the risk of this emergency and recognize that fever is often the sole indicator of an infection in this vulnerable patient population.

Introduction

Febrile neutropenia (FN) is one of the most common oncologic emergencies (Barre et al., 2022; Seltzer et al., 2022). This life-threatening condition has been documented in up to 50% of patients with solid tumors and in more than 80% of patients with hematologic malignancies receiving cytotoxic chemotherapy (Barre et al., 2022; Seltzer et al., 2022; Stephens, 2020).

FN and its subsequent complications can significantly affect patient outcomes, including delayed cancer therapy and diminished quality of life (Zhu et al., 2023). It is a common cause of hospitalization in patients receiving chemotherapy and may be fatal if not addressed in a timely manner (Atallah-Yunes, 2021; Foley & Hoffman, 2023). The morbidity and mortality of FN are primarily attributed to increased susceptibility to infectious processes associated with decreased immune system function, mucosal barrier disruptions, gastrointestinal colonization, and previous antimicrobial exposure (Keck et al., 2022).

Patients with FN are especially at risk for sepsis (50% of patients) and septic shock (10%) (Seltzer et al., 2022; Stephens, 2020). Urgent evaluation and treatment of neutropenic fevers are required for this vulnerable patient population. Prompt administration of empirical antibiotics has been shown to be beneficial for patient outcomes, with mortality rates ranging from 4%– 20% (Zimmer & Freifeld, 2019). In contrast, mortality rates have been noted up to 50% in patients with shock, and as high as 70% for patients who do not receive antibiotics (Gould Rothberg et al., 2022; Zimmer & Freifeld, 2019).

Studies have identified a lack of adherence to risk assessment and management guidelines when clinicians treat patients with cancer and FN, with deadly consequences reported. Cossey and Cote (2024) described how the risk of unnecessary hospitalization, nosocomial infection, and antibiotic resistance increased when clinician guideline adherence was low. The authors emphasized that a comprehensive understanding of evaluation and management guidelines for FN is essential for clinicians caring for patients with cancer (Cossey & Cote, 2024).

In normal hematopoiesis, or the formation of new blood cells, the myeloid stem cell produces neutrophils, eosinophils, basophils, and monocytes. These cells are collectively known as granulocytes or polymorphonuclear leukocytes, which are a type of white blood cell (WBC) (Ferraro, 2022). Granulocytes play a fundamental role in the immune system by ingesting and destroying microorganisms, as well as releasing chemical mediators that enhance the inflammatory response. Neutrophils typically represent the largest number of WBCs in the body, encompassing 50%–60% of the total number found in circulation (Ferraro, 2022). The reference range for WBCs varies from 4,000–10,000 cells/mcl, with 5% of the human population falling outside of these parameters (Ferraro, 2022). Neutrophils are formed in the bone marrow and serve as the first responders to acute inflammation related to pathogen invasion (Foley & Hoffman, 2023). They are mobilized to the site of infection and use several methods to break down and destroy pathogens, including chemical release and phagocytosis (Foley & Hoffman, 2023; Zimmer & Freifeld, 2019). Neutrophils also contribute to injury healing, tissue repair, and adaptive immune response regulation (Stephens, 2020).

Neutropenia is defined as a decrease in the absolute number of circulating neutrophils in the peripheral blood (Ferraro, 2022). The absolute neutrophil count (ANC) is typically used to grade the severity of neutropenia (Copelan et al., 2025). ANC can be calculated by multiplying the total WBC count by the percentage of polymorphonuclear leukocytes and bands, an immature form of WBCs (Cossey & Cote, 2024) (see Figure 14-1).

Patients are generally considered neutropenic when their ANC is less than 1,500 cells/mcl. The severity of neutropenia can be further categorized as follows (Copeland et al., 2025):

- Mild: ANC 1,000–1,500 cells/mcl
- Moderate: ANC 500–1,000 cells/mcl

FIGURE 14-1. Absolute Neutrophil Count Calculation

Formula
White blood cell count (cells/mcl) × [% of neutrophils + % of bands)] ÷ 100 = absolute neutrophil count

Example
White blood cell count = 1.5 (1,500 cells/mcl)
% of neutrophils = 72.3
% of bands = 4
1,500 × [(72.3 + 4) ÷ 100] =
1,500 × [76.3 ÷ 100]
1,500 × 0.763 = 1,144.5 cells/mcl

Note. Based on information from Silvestre-Roig et al., 2016.

- Severe: ANC 200–500 cells/mcl
- Very severe: ANC < 200 cells/mcl

When ANC is less than 100 cells/mcl, it is commonly referred to as profound neutropenia (Taplitz et al., 2018). Although the degree and length of neutropenia can vary, higher degrees of neutropenia are associated with increased rates of infection and infection-related death (Ferraro, 2022).

Patients who are neutropenic with a fever are considered to have FN (Foley & Hoffman, 2023). Prompt identification of a neutropenic fever is critical. Fever may be the only indicator of an infection in this vulnerable population because of their inability to produce an inflammatory response (Barre et al., 2022). A diagnosis of FN is defined as a single oral temperature greater than or equal to 101°F (38.3°C) or a sustained temperature of greater than or equal to 100.4°F (38°C) for one hour with an ANC of less than 500 cells/mcl or an ANC that is expected to decrease below 500 cells/mcl within 48 hours (Taplitz et al., 2018; Zimmer & Freifeld, 2019).

Incidence

In the past 20 years, the overall incidence of FN has decreased because of advances in chemotherapy treatments and supportive care (Molina, 2023). In the United States, FN is estimated to affect approximately 60,294 patients annually, including 7.83 cases per 1,000 patients with cancer (Boccia et al., 2022). FN occurrences have been shown to vary by malignancy. Approximately 50% of patients with solid tumors who receive chemotherapy develop FN, and the number rises to more than 80% in those with hematologic disease receiving chemotherapy or transplants (Stephens, 2020).

In addition to cancer type, the incidence of FN has been noted to vary based on several other factors, including the type and cycle of cancer therapy, age, and sex (Rasmy et al., 2016). The type of cancer treatment, specifically chemotherapy, has also been shown to affect the likelihood of patients developing neutropenic fevers. Up to 30% of patients with cancer receiving cytotoxic chemotherapy can experience a neutropenic fever (Boccia et al., 2022; Rasmy et al., 2016). The incidence rates for neutropenia related to chemotherapy are approximately 2.4–15.4 cases per million annually in the United States (Boccia et al., 2022). The onset of neutropenia can occur within 5–10 days after chemotherapy, which is often when patients are reaching nadir, the point at which the WBC count is at its lowest (Zimmer & Freifeld, 2019).

FN is among the most common chemotherapy-related emergencies resulting in hospital admission and death (Keck et al., 2022). Patients receiving chemotherapy treatment for a solid tumor malignancy are typically neutropenic for less than seven days, with the highest rates of FN occurring during the first cycle of therapy. In contrast, hematologic malignancy chemotherapy treatments and hematopoietic stem cell transplantation conditioning regimens are associated with a more prolonged neutropenia that may last 14 days or longer (Zimmer & Freifeld, 2019).

Clinical Manifestations

Fever is often the only sign or symptom of infection in patients with neutropenia and may go undetected (Barre et al., 2022; Ferraro, 2022; Taplitz et al., 2018). This is due to the patient's decreased ability to mount an inflammatory response. Clinicians should be aware that patients who are severely or profoundly neutropenic with a suspected infection may be afebrile or in a hypothermic state (Taplitz et al., 2018).

The lack of typical infectious signs and symptoms represents a significant challenge in identifying FN (Barre et al., 2022). An absence of infection signs and symptoms commonly seen in patients without neutropenia cannot exclude the possibility of infection. Diagnosis may be particularly challenging, as chest radiography may not reveal an infiltrate because of the lack of circulating neutrophils (Cantwell & Perkins, 2018; Cossey & Cote, 2024). Skin and soft tissue infections in patients with neutropenia may not present with erythema, warmth, pain, or edema (Cantwell & Perkins, 2018; Cossey & Cote, 2024).

When patients with neutropenia present with any infection-associated symptoms, clinicians should be highly suspicious of their origin and perform additional symptom assessments. Common infectious signs or symptoms are fatigue, chills, productive cough, headache, dysuria, diarrhea, sore throat, and abscesses (Ferraro, 2022).

Risk Factors and Etiology

Multiple factors should be considered when assessing a patient's risk for FN. Clinicians need to consider patient-, disease-, and treatment-related subcategories that can be predictive of patients developing neutropenic fever (Ferraro, 2022; Molina, 2023) (see Figure 14-2).

The source of a fever in patients with cancer may be infectious or noninfectious. It is important to differentiate the root cause to administer appropriate treatment

FIGURE 14-2. Febrile Neutropenia Risk Factors

Patient-Related Factors	Disease-Related Factors	Treatment-Related Factors
• Age, particularly 65 years or older • Female sex • Reduced body surface area • Lowered performance status • Poor nutrition • Recent surgery or open wounds • Diminished immune function • Multiple comorbidities, including cardiovascular disease, liver disease, renal insufficiency, diabetes mellitus, chronic obstructive pulmonary disease	• Cancer tumor invasion of the bone marrow • Advanced stage of underlying malignancy • Certain malignancies: leukemia, lung cancer, lymphoma, myelodysplastic syndrome • Hematologic laboratory abnormalities	• Multiple cancer treatment therapies • Chemotherapy regimen history • Chemotherapy dose intensity • History of or current bone marrow irradiation • Current neutropenia

Note. Based on information from Ferraro, 2022; Molina, 2023.

(Foley & Hoffman, 2023). Determining the etiology of the fever may be complicated by treatment-related bone marrow suppression or myelosuppression, resulting in an overall lower blood cell concentration, including decreased neutrophils (Foley & Hoffman, 2023).

An infectious source is identified in 30%–50% of FN cases with either a microbiologically or clinically documented infection (Punnapuzha et al., 2023). Insufficient neutrophil reserves leave patients more vulnerable without the immune system's first responders, increasing susceptibility to pathogenic invasion (Cossey & Cote, 2024). Up to 50% of patients with FN will develop an infection that can lead to sepsis; this is significant because sepsis is a leading cause of death in patients undergoing myelosuppressive treatment. Although there are a multitude of potential sources of infection in FN, most initial infections are related to bacteria (Barre et al., 2022; Stephens, 2020). Bacterial infections are noted in the earlier phases of neutropenia. They are commonly associated with Gram-positive organisms, such as Staphylococcus and Streptococcus, as well as Gram-negative rods, including *Escherichia coli*, *Klebsiella*, *Enterobacter*, and *Pseudomonas aeruginosa* (Barre et al., 2022; Ferraro, 2022; Zimmer & Freifeld, 2019).

Gram-positive organisms are generally responsible for most FN cases and have been associated with up to 60% of documented infections (Molina, 2023). Estimates of up to 25% of patients with FN have documented bacteremia (Freifeld et al., 2011; Stephens, 2020). The increase in Gram-positive versus Gram-negative cultures has been attributed to the extended use of long-term vascular catheters and Gram-negative prophylaxis. Clinicians need to recognize that although Gram-positive infections have been diagnosed more frequently, Gram-negative infections have been associated with a higher mortality rate (Stephens, 2020). Dependent on the prophylaxis regimens used by clinicians, the etiology of infections in patients with FN has continued to shift (Keck et al., 2022; Mikulska et al., 2014). Accordingly, a global increase in the incidence of Gram-negative resistance is particularly concerning in patients with FN (Keck et al., 2022).

Overall, bacterial infections related to FN most commonly result from the translocation of organisms from the gut (Zimmer & Freifeld, 2019). Gastrointestinal mucosa is a rapidly dividing tissue adversely affected by cytotoxic chemotherapy, leading to varying mucosal injuries and allowing enteric organisms to enter the bloodstream (Barre et al., 2022). Compromised oral mucosa can become a portal of entry for bacteria (Cossey & Cote, 2024). Additional sources of bacterial infection include the respiratory tract, genitourinary tract, indwelling catheter insertion sites, skin, and soft tissue (Barre et al., 2022; Stephens, 2020).

In contrast to bacterial sources, viral and fungal infections are less commonly identified in patients with FN (Long & Koyfman, 2019). Respiratory viruses have been identified in up to 20% of patients with neutropenic fever (Stephens, 2020). However, due to the lack of rapid testing use, previously reported viral illness rates were likely underestimated (Pochon & Voigt, 2019). Viral organisms can include respiratory viruses, such as influenza, respiratory syncytial virus, rhinovirus, coronavirus, adenovirus, and herpes viruses (e.g., herpes simplex, Epstein-Barr) (Stephens, 2020). Fungal infections, particularly *Candida* and *Aspergillus*, are generally seen in patients with severe and prolonged neutropenia for longer than seven days (Ferraro, 2022; Stephens, 2020). Infections with fungal etiologies are more likely to occur in patients receiving multiple courses of broad-spectrum antibiotics, especially following seven days of empirical antibiotics (Ferraro, 2022; Freifeld et al., 2011; Stephens, 2020). Fungal infections have been particularly associated with gut translocation, fungal pneumonias (e.g., aspergillosis), and vascular catheters (Stephens, 2020).

Noninfectious fevers are typically diagnosed by exclusion and have been associated with approximately 3%–5% of FN cases (Freifeld et al., 2011; Pasikhova et al., 2018; Stephens, 2020). Noninfectious etiologies vary and may include cytokine release syndrome, mucositis, radiation, surgery, medications, and tumor fever. Although nearly all cancer types may cause a fever, tumor fevers are typically associated with specific malignancies, such as acute leukemias, lymphomas, and renal cell carcinoma (Pasikhova et al., 2018). The underlying process resulting in a tumor fever has not been clearly identified. However, it is theorized that the tumor releases endogenous cytokines, which act as pyrogens that result in an inflammatory response and an associated fever (Foley & Hoffman, 2023). Select medications, including chemotherapy agents and immunosuppressants, are associated with a high risk of developing neutropenia and may also cause fevers (Ferraro, 2022; Foley & Hoffman, 2023). Drug-induced neutropenia mechanisms include antibody-mediated and direct toxic effects on bone marrow (Ferraro, 2022).

No causative organism could be identified in neutropenic fever cases in 45%–50% of patients (Molina, 2023; Stephens, 2020). Cases in which the infectious etiology cannot be identified either clinically or microbiologically are commonly referred to as fevers of unknown origin (Punnapuzha et al., 2023). Nonetheless, clinicians are strongly advised to treat fevers as infectious in origin until proven otherwise; this recommendation is rooted in the life-threatening nature of neutropenic fevers and the fact that infections are the primary cause of morbidity and mortality in patients with cancer and FN (Stephens, 2020).

Pathophysiology and Patient Evaluation

Contributing factors to the pathogenesis of FN are multifactorial. Neutropenia in patients with cancer can be related to an underlying malignancy directly interfering with hematopoiesis, which occurs in primary bone marrow diseases such as leukemia (Barre et al., 2022). Neutropenia can also occur due to the metastatic replacement of bone marrow associated with a primary malignancy, such as solid tumor metastases (Sereeaphinan et al., 2021).

Although neutropenia can be related to an underlying malignancy, this condition can also be a result of cytotoxic therapy in patients with cancer (Barre et al., 2022; Sereeaphinan et al., 2021). Myelosuppressive therapies, including chemotherapy and radiation, cause neutropenia by damaging or destroying hematopoietic precursor cells, in addition to injuring the structure of the bone marrow (Stephens, 2020). Decreased bone marrow production of neutrophils and ineffective granulopoiesis fail to replace circulating leukocytes at the end of their life span, resulting in neutropenia. Given the short life span of circulating neutrophils in the peripheral blood, neutropenia develops rapidly after myelosuppressive treatment regimens The neutrophil count typically nadirs around 5–10 days following chemotherapy administration (Brock & Cruz-Carreras, 2020). Circulating neutrophils may be further damaged or destroyed by certain chemotherapy agents, resulting in a more rapid decline in ANC (Stephens, 2020).

Given that cytotoxic chemotherapy is nonselective, patients with neutropenia also experience lymphopenia and thrombocytopenia. Lymphocytes, including T cells, B cells, and natural killer cells, play a significant role in the immune system and have an overall effect on infection response (Stephens, 2020). Although the precise effect of lymphopenia on the pathophysiology of FN has yet to be clearly determined, clinicians should understand that lymphopenia has been associated with an increased mortality risk (Stephens, 2020).

In addition to lymphopenia, most patients with neutropenia are thrombocytopenic. Platelets have largely been recognized as an essential component of the immune system. They play a multifactorial role in infection response, including the secretion of inflammatory mediators and regulators. Platelets are also crucial in the development and resolution of organ failure in inflammatory states such as sepsis. Thrombocytopenia has been associated with poor outcomes in patients experiencing a critical illness (Stephens, 2020).

Cytotoxic chemotherapy can affect most organ systems, given that this treatment targets all rapidly dividing cells, including healthy and malignant cells (Stephens, 2020; Zimmer & Freifeld, 2019). The most affected organ system is the gastrointestinal tract, specifically injury to the mucosal barrier. This is particularly concerning because gut mucosa cells act as an anatomic barrier to the colonized organisms in the gastrointestinal tract (Barre et al., 2022; Zimmer & Freifeld, 2019). Disruption of this gut barrier creates entryways through which enteric pathogens, including bacteria and yeast, can cross into the bloodstream. This entryway represents a significant source of Gram-negative, Gram-positive, and fungal infections in patients with neutropenia. Infections in these individuals are more commonly related to opportunistic pathogens that inhabit the skin, oral cavity, and gastrointestinal tract (Punnapuzha et al., 2023). Neutropenia has also been shown to affect the respiratory system, specifically by decreasing cell counts of alveolar macrophages, lymphocytes, and neutrophils (Stephens, 2020).

A febrile episode in patients with neutropenia typically arises when an infectious pathogen is encountered (Punnapuzha et al., 2023; Rasmy et al., 2016). Given their immunocompromised state, patients with cancer have a hindered ability to fight off an infection and are more vulnerable to pathogen invasion due to host barrier damage, such as the mucosal lining of the gastrointestinal tract (Punnapuzha et al., 2023; van der Velden et al., 2014). The fever response is thought to be related to the production of cytokines responsible for activating the immune system. Cytokine production is facilitated by exogenous pyrogens that result in an inflammatory response (El-Radhi, 2018). Any patient with neutropenia can develop a febrile condition; however, patients with cancer receiving cytotoxic therapy are especially vulnerable due to treatment-related bone marrow suppression (Dale, 2025).

Patient Assessment

Nurses should obtain a thorough patient history to identify symptoms that may help determine the site of infection. An initial evaluation should focus on assessing a patient's risk for developing serious complications.

A comprehensive history includes the following (Cossey & Cote, 2024; Ferraro, 2022; Klastersky et al., 2016; Long & Koyfman, 2019; Sereeaphinan et al., 2021):

- A history of cancer and cancer treatment, including the date of the most recent therapy. Patients who have received chemotherapy in the past six weeks who are experiencing a fever should be assumed to be neutropenic until proven otherwise.
- Current medications (e.g., prescribed, over the counter, herbal products)
- History of presenting illness (e.g., precipitating factors, onset, duration)
- Changes in activities of daily living or functional status
- Past medical history (e.g., tuberculosis exposure, comorbidities, history of prior infections, recent antibiotic use, HIV status, recurrent episodes of neutropenia)
- Social history (e.g., tobacco use, alcohol use, sexual activity, recent travel, sick contacts, occupational exposure to toxic agents)
- Family history (e.g., recent infections, unexplained deaths)

Nurses should perform a comprehensive physical examination, focusing on sites most likely to be infected, such as the skin, oral mucosa, catheter insertion sites, lungs, abdomen, and perirectal area, to evaluate for signs of infection (Cossey & Cote, 2024) (see Table 14-1).

TABLE 14-1
Physical Examination for Patients With Febrile Neutropenia

Type of Examination	Assessment
Neurologic	• Assess orientation status and note any change in mental status. • The presence of restlessness, irritability, somnolence, or confusion is concerning for sepsis.
Integumentary	• Inspect and palpate skin. • The presence of rash, pallor, edema, erythema, and tenderness increases suspicion for infection.
Head, eyes, ears, nose, and throat	• Assess oral mucosa, especially noting any signs of mucositis. • The presence of oral mucositis can provide potential insight into the overall gastrointestinal mucosa condition. • Evaluate for sinus tenderness.
Pulmonary	• Auscultate lungs. • Diminished breath sounds increase suspicion for pneumonia. • Crackles and wheezing increase suspicion for congestive heart failure or pulmonary edema.
Lymphatic	• Inspect and palpate for enlarged lymph nodes, especially surrounding the suspected site of infection.
Abdominal	• Auscultate for bowel sounds, noting hypoactive bowel sounds. • Palpate for tenderness. Positive tenderness increases concern for infection. • Presence of costovertebral angle tenderness may suggest a renal infection.
Rectal	• Inspect the perineum and perianal areas for signs of inflammation. • Digital examination is contraindicated, given the sensitivity of the perirectal mucosa.

Note. Based on information from Cossey & Cote, 2024; Ferraro, 2022.

Advanced Practice Considerations

Diagnostics and Laboratory Tests

A complete set of vital signs should be performed on presentation, including pulse oximetry and temperature (Cossey & Cote, 2024). Temperature elevation of a single temperature greater than 100.4°F–101°F (38°C–38.3°C) over one hour in patients with an ANC less than or equal to 500 cells/mcl is considered an emergency (Ferraro, 2022). Hypotension and tachycardia increase concern for sepsis (Ferraro, 2022).

Clinicians are advised to avoid rectal temperatures due to the potential risk of infection and avoid axillary temperatures, as accuracy in relation to core body temperature may be suspect (Cossey & Cote, 2024).

A complete blood count with differential is required to assess and grade neutropenia; ANC should be calculated. An elevated WBC with segmental (immature) neutrophils and elevated band neutrophils, or a noted shift to the left, can be indicative of bacterial infection (Ferraro, 2022). Monitoring the left shift (abnormal increase of neutrophils) can be helpful in tracking the course of an infection (Preethi, 2023). At least two sets of blood cultures (aerobic and anaerobic) should be drawn from different sites. Typically, this means two peripheral sets or one peripheral set and one set from each lumen of a central venous catheter (if present) (Ferraro, 2022; Gudiol et al., 2020). Rapid diagnostic tests and technologies, such as polymerase chain reaction panels, are gaining utility in decreasing the time to pathogen identification. Blood culture polymerase chain reaction panels can detect Gram-positive and Gram-negative resistance patterns, reducing the time to escalate or add antimicrobials (Keck et al., 2022).

Next-generation sequencing assays have been assessed in small studies and found helpful in the rapid identification of pathogens; however, the cost and technology may be prohibitive to many, and larger studies need to be conducted (Keck et al., 2022). Additional cultures should be considered, such as existing wounds, sputum analyses if respiratory symptoms are present, and stool culture if diarrhea is present. Viral testing studies, including nasopharyngeal swab testing, are recommended during the influenza season and for patients presenting with flu-like symptoms (Cossey & Cote, 2024; Gudiol et al., 2020; Stephens, 2020).

Electrolytes, renal, and hepatic studies (e.g., blood urea nitrogen, creatinine, total bilirubin, transaminase enzymes) are important markers of organ function. If the clinical scenario warrants, arterial blood gases and coagulation studies should be drawn. Lactate levels may also be justified, as an increased level may help detect early sepsis-induced malperfusion. In a study of individuals with cancer aged 3 months to 18 years, serum lactate levels drawn at the time of FN presentation served as a surrogate marker for developing septic shock within 48 hours among those who were hemodynamically stable (Suwanpakdee et al., 2021). In those with a lactate level greater than 2.5 mmol/L, preemptive aggressive hemodynamic monitoring and treatment were needed to ensure adequate tissue perfusion. Similar findings have been noted in adult patients with cancer, specifically highlighting that a lactate level greater than 2.5 mmol/L and greater than 3.5 mmol/L at 24 hours were predictors of mortality (Gicheru et al., 2023; Nazer et al., 2020). Procalcitonin levels have also been used for risk stratification for mortality in patients with FN. Coyne et al. (2022) found that a procalcitonin cutoff of < 0.25 ng/ml was associated with a negative predictive value of 98.7% with respect to mortality. Their findings suggested that procalcitonin may be helpful to identify low-risk patients appropriate for discharge from cancer emergency departments (EDs) (Coyne et al., 2022). Similarly, elevated C-reactive protein levels (> 20–30 mg/dl) have been correlated to increased mortality (Gudiol et al., 2020). However, additional larger studies are needed to validate these tests as predictive markers.

Urinalysis and urine culture analyses, regardless of urinary symptoms, may help diagnose urinary tract infections in patients with FN; however, in patients already receiving broad-spectrum antibiotics, it rarely affects antibiotic treatment strategies (Grigg et al., 2019; Hata & Ihara, 2024). Antimicrobial and diagnostic stewardship approaches are growing as resistance rates rise and may be a consideration (Tran et al., 2023). Although urine tests are inexpensive and noninvasive, routine testing, especially in patients who are asymptomatic, can also create unnecessary financial burdens and may affect or delay antibiotic management (Zgheib et al., 2021). Urinalysis may only be indicated in patients with FN who have urinary signs and symptoms and in those with a history of urinary tract disease. Urine cultures should be analyzed regardless of the urinalysis result (Alonso-Cadenas et al., 2023). If respiratory symptoms are present, a chest radiograph should be obtained, and if abdominal symptoms or distention are present, abdominal x-rays may be performed if typhlitis is suspected (Ferraro, 2022; Olsen et al., 2023).

Risk Assessment and Prevention

Awareness of low- and high-risk categories for developing FN helps guide diagnosis and infection prevention strategies in this patient population. These risk categories have also been used to assess the risk of medical complications in patients diagnosed with FN and have been referenced in clinical predictive models to assist clinicians in determining the appropriate care setting to treat these patients.

Low-risk patient characteristics include the following (Ferraro, 2022):

- Anticipated neutropenia period to be less than seven days
- Few comorbidities
- No previous fungal infections
- Age younger than 60 years
- Mild to moderate symptoms
- Stable physiologic status

High-risk patient indicators include the following (Ferraro, 2022):

- Anticipated neutropenic period to be longer than seven days
- Profoundly neutropenic with ANC $\leq$ 100 cells/mcl
- Multiple medical conditions (e.g., hypotension, pneumonia, abdominal pain, neurologic changes)
- Compromised mucosal and skin barriers

Additional identified high-risk factors include the following (Tsuchihashi et al., 2024):

- Age older than 65 years
- Uncontrolled primary disease
- History of invasive fungal infections

The National Comprehensive Cancer Network (NCCN) (2025a) classifies common chemotherapy regimens based on FN risk. It defines high-risk regimens as those that have reported an incidence of FN in greater than 20% of patients (NCCN, 2025a). NCCN clearly notes that its classifications are not comprehensive and reminds clinicians that the type of chemotherapy regimen is only one factor that should be considered when assessing patients' FN risk.

Adding monoclonal antibodies to chemotherapy regimens may increase the risk of FN (NCCN, 2025a). A specific concern has been identified regarding rituximab, which is an anti–cluster of differentiation 20 (CD20) monoclonal antibody primarily used for CD20+ hematologic malignancies. Rituximab has the capability of inducing severe neutropenia and has been associated with prolonged neutropenia with a delayed onset, even without concurrent chemotherapy administration. Attention should be paid to monoclonal antibodies that cause prolonged neutropenia with delayed onset, or to other drugs targeting CD20 (NCCN, 2025a).

Infection prevention measures include preemptive or prophylaxis therapy using broad-spectrum antimicrobial agents aimed at the most common viral, fungal, and bacterial pathogens in patients at high risk for complications from infections. Antibacterial prophylaxis is not recommended for low-risk patients, as the primary benefit of antibacterial prophylaxis is reducing fever rather than reducing infection (NCCN, 2025b). For patients with nonmyeloid malignancies at high risk for FN, clinicians should also consider prophylactic subcutaneous administration of granulocyte–colony-stimulating factors, which have been approved to reduce the incidence of FN in patients with nonmyeloid malignancies receiving chemotherapy. Prophylaxis recommendations include administration of daily doses (5 mcg/kg) of filgrastim after myelosuppressive therapy until recovery of ANC post-nadir, or one 6 mg dose of pegfilgrastim (NCCN, 2025b; Tsuchihashi et al., 2024). A U.S. Food and Drug Administration–approved biosimilar or delivery device can also be used.

Treatment Modalities

Prediction Models to Determine Treatment Care Setting

Several clinicians and organizations have developed tools to assess the risk of medical complications in patients with cancer and FN and determine the appropriate care setting for administering treatment. Talcott et al. (1992) developed a clinical risk model classifying patients into four categories of risk:

- Group 1: patients who developed FN in the inpatient setting
- Group 2: outpatients with serious concurrent comorbidity within 24 hours of presentation
- Group 3: outpatients without serious concurrent comorbidity but with uncontrolled cancer
- Group 4: remaining patients who had no high-risk features

The goal of this prediction model was to identify patients with FN who were at low risk for complications that could be treated in the outpatient setting or with oral antibiotics. The authors concluded the prediction model should not preclude clinical judgment and vigilance because patients at low risk still have risk (Talcott et al., 1992).

The Clinical Index of Stable Febrile Neutropenia is a risk predictive model for triage use within an ED setting. Four hundred patients with FN presenting to the ED within a single institution were retrospectively classified into three risk groups: low, intermediate, and high. However, despite the risk score, researchers noted that most ED physicians tended to overtreat and hospitalize patients (Heo et al., 2023). The developers concluded that the ED clinicians can use the Multinational Association of Supportive Care in Cancer (MASCC) Risk Index to quickly screen patients at high risk, and then use the Clinical Index of Stable Febrile Neutropenia model to plan for outpatient treatment (Moon et al., 2018). Notably, through this analysis, three variables were identified related to a return ED visit following discharge: high shock index (pulse rate divided by systolic blood pressure), presence of thrombocytopenia (platelets < 100,000 cells/mcl), and an elevated lactic acid value (≥ 2 mmol/L) (Heo et al., 2023).

The MASCC Risk Index was developed to classify risk factors and determine or stratify patient management, the need for IV antibiotics, and the need for hospitalization (Chaftari et al., 2021; Klastersky et al., 2000). It incorporates a scoring system with several characteristics contributing to a total maximum score of 26, with a score of 21 or greater indicating a low risk (see Figure 14-3). Scoring criteria include the burden of symptoms, hypotension, presence of chronic obstructive pulmonary disease, history of previous fungal infections, dehydration requiring IV fluids, and inpatient versus outpatient status. Critics of the MASCC Risk Index have noted that it does show high sensitivity but low specificity within patients with solid tumors (Moon et al., 2018). The developers have also identified a critical omission with differences in

FIGURE 14-3. Multinational Association of Supportive Care in Cancer Risk Assessment Tool

Assessment	Score Weight
No hypotension (systolic blood pressure > 90)	5
No chronic obstructive pulmonary disease, defined as active chronic bronchitis, emphysema, the need for oxygen therapy, corticosteroids, and/or bronchodilators, or a decrease in forced expiratory volume	4
Solid tumor	4
No history of fungal infection in those with hematologic malignancy	4
No dehydration requiring IV fluid resuscitation	3
Current status as an outpatient	3
Age < 60 years	2
Total: low risk > 21	

Burden of illness/amount of symptoms score is weighted as 5 for mild or no symptoms, 3 for moderate symptoms, and 0 for moribund or severe symptoms.

Note. Based on information from Klastersky et al., 2000.

the severity and duration of neutropenia with respect to the underlying malignancy (hematologic vs. solid tumors) (Klastersky et al., 2000).

To counter criticism, the developers noted that the model was extensively studied with worldwide clinician participation (20 institutions within 15 countries), was created to be generalizable, and has external and internal validity. Nevertheless, the model may need to be retested and adapted to meet changes in the care and management of patients with cancer and FN (Klastersky et al., 2000).

Regardless of the risk assessment tool used, patients should have access to a thermometer, phone, caregiver, transportation, and readiness to close follow-up. Additionally, patients are recommended to be within 30 miles or one hour from the hospital (Cossey & Cote, 2024; Foley & Hoffman, 2023; Taplitz et al., 2018). Many tools exist to help clinicians consider outpatient management, especially for those at low risk, to reduce potential exposure to nosocomial infections. However, no tool should replace clinician judgment or supersede patient presentation, laboratory results, and the presence of comorbid conditions (Cossey & Cote, 2024).

Pharmacologic Interventions

The type and duration of antibiotics and other anti-infectious agents vary depending on the disease, expected duration of neutropenia, risk stratification, and clinical signs or symptoms of infection (Keck et al., 2022; NCCN, 2025b). A preemptive approach (waiting for culture results before prescribing) compared to empiric therapy (starting when suspicious of fungal infection) may reduce the duration and rate of antifungal medication use without increasing mortality (Uneno et al., 2022). Usual first-line therapies include beta-lactam therapy with medications, such as piperacillin/tazobactam or cefepime, or an antipseudomonal carbapenem, such as imipenem/cilastin or meropenem (Cossey & Cote, 2024; Gudiol et al., 2020; Taplitz et al., 2018). For those at low risk for complications, oral antimicrobial therapies may be considered; however, high-risk patients should be admitted to the hospital with IV medication administration (Gudiol et al., 2020).

For intermediate or high-risk patients with an expected duration of neutropenia greater than seven days, fluoroquinolone prophylaxis can be prescribed (NCCN, 2025b). If patients are intolerant, a third-generation cephalosporin or trimethoprim/sulfamethoxazole can be administered as an alternative. Vancomycin is used to treat possible *Staphylococcus aureus*, and therapy should be modified based on a patient history of infection or when colonization with resistant organisms occurs (Cossey & Cote, 2024).

Antimicrobial stewardship clinicians have suggested shorter antibiotic courses because continued empirical administration without identification of the specific offender may encourage bacterial resistance (Hata & Ihara, 2024). Gudiol et al. (2020) outlined other empirical treatments when a source of infection was apparent, such as oropharyngeal mucositis, skin and soft tissue, catheter-related, central nervous system, or urinary tract infection. The authors suggested stopping empirical antibiotic therapy in those with FN who are asymptomatic, hemodynamically stable, and without a documented infection, despite the result of the neutrophil count (Gudiol et al., 2020).

Nonpharmacologic Interventions

Handwashing is an easy, low-cost, and efficacious intervention for basic infection prevention. Xun et al. (2021) performed a systematic review with a meta-analysis and concluded that dirty hands are a vector for several gastrointestinal infections (e.g., diarrhea) and respiratory infections. These infections can cause serious complications, especially for those who are immunocompromised. The more frequently hands were washed, the lower the risk of disease. The frequency of handwashing can be influenced and is improved by a number of factors, including sex (female), age (middle-aged vs. older or younger), education level (more educated), religious culture, and economic conditions (more frequent in higher economic countries when exposed to pollutants). High-quality evidence that indicated the best range for the number of washings per day was not found (Xun et al., 2021).

It was thought that a specific diet, notably a neutropenic or low bacterial diet, would reduce the risk of bacterial contamination from foodborne infections in those who were immunocompromised. This diet typically excluded raw or uncooked foods, deli meats, foods served buffet style, and yogurt with live or active cultures. It only allowed thoroughly cooked food, pasteurized dairy products, and boiled or filtered water. However, evidence from multiple studies and systematic reviews has shown that this diet has no benefit in mortality or infection prevention, and further suggested that following this regimen may negatively impact nutritional status and quality of life (Matteucci et al., 2023; Radhakrishnan et al., 2022; Ramamoorthy et al., 2020; Sonbol et al., 2019). Most clinicians have concluded that education and guidance on safe food handling and good hygiene practices are more important.

The U.S. Food and Drug Administration (2024) has safe food handling guidelines that encourage four simple steps: clean, separate, cook, and chill. To clean, hands should be washed with warm water and soap before and after handling food, and after using the bathroom, changing any diapers, or handling pets. Cutting boards, dishes, utensils, and countertops should be washed with hot, soapy water after preparing any food. Disposable paper towels are preferred over kitchen towels to clean surfaces (when cloth towels are used, they should be laundered often in the hot cycle). Fruits and vegetables should be rinsed and scrubbed under running water, including those with skins and rinds. If eating canned goods, the lids should be cleaned before opening. The U.S. Food and Drug Administration (2024) also encourages the separation of raw meat, seafood, and poultry from other food items; these proteins should not interact in grocery bags or on cutting boards. Food should be cooked thoroughly using a thermometer to ensure the proper temperature, and cold items should be kept in a refrigerator or freezer. By educating patients and caregivers, unnecessary dietary restrictions can be minimized and nutritional intake can be enhanced (Matteucci et al., 2023).

Nursing Management

Oncology nurses play an important role in the diagnosis and management of FN. Nurses should know the myelosuppressive capability of different chemotherapy, biotherapy, and radiation therapy regimens and the expected time frame of the nadir. NCCN (2025a) details various regimens with an increased risk of FN within its guidelines. Monitoring complete blood count and assessing for signs and symptoms of infection are within the scope of nursing practice and especially important if patients have an indwelling device, such as a central venous or urinary catheter (Miller, 2022). Accordingly, clinicians performing critical activities such as catheter maintenance should receive updated nosocomial infection prevention training (Commission for Hospital Hygiene and Infection Prevention, 2022).

Once diagnosed, prompt workup and administration of antibiotics are crucial. The American Society of Clinical Oncology and the Infectious Diseases Society of America recommend IV antibiotics be administered within one hour of evaluation and preferably after cultures have been obtained (Cossey & Cote, 2024). Koenig et al. (2020) performed a systematic review assessing prompt antibiotic therapy in patients with cancer and fever and neutropenia during chemotherapy. They noted an association between a longer time to antibiotic administration and impaired safety (Koenig et al., 2020).

Nurses should educate patients, caregivers, and visitors on the importance of adhering to meticulous hygiene practices, including frequent handwashing and good oral care. Patients with neutropenia should be instructed not to share food or cutlery with others, follow food safety guidelines, and avoid large crowds and sick contacts (Miller, 2022). Patients and caregivers need to recognize the signs and symptoms of infection and avoid activities that may affect the integrity of their skin while neutropenic. Gloves are recommended to be worn while gardening, and patients should be discouraged from providing direct care for reptiles, birds, fish, and farm animals (Olsen et al., 2023). If needed, shaving should be performed using an electric razor. Patients considering procedures such as manicures, pedicures, waxing, and tattoos should defer to their healthcare providers. Patients and household members are generally recommended to remain current on vaccinations, particularly influenza, COVID-19, and pneumococcal, although the decision to receive vaccinations should be discussed with the healthcare team (Commission for Hospital Hygiene and Infection Prevention, 2022; NCCN, 2025b). Patients should also speak with their healthcare team about participation in sexual activity and the use of tampons, enemas, suppositories, and dental floss.

Nurses should emphasize that FN is an emergency and that prompt intervention is necessary (Miller, 2022). Ensuring that patients have access to a thermometer to check for fevers is important. Additionally, patients must understand their potential for neutropenia in relation to their disease as well as their anticancer regimen.

Summary

FN is a common oncologic emergency that presents a significant burden on patients with cancer regarding morbidity, mortality, financial cost, and quality of life (Boccia et al., 2022). Clinicians working in the oncology specialty need to be knowledgeable of factors that may increase the risk of this emergency and recognize that fever is often the sole indicator of an infection in this vulnerable patient population. Nurses are critical in managing and treating patients with FN through administering timely antibiotic treatment and providing comprehensive education.

References

Alonso-Cadenas, J.A., Sancosmed Ron, M., Herrero, B., Lera Carballo, E., Lassaletta, A., Rodrigo, R., & de la Torre, M. (2023). Role of urine culture in paediatric patients with cancer with fever and neutropenia: A prospective observational study. *Archives of Disease in Childhood, 108*(12), 982–986. https://doi.org/10.1136/archdischild-2023-325992

Atallah-Yunes, S.A., Kadado, A.J., Haddadin, F., Sawalha, K., Hernandez-Montfort, J., & Ali, S.S. (2021). Impact of cardiovascular comorbidities on inpatient mortality in patients hospitalized with neutropenic fever. *Supportive Care in Cancer, 29*(1), 509–513. https://doi.org/10.1007/s00520-020-05518-6

Barre, S., McElwee, J., Calhoun, C., Weant, K.A., Maldonado, A., & Bell, C.M. (2022). Review of hematological and oncological emergencies. *Advanced Emergency Nursing Journal, 44*(2), 84–102. https://doi.org/10.1097/TME.0000000000000399

Boccia, R., Glaspy, J., Crawford, J., & Aapro, M. (2022). Chemotherapy-induced neutropenia and febrile neutropenia in the US: A beast of burden that needs to be tamed? *Oncologist, 27*(8), 625–636. https://doi.org/10.1093/oncolo/oyac074

Brock, P., & Cruz-Carreras, M.T. (2020). Emergency complications of malignancy. In J.E. Tintinalli & O.J. Ma (Eds.), *Tintinalli's emergency medicine: A comprehensive study guide* (9th ed., pp. 9–11). McGraw-Hill Education.

Cantwell, L., & Perkins, J. (2018). Infectious disease emergencies in oncology patients. *Emergency Medicine Clinics of North America, 36*(4), 795–810. https://doi.org/10.1016/j.emc.2018.06.009

Chaftari, P., Chaftari, A.-M., Hachem, R., Yeung, S.-C.J., Dagher, H., Jiang, Y., ... Raad, I. (2021). The role of procalcitonin in identifying high-risk cancer patients with febrile neutropenia: A useful alternative to the Multinational Association for Supportive Care in Cancer score. *Cancer Medicine, 10*(23), 8475–8482. https://doi.org/10.1002/cam4.4355

Commission for Hospital Hygiene and Infection Prevention. (2022). Infection prevention requirements for the medical care of immunosuppressed patients: Recommendations of the Commission for Hospital Hygiene and Infection Prevention (KRINKO) at the Robert Koch Institute. *GMS Hygiene and Infection Control, 17,* Doc 07. https://doi.org/10.1007/s00103-020-03265-x

Copelan, E., Avalos, B., & Friend, R. (2025). Evaluation of neutropenia. *BMJ Best Medical Practice.* Retrieved September 25, 2025, from https://bestpractice.bmj.com/topics/en-gb/893

Cossey, J., & Cote, M.C.B. (2024). Evaluation and management of febrile neutropenia in patients with cancer. *JAAPA, 37*(8), 16–20. https://doi.org/10.1097/01.JAA.0000000000000054

Coyne, C.J., Castillo, E.M., Shatsky, R.A., & Chan, T.C. (2022). Procalcitonin as a predictive tool for death and ICU admission among febrile neutropenic patients visiting the emergency department. *Medicina, 58*(8), 985. https://doi.org/10.3390/medicina58080985

Dale, D.C. (2025). Neutropenia. In J.L. Spivak (Ed.), *Merck manual professional version: Hematology and oncology: Leukopenias.* Merck. https://www.merckmanuals.com/professional/hematology-and-oncology/leukopenias/neutropenia

El-Radhi, A.S. (2018). Pathogenesis of fever. In A.S. El-Radhi, J. Carroll, & N. Klein (Eds.), *Clinical manual of fever in children* (pp. 53–68). Springer. https://doi.org/10.1007/978-3-319-92336-9_3

Ferraro, C. (2022). Neutropenia. In D. Camp-Sorrell, R.A. Hawkins, & D.G. Cope (Eds.), *Clinical manual for the oncology advanced practice nurse* (pp. 845–852). Oncology Nursing Society.

Foley, A.M., & Hoffman, M. (2023). CE: Febrile neutropenia in the chemotherapy patient. *American Journal of Nursing, 123*(5), 36–42. https://doi.org/10.1097/01.NAJ.0000931888.96896.a1

Freifeld, A.G., Bow, E.J., Sepkowitz, K.A., Boeckh, M.J., Ito, J.I., Mullen, C.A., ... Wingard, J.R. (2011). Executive summary: Clinical practice guideline for the use of antimicrobial agents in neutropenic patients with cancer: 2010 update by the Infectious Diseases Society of America. *Clinical Infectious Diseases, 52*(4), 427–431. https://doi.org/10.1093/cid/ciq147

Gicheru, B., Shah, J., Wachira, B., Omuse, G., & Maina, D. (2023). The diagnostic accuracy of an initial point-of-care lactate at the emergency department as a predictor of in-hospital mortality among adult patients with sepsis and septic shock. *Frontiers in Medicine, 10,* 1173286. https://doi.org/10.3389/fmed.2023.1173286

Gould Rothberg, B.E., Quest, T.E., Yeung, S.-C.J., Pelosof, L.C., Gerber, D.E., Seltzer, J.A., ... Kyriacou, D.N. (2022). Oncologic emergencies and urgencies: A comprehensive review. *CA: A Cancer Journal for Clinicians, 72*(6), 570–593. https://doi.org/10.3322/caac.21727

Grigg, S.E., Date, P., Loh, Z., Estacio, O., Johnson, D.F., Hawkes, E.A., & Grigg, A. (2019). Urine cultures at the onset of febrile neutropenia rarely impact antibiotic management in asymptomatic adult cancer patients. *Supportive Care in Cancer, 27*(4),1223–1227. https://doi.org/10.1007/s00520-018-4476-7

Gudiol, C., Aguilar-Guisado, M., Azanza, J.R., Candel, F.J., Cantón, R., Carratalà, J., ... de la Cámara, R. (2020). Executive summary of the consensus document of the Spanish Society of Infectious Diseases and Clinical Microbiology (SEIMC), the Spanish Network for Research in Infectious Diseases (REIPI) and the Spanish Society of Haematology and Haemotherapy (SEHH) on the management of febrile neutropenia in patients with hematological malignancies. *Enfermedades Infecciosas y Microbiología Clínica, 38*(4), 174–181. https://doi.org/10.1016/j.eimc.2019.01.013

Hata, N., & Ihara, T. (2024). Impact of urinary culture on diagnosis and treatment strategy after empiric therapy in febrile neutropenic patients. *Acute Medicine and Surgery, 11*(1), e70012. https://doi.org/10.1002/ams2.70012

Heo, S., Jeon, K., Park, B., Ko, R.-E., Kim, T., Hwang, S.Y., ... Lee, S.U. (2023). Clinical factors predicting return emergency department visits in chemotherapy-induced febrile neutropenia patients. *American Journal of Emergency Medicine, 67,* 90–96. https://doi.org/10.1016/j.ajem.2023.02.012

Keck, J.M., Wingler, M.J.B., Cretella, D.A., Vijayvargiya, P., Wagner, J.L., Barber, K.E., ... Stover, K.R. (2022). Approach to fever in patients with neutropenia: A review of diagnosis and management. *Therapeutic Advances in Infectious Disease, 9.* https://doi.org/10.1177/20499361221138346

Klastersky, J., de Naurois, J., Rolston, K., Rapoport, B., Maschmeyer, G., Aapro, M., & Herrstedt, J. (2016). Management of febrile neutropenia: ESMO Clinical Practice Guidelines. *Annals of Oncology, 27*(5, Suppl.), v111–v118. https://doi.org/10.1093/annonc/mdw325

Klastersky, J., Paesmans, M., Rubenstein, E.B., Boyer, M., Elting, L., Feld, R., ... Talcott, J. (2000). The Multinational Association for Supportive Care in Cancer risk index: A multinational scoring system for identifying low-risk febrile neutropenic cancer patients. *Journal of Clinical Oncology, 18*(16), 3038–3051. https://doi.org/10.1200/JCO.2000.18.16.3038

Koenig, C., Schneider, C., Morgan, J.E., Ammann, R.A., Sung, L., & Phillips, B. (2020). Association of time to antibiotics and clinical outcomes in patients with fever and neutropenia during chemotherapy for cancer: A systematic review. *Supportive Care in Cancer, 28*(3), 1369–1383. https://doi.org/10.1007/s00520-019-04961-4

Long, B., & Koyfman, A. (2019). Oncologic emergencies: The fever with too few neutrophils. *Journal of Emergency Medicine, 57*(5), 689–700. https://doi.org/10.1016/j.jemermed.2019.08.009

Matteucci, S., De Pasquale, G., Pastore, M., Morenghi, E., Pipitone, V., Soekeland, F., ... Mancin, S. (2023). Low-bacterial diet in cancer patients: A systematic review. *Nutrients, 15*(14), 3171. https://doi.org/10.3390/nu15143171

Mikulska, M., Viscoli, C., Orasch, C., Livermore, D.M., Averbuch, D., Cordonnier, C., & Akova, M. (2014). Aetiology and resistance in bacteraemias among adult and paediatric haematology and cancer patients. *Journal of Infection, 68*(4), 321–331. https://doi.org/10.1016/j.jinf.2013.12.006

Miller, K. (2022). Hematologic complications. In J.A. Eggert, K.L. Byar, & L.S. Parks (Eds.), *Cancer basics* (3rd ed., pp. 333–356). Oncology Nursing Society.

Molina, K.C. (2023). Best practices in the management of infectious complications for patients with cancer: Management of febrile neutropenia. *Journal of the Advanced Practitioner in Oncology, 14*(3), 201–206. https://doi.org/10.6004/jadpro.2023.14.3.4

Moon, H., Choi, Y.J., & Sim, S.H. (2018). Validation of the Clinical Index of Febrile Neutropenia (CISNE) model in febrile neutropenia patients visiting the emergency department. Can it guide emergency physicians to a reasonable decision on outpatient vs. inpatient treatment? *PLOS ONE, 13*(12), e0210019. https://doi.org/10.1371/journal.pone.0210019

National Comprehensive Cancer Network. (2025a). *NCCN Clinical Practice Guidelines in Oncology (NCCN Guidelines®): Hematopoietic growth factors* [v.1.2025]. https://www.nccn.org

National Comprehensive Cancer Network. (2025b). *NCCN Clinical Practice Guidelines in Oncology (NCCN Guidelines®): Prevention and treatment of cancer-related infections* [v.1.2025]. https://www.nccn.org

Nazer, L.H., Rimawi, D., & Hawari, F.I. (2020). Evaluating the predictive value of lactate in patients with cancer having septic shock. *Journal of Intensive Care Medicine, 35*(8), 789–796. https://doi.org/10.1177/0885066618788821

Olsen, M., LeFebvre, K.B., Walker, S.L., & Dunphy, E.P. (Eds.). (2023). *Chemotherapy and immunotherapy guidelines and recommendations for practice* (2nd ed.). Oncology Nursing Society.

Pasikhova, Y., Ludlow, S., & Baluch, A. (2018). Fever in patients with cancer. *Cancer Control, 24*(2), 193–197. https://doi.org/10.1177/107327481702400212

Pochon, C., & Voigt, S. (2019). Respiratory virus infections in hematopoietic cell transplant recipients. *Frontiers in Microbiology, 9,* 3294. https://doi.org/10.3389/fmicb.2018.03294

Preethi, R. (2023). Left shift indices in blood cell count—Clinical significance. *iCliniq*. https://www.icliniq.com/articles/blood-health/left-shift-indices-in-blood-cell-count

Punnapuzha, S., Edemobi, P.K., & Elmoheen, A. (2023). Febrile neutropenia. In *StatPearls*. StatPearls Publishing. https://www.ncbi.nlm.nih.gov/books/NBK541102

Radhakrishnan, V., Lagudu, P.B.B., Gangopadhyay, D., Vijaykumar, V., Rajaraman, S., Perumal Kalaiyarasi, J., ... Ganesan, T.S. (2022). Neutropenic versus regular diet for acute leukaemia induction chemotherapy: Randomised controlled trial. *BMJ Supportive and Palliative Care, 12*(4), 421–430. https://doi.org/10.1136/spcare-2022-003833

Ramamoorthy, V., Rubens, M., Appunni, S., Saxena, A., McGranaghan, P., Veledar, E., ... Kotecha, R. (2020). Lack of efficacy of the neutropenic diet in decreasing infections among cancer patients: A systematic review. *Nutrition and Cancer, 72*(7), 1125–1134. https://doi.org/10.1080/01635581.2019.1675723

Rasmy, A., Amal, A., Fotih, S., & Selwi, W. (2016). Febrile neutropenia in cancer patients: Epidemiology, microbiology, pathophysiology and management. *Journal of Cancer Prevention and Current Research, 5*(3), 273–278. https://doi.org/10.15406/jcpcr.2016.05.00165

Seltzer, J.A., Frankfurt, O., & Kyriacou, D.N. (2022). Association of an emergency department febrile neutropenia intervention protocol with time to initial antibiotic treatment. *Academic Emergency Medicine, 29*(1), 73–82. https://doi.org/10.1111/acem.14335

Sereeaphinan, C., Kanchanasuwan, S., & Julamanee, J. (2021). Mortality-associated clinical risk factors in patients with febrile neutropenia: A retrospective study. *International Journal of Infectious Diseases, 1,* 5–11. https://doi.org/10.1016/j.ijregi.2021.09.002

Silvestre-Roig, C., Hidalgo, A., & Soehnlein, O. (2016). Neutrophil heterogeneity: Implications for homeostasis and pathogenesis. *Blood, 127*(18), 2173–2181. https://doi.org/10.1182/blood-2016-01-688887

Sonbol, M.B., Jain, T., Firwana, B., Hilal, T., Deleon, T., Murad, A., ... Khera, N. (2019). Neutropenic diets to prevent cancer infections: Updated systematic review and meta-analysis. *BMJ Supportive and Palliative Care, 9*(4), 425–433. https://doi.org/10.1136/bmjspcare-2018-001742

Stephens, R.S. (2020). Neutropenic fever in the intensive care unit. In J.L. Nates & K.J. Price (Eds.), *Oncologic critical care* (pp. 1297–1311). Springer. https://doi.org/10.1007/978-3-319-74588-6_118

Suwanpakdee, D., Prasertsin, W., Traivaree, C., & Rujkijyanont, P. (2021). Serum lactate: A predictor of septic shock in childhood cancers with febrile neutropenia. *Global Pediatric Health, 8*. https://doi.org/10.1177/2333794X211022711

Talcott, J.A., Siegel, R.D., Finberg, R., & Goldman, L. (1992). Risk assessment in cancer patients with fever and neutropenia: A prospective, two-center validation of a prediction rule. *Journal of Clinical Oncology, 10*(2), 316–322. https://doi.org/10.1200/JCO.1992.10.2.316

Taplitz, R.A., Kennedy, E.B., Bow, E.J., Crews, J., Gleason, C., Hawley, D.K., ... Flowers, C.R. (2018). Outpatient management of fever and neutropenia in adults treated for malignancy: American

Society of Clinical Oncology and Infectious Diseases Society of America Clinical Practice Guideline update. *Journal of Clinical Oncology, 36*(14), 1443–1453. https://doi.org/10.1200/JCO.2017.77.6211

Tran, M., Palmer, S., Moore, D.T., Bartelt, L., Friedland, A., Grgic, T., ... Shaw, R. (2023). Utility of urine cultures during febrile neutropenia workup in hematopoietic stem cell transplantation recipients without urinary symptoms. *Open Forum Infectious Diseases, 10*(5). https://doi.org/10.1093/ofid/ofad236

Tsuchihashi, K., Ito, M., Okumura, Y., Nio, K., Ozaki, Y., Nishio, H., ... Baba, E. (2024). Therapeutic use of granulocyte colony-stimulating factor (G-CSF) in patients with febrile neutropenia: A comprehensive systematic review for clinical practice guidelines for the use of G-CSF 2022 from the Japan Society of Clinical Oncology. *International Journal of Clinical Oncology, 29*(6), 700–705. https://doi.org/10.1007/s10147-024-02541-z

Uneno, Y., Imura, H., Makuuchi, Y., Tochitani, K., & Watanabe, N. (2022). Pre-emptive antifungal therapy versus empirical antifungal therapy for febrile neutropenia in people with cancer. *Cochrane Database of Systematic Reviews, 11,* CD013604. https://doi.org/10.1002/14651858.CD013604.pub2

U.S. Food and Drug Administration. (2024). *Safe food handling.* https://www.fda.gov/food/buy-store-serve-safe-food/safe-food-handling

van der Velden, W.J., Herbers, A.H., Netea, M.G., & Blijlevens, N.M. (2014). Mucosal barrier injury, fever and infection in neutropenic patients with cancer: Introducing the paradigm febrile mucositis. *British Journal of Haematology, 167*(4), 441–452. https://doi.org/10.1111/bjh.13113

Xun, Y., Shi, Q., Yang, N., Yang, N., Li, Y., Si, W., ... Chen, Y. (2021). Associations of hand washing frequency with the incidence of illness: A systematic review and meta-analysis. *Annals of Translational Medicine, 9*(5), 395. https://doi.org/10.21037/atm-20-6005

Zgheib, H., El Zakhem, A., Wakil, C., Cheaito, M.A., Cheaito, R., Finianos, A., ... El Majzoub, I. (2021). Role of urine studies in asymptomatic febrile neutropenic patients presenting to the emergency department. *World Journal of Emergency Medicine, 12*(2), 99–104. https://doi.org/10.5847/wjem.j.1920–8642.2021.02.003

Zhu, X., Zhang, W., Zhang, Y., Wang, Y., Hu, H., Li, J., ... Huang, D. (2023). Pegfilgrastim on febrile neutropenia in pediatric and adolescent cancer patients: A systematic review and meta-analysis. *Hematology, 28*(1), 2172292. https://doi.org/10.1080/16078454.2023.2172292

Zimmer, A.J., & Freifeld, A.G. (2019). Optimal management of neutropenic fever in patients with cancer. *Journal of Oncology Practice, 15*(1), 19–24. https://doi.org/10.1200/JOP.18.00269

Luciana Lopes Manfredini, PhD, BSN,
and Katie Dombrowski, DNP, AGNP-C

CHAPTER 15

Sepsis and Septic Shock

FAST FACTS

- **Description:** Sepsis is a life-threatening organ dysfunction caused by a dysregulated response to infection. It can progress to septic shock if left untreated.
- **Incidence:** Sepsis is a significant cause of death and hospital costs worldwide, with exceptionally high risk and poor survival rates among patients with cancer.
- **Clinical Manifestations:** In immunosuppressed patients with cancer, hypotension, tachycardia, and tachypnea are often early signs of sepsis and may occur with or without fever.
- **Risk Factors and Etiology:** Sepsis is primarily caused by infections, with patients with cancer being at higher risk due to compromised immune systems. Additional risk factors include comorbidities, age extremes, recent surgeries, and prolonged neutropenia.
- **Pathophysiology and Patient Evaluation:** Assessment includes vital signs, blood samples, cultures (e.g., blood, urine, secretions), and consideration of radiologic imaging to identify the source of infection.
- **Advanced Practice Considerations:** Advanced practice considerations for sepsis include timely and comprehensive laboratory and diagnostic tests, which are essential for early identification, therapy guidance, and monitoring response in sepsis management.
- **Treatment Modalities:** Treatment involves prompt, broad-spectrum antibiotics, fluid resuscitation, and hemodynamic and oxygen support as needed. Antimicrobials should be administered within one hour of recognizing sepsis or septic shock.
- **Nursing Management:** Early recognition using evidence-based tools and prompt interventions, such as obtaining blood samples and cultures before administering antimicrobials, enables oncology nurses to respond swiftly and effectively, collaborating with the interprofessional team to ensure optimal outcomes for patients with sepsis or septic shock.
- **Outcomes:** Sepsis and septic shock are life-threatening oncologic emergencies requiring early detection and intervention. Oncology nurses play a critical role in recognizing, reporting, and helping to prevent these conditions.

Introduction

Sepsis is a life-threatening organ dysfunction caused by a dysregulated inflammatory host response to infection (Brent, 2021). If not promptly controlled or treated, it can progress to septic shock and ultimately lead to circulatory collapse, resulting in cellular and metabolic dysfunction, multiple organ failure, and a high risk of mortality (Jarczak et al., 2021). Identification of risk factors and symptoms is essential to reduce the morbidity and mortality of this disorder, and management of sepsis requires prompt assessment and treatment. Patients with cancer should be stratified by their unique risks and treated accordingly.

Nursing management of sepsis and septic shock requires knowledge of the risk factors of infection, the predictors for progression, and the pathophysiology of the disorders while instituting preventive measures, recognizing the early manifestations, and ensuring prompt enactment of appropriate interventions.

Incidence

In 1992, sepsis was first defined as an excessive inflammatory response to infection, identified by meeting at least two systemic inflammatory response syndrome (SIRS) criteria: abnormal temperature, heart rate, respiratory rate, or white blood cell count. The definition has since evolved, as sepsis is now recognized as life-threatening organ dysfunction caused by a dysregulated response to infection. Although SIRS is no longer part of the official definition, it can still help identify possible infections (Meyer & Prescott, 2024).

Each year, approximately 1.7 million adults in the United States will develop sepsis, resulting in 350,000 deaths (Dantes et al., 2023). Globally, an estimated 48.9 million sepsis cases and 11 million associated deaths occur annually, with approximately 85% occurring in low- and middle-income countries (Rudd et al., 2020). Sepsis is the leading cause of in-hospital mortality and the most expensive condition treated during hospitalization (Meyer & Prescott, 2024; Rhee et al., 2019). The Agency for Healthcare Research and Quality reported an excess of $52 billion in sepsis-related medical costs in the United States (Owens et al., 2024).

Nazer et al. (2022) evaluated more than 6,000 patients with cancer and sepsis, severe sepsis, or septic shock. Results indicated poor survival, with in-hospital death reported in approximately two-thirds of those studied. In addition, they reported high rates of hospital admission (62%), 28–30 day mortality (50%), and intensive care unit (ICU) admission (48%) (Nazer et al., 2022).

The National Comprehensive Cancer Network (NCCN, 2025) identified infection, a major cause of sepsis, as the most common cause of death not directly related to malignancy. Sepsis is considered the leading cause of mortality in patients with hematologic malignancies, as well as in those with solid tumors undergoing neutropenia-inducing chemotherapy treatments (Kochanek et al., 2019). Up to 30% of patients with hematologic malignancies develop sepsis within the first year of diagnosis and treatment (Orhin et al., 2024).

Patients with cancer are inherently at higher risk for developing sepsis. Additional risk factors include comorbidities and chronic illnesses, poor performance status or nutrition, age extremes (aged younger than 5 years or older than 60 years), immunosuppression, use of prophylactic antibiotics or corticosteroids, recent surgeries or invasive procedures (e.g., indwelling catheters, central lines, feeding tubes), and hospitalizations, especially in ICUs.

Prolonged neutropenia, particularly in patients with hematologic malignancies or those undergoing stem cell transplantation, is another significant risk factor. The duration (> 7 days) and severity of the neutropenia—defined as an absolute neutrophil count (ANC) less than 100–500 cells/mcl—can lead to infections that result in sepsis (NCCN, 2025; Rudd et al., 2020). If the infection is not eliminated or the pathologic immune response is not reversed, patients will progress to multiorgan failure syndrome, which carries a mortality rate up to 75% (Al-Khafaji & Sharma, 2024).

Common Pathogens

Many pathogens can cause infection, including bacteria (Gram-positive or Gram-negative), fungi, viruses, and parasites. These pathogens can enter the body via invasive IV lines or catheters (e.g., indwelling urinary catheters) through the skin, bloodstream, respiratory tract, gastrointestinal (GI) tract, and urinary tract (see Table 15-1). The most common sites of infection are the lung (37%), genitourinary (27%–37%), abdominal/GI (5%–13%), skin (8%), and primary bacteremia (7%) (Chou et al., 2020). The pathogens that cause infections can enter the body either actively, by exposure to infectious organisms, or passively, via penetration of normal flora into areas where they do not usually occur. Once they evade healthy host defense mechanisms, the pathogens can initiate the cascade of events characteristic of sepsis.

Although infections caused by Gram-positive organisms have increased over the past decades, primarily from the use of intravascular devices and broad-spectrum antibiotics, Gram-negative organisms, often originating from the gut, continue to be a significant and virulent cause of sepsis in adult patients with cancer (Neviere, 2024). Accurate identification of the infectious pathogen is crucial for selecting the appropriate antibiotic therapy based on pathogen susceptibility. However, the causative organism is never identified in up to 40% of all septic shock cases (Li et al., 2022).

Clinical Manifestations

Sepsis presents with a broad spectrum of clinical manifestations because of its complex and multifactorial nature (see Table 15-2). The combination of infection site, pathogen type, acute dysfunction of one or more organs, and baseline health status contributes to the substantial heterogeneity in presentation. Recognizing sepsis in a timely manner remains challenging, as early signs are often nonspecific and can mimic other conditions. Additionally, these manifestations may be masked in patients who are immunosuppressed or by medications such as beta-blockers or antipyretics. Patients can exhibit general, nonspecific signs and symptoms of infection, including the following (Meyer & Prescott, 2024; Neviere, 2025):

- Temperature > 100.94°F (38.3°C) or < 96.8°F (36°C)
- Heart rate > 90 beats/minute or more than two standard deviations above the normal value for age (cutoff = mean + 2 × standard deviation)
- Tachypnea, respiratory rate > 20 breaths/minute
- Arterial hypotension (e.g., systolic blood pressure < 90 mm Hg or mean arterial pressure < 70 mm Hg)

Clinical signs and symptoms that localize to a specific infectious source can aid in diagnosis. For example, cough and dyspnea may indicate pneumonia, whereas localized pain and purulent discharge from a surgical wound may suggest the presence of an underlying abscess (Neviere, 2025).

TABLE 15-1
Portals of Entry and Common Microbial Organisms Associated With Sepsis Risk

Portal of Entry	Examples
Central nervous system (surgically/procedurally induced and nonsurgically induced)	Gram-negative: *Pseudomonas aeruginosa* Gram-positive: *Staphylococcus aureus*, *Propionibacterium* species, *Haemophilus influenzae*, pneumococcal meningitis Viral: varicella zoster, human herpesvirus 6, cytomegalovirus, Epstein-Barr virus, West Nile virus, Zika virus, arbovirus Fungal: *Candida*, mucormycosis, Zygomycetes, *Fusarium* species, cryptococcal toxoplasmosis
Central venous catheter	Gram-negative: *Stenotrophomonas maltophilia*, *Acinetobacter* species, *Pseudomonas aeruginosa* Gram-positive: coagulase-negative *Staphylococcus*, coryneform bacteria, *Propionibacterium* species, *Enterococcus* species Fungal: *Candida*
Soft tissue (skin)	Gram-negative: *Pseudomonas aeruginosa* Gram-positive: *Staphylococcus aureus*, streptococci Viral: varicella-zoster Fungal: *Candida*, mucormycosis, Zygomycetes, *Fusarium* species
Respiratory tract (nasal sinus, lungs)	Gram-negative: *Pseudomonas aeruginosa*, *Acinetobacter* species, *Neisseria meningitides*, pertussis, *Escherichia coli*, *Klebsiella* species Gram-positive: *Streptococcus pneumoniae* (pneumococcus), viridans (alpha-hemolytic) streptococci, *Staphylococcus aureus* Viral: cytomegalovirus, herpes simplex virus, upper respiratory virus (e.g., influenza, parainfluenza, metapneumovirus, rhinovirus), *Legionella*, adenovirus, respiratory syncytial virus Fungal: *Candida*, mucormycosis, *Aspergillus*, Zygomycetes, *Cryptococcus*, *Nocardia*, *Mycobacterium tuberculosis*, *Pneumocystis jiroveci*
Gastrointestinal mucosa (mouth, esophagus, intestine, stomach, rectum)	Gram-negative: *Escherichia coli*, *Klebsiella* species, *Pseudomonas aeruginosa* Gram-positive: *Enterococcus* species, *Clostridium* species Viral: cytomegalovirus, herpes simplex virus Fungal: *Candida*
Urogenital (bladder, urinary tract, vagina)	Gram-negative: *Pseudomonas aeruginosa*, *Escherichia coli*, *Klebsiella* species Viral: herpes simplex virus Fungal: *Candida*

This list presents the most common pathogens noted in the literature. However, any organism can act as a pathogen if it gains access to body tissues.

Note. Based on information from Dellinger et al., 2013; Lewis et al., 2011; National Comprehensive Cancer Network, 2025; Penack et al., 2014.

TABLE 15-2
Clinical Manifestations of Sepsis by System

System Affected	Signs and Symptoms
General or systemic	Fever or hypothermia Malaise, fatigue, lethargy Hyperglycemia due to insulin resistance Leukocytosis (> 12,000 cells/mcl) or leukopenia (< 4,000 cells/mcl)
Dermatologic or peripheral vascular	Cold, clammy skin Cyanosis, acrocyanosis Tissue necrosis, poor wound healing, stasis ulcers
Neurologic	Mild confusion, agitation, anxiety, disorientation Delirium, stupor, coma Septic encephalopathy Mental status changes that may precede fever or hypotension
Cardiovascular	Hypotension Lactate > 5 mmol/L Requirement for vasopressor therapy High cardiac output, low systemic vascular resistance, myocardial depression
Pulmonary	Dyspnea, tachypnea Respiratory alkalosis due to hyperventilation Progression to acute respiratory distress syndrome
Hepatic	Elevated liver function tests Mild hepatic dysfunction
Gastrointestinal	Ileus and gut ischemia Neutropenic enterocolitis (typhlitis): abdominal pain, bloating, hypoactive/absent bowel sounds, watery or bloody diarrhea, nausea, vomiting
Renal	Oliguria Elevated creatinine and blood urea nitrogren Acute kidney injury due to hypoperfusion, vasoconstriction, cytokine release, neutrophil activation

Note. Based on information from Evans et al., 2021; Meyer & Prescott, 2024.

Cutaneous findings may vary with the progression of sepsis. In early stages, patients may exhibit warm, flushed skin due to peripheral vasodilation. As sepsis advances to septic shock, skin perfusion typically decreases, resulting in cool extremities as blood flow is redirected to vital organs. Clinical signs such as delayed capillary refill, cyanosis, and mottling are indicative of impaired perfusion and may signal the onset of shock. Additional manifestations of tissue hypoperfusion include altered mental status, ranging from restlessness to obtundation, and reduced urine output, such as oliguria or anuria. In severe or prolonged shock, GI perfusion may also be compromised, leading to ileus and absent bowel sounds, often considered late findings of systemic hypoperfusion (Neviere, 2025).

Risk Factors and Etiology

Background and Definition

Sepsis is characterized by life-threatening dysfunction of one or more organs in the presence of a suspected or confirmed infection. This organ dysfunction may impact the respiratory, cardiovascular, coagulation, or neurologic systems. The term *severe sepsis* is no longer used because acute organ dysfunction is required for sepsis.

Septic shock is defined as sepsis with cardiovascular organ dysfunction as indicated by severe hypotension; venous or arterial blood lactate level greater than 5 mmol/L (> 45.05 mg/dl), or need for vasoactive medication (Meyer & Prescott, 2024; Schlapbach et al., 2024).

Patients with cancer have an inherently compromised immune system and respond differently to infections compared to the general population.

Recipients of stem cell or bone marrow transplants are particularly vulnerable to infections due to the use of myeloablative and lymphodepleting conditioning regimens, which can severely impair immune reconstitution for up to two years or more. Both autologous and allogeneic transplantation result in prolonged myelosuppression, often reducing ANC below 100 cells/mcl for several days to weeks, depending on the intensity of the conditioning protocol (Akhmedov, 2021; NCCN, 2025). Recovery of B and T lymphocytes may take months to years, substantially increasing the risk of fatal opportunistic infections in the absence of timely intervention. Early post-transplant lymphocyte counts below 300–500 cells/mcl have been associated with decreased overall survival. Additionally, recipients of allogeneic transplants face heightened risk because of the need for sustained immunosuppressive therapy to prevent or control graft-versus-host disease (Akhmedov, 2021; NCCN, 2025).

Numerous chimeric antigen receptor T-cell therapies directed against biomarkers used in the treatment of hematologic malignancies, such as cluster of differentiation 19 or B-cell maturation antigen, are associated with significant immunologic toxicities. Adverse effects, most notably neutropenia, lymphopenia, and hypogammaglobulinemia, substantially elevate the risk of infections, particularly within the first 30 days following therapy initiation. Bacterial infections are most common early on, whereas opportunistic infections tend to occur later, often weeks to months following treatment, especially if prolonged neutropenia persists (NCCN, 2025).

The Surviving Sepsis Campaign (SSC) provides international guidelines for the management of sepsis and septic shock (Evans et al., 2021). These recommendations emphasize improving care after ICU discharge, address the long-term effects of sepsis and the challenges these effects pose for recovery and rehabilitation, and highlight the importance of including patients and caregivers in goals-of-care discussions and discharge planning.

Risk Models

Sepsis can be challenging to detect, as it often presents with nonspecific symptoms that may be easily mistaken for other conditions, and its clinical presentation can vary widely among patients. Prompt and accurate identification is critical, as each hour of delayed treatment significantly increases the risk of mortality (Evans et al., 2021; Multinational Association of Supportive Care in Cancer, 2015).

Traditional scoring systems, such as the Sequential Organ Failure Assessment (SOFA), the Quick Sequential Organ Failure Assessment (qSOFA), the National Early Warning Score (NEWS), the Modified Early Warning Score (MEWS), and the Emergency Oncology Scale (EMOnco), have contributed meaningfully to clinical decision-making, particularly by helping to reduce cognitive biases. Despite their utility, these tools have demonstrated limited sensitivity in accurately predicting sepsis, with qSOFA showing limitations in early detection compared to NEWS and MEWS (Liu et al., 2025). Recognizing these shortcomings, studies advocate for the use of more comprehensive and dynamic screening strategies, especially in high-risk patient populations (Evans et al., 2021; Giacobbe et al., 2021).

Sequential Organ Failure Assessment

SOFA was developed as an objective tool to quantify organ dysfunction or failure in intensive care settings (Vincent et al., 2019). It is a seven-item scoring system that numerically quantifies the number and severity of organ dysfunction in six organ systems: respiratory, coagulation, liver, cardiovascular, renal, and neurologic. The SOFA score has been validated in patients in the ICU to predict sepsis more accurately than the previous SIRS criteria. Particularly in low-income countries, SOFA can be employed as a screening tool to predict 28–30-day mortality among patients with sepsis (Qiu et al., 2023). Because staff in acute care and outpatient settings may not have all the information needed to perform the complete SOFA scoring method, a modified version of SOFA was developed, the qSOFA.

Quick Sequential Organ Failure Assessment

The qSOFA is a three-item scoring system that allots points for respiratory rate, mental status, and systolic blood pressure and can be used easily by any clinician in any setting. However, SSC guidelines have been updated to strongly discourage relying solely on qSOFA for sepsis screening because of its limited sensitivity (Evans et al., 2021). Studies have shown that qSOFA is more specific but less sensitive than having two of four SIRS criteria for early identification of infection-induced organ dysfunction (Evans et al., 2021; Herwanto et al., 2019).

National Early Warning Score

NEWS was developed in 2012 by the Royal College of Physicians and updated in 2017 to NEWS2 to standardize the assessment and response to acute illness. This screening tool encompasses an aggregate scoring system derived from six physiologic parameters: respiration rate, oxygen saturation, systolic blood pressure, pulse rate, level of consciousness or new confusion, and temperature (Royal College of

Physicians, 2017). The scoring system ranges from aggregate scores of zero to seven or greater. It is associated with a clinical risk of low to high, as well as the urgency of clinical responses.

Modified Early Warning Score

MEWS is a clinical tool designed to identify early signs of physiologic deterioration in hospitalized patients. It is based on routinely measured vital signs: respiratory rate, heart rate, systolic blood pressure, temperature, and level of consciousness. The total score reflects the degree of physiologic instability, guiding escalation of care and timely intervention (Subbe et al., 2001).

Initially validated by Subbe et al. (2001), MEWS demonstrated substantial predictive value for unexpected ICU admissions, cardiac arrests, and in-hospital mortality. In subsequent years, its application expanded to various hospital settings as a track-and-trigger system, particularly for detecting sepsis and other acute clinical deteriorations.

Emergency Oncology Scale

EMOnco is a tool for screening patients with cancer in emergency departments. The protocol has five levels and suggests that patients with risk criteria for sepsis be triaged as level 1 and treated immediately. These criteria include the following (Manfredini et al., 2024):

- Presenting or reporting fever (axillary > 100.04°F [37.8°C] or oral > 100.94°F [38.3°C])
- Undergoing antineoplastic chemotherapy
- Having active hematologic disease
- Receiving a postallogeneic bone marrow transplantation
- Having suspected neutropenia
- Being associated with tremors
- Experiencing changes in mental status or oliguria
- Presenting with suspected or confirmed infectious focus

Implementation of integrated electronic health record clinical decision support tools to identify sepsis early and aid with management is crucial. The development of artificial intelligence tools can also support the early detection of sepsis. Machine learning models that use historical data have shown superior accuracy in predicting critical illness when compared to traditional scoring systems. These models use algorithms that consider body temperature, heart rate, respiratory rate, systolic and diastolic blood pressure, pain, sex, and age (Liu et al., 2025). These systems are under development and could be applied to electronic health records to help decision-making.

Pathophysiology and Patient Evaluation

Sepsis is a progressive disorder that involves complex interactions between a pathogen and a host's immune system. Infection occurs when an organism or microbe evades the healthy immune response of the host and enters sterile sites within the body, such as the bloodstream and internal organs, and colonizes and reproduces within host cells.

The Healthy Immune Response to Infection

When bacterial pathogens enter a sterile site in the body, resident immune cells, especially macrophages, detect and respond to the threat. This response involves the recognition of microbial components by surface receptors on innate immune cells, triggering phagocytosis, bacterial killing, and the clearance of tissue debris. Macrophages also release proinflammatory cytokines, which recruit additional immune cells like leukocytes to the site. Both proinflammatory and anti-inflammatory mediators tightly regulate this response. In most cases, localized infections are effectively cleared, leading to tissue repair and healing (Neviere, 2024).

Transition to Sepsis

Sepsis develops when the immune response to infection becomes systemic rather than remaining localized. This generalized inflammatory reaction may result from microbial toxins, excessive cytokine release, or complement system activation. Although anti-inflammatory responses may help reduce inflammation-related damage, they can also impair the body's ability to fight the infection. Genetic factors may predispose some individuals to developing sepsis. Variations in genes encoding innate immune receptors, such as toll-like receptor 4 and nucleotide-binding oligomerization domain containing 2, can alter pathogen recognition and trigger an exaggerated inflammatory response. Polymorphisms in cytokine genes, including tumor necrosis factor-alpha, interleukin (IL)-1 beta, IL-6, and the anti-inflammatory mediator IL-10, have also been linked to differences in susceptibility and disease severity. In addition, genetic variations affecting coagulation and complement pathways, such as protein C and mannose-binding lectin deficiencies, may impair host defense mechanisms. Differences in human leukocyte antigen haplotypes and genes regulating endothelial function further contribute to individual variability in the risk of developing sepsis and its clinical outcomes (Neviere, 2024).

Although the early inflammatory and coagulation pathways in sepsis are well understood, the precise cellular mechanisms leading to organ dysfunction and death remain unclear, highlighting the complexity and severity of systemic sepsis (Neviere, 2024).

Patient Assessment

History

A comprehensive and systematic patient history is an essential component of the nursing assessment, enabling the identification of potential risk factors for infection and informing a clinical management plan. Major comorbid illnesses (e.g., diabetes mellitus, chronic obstructive pulmonary disease, renal insufficiency, cardiovascular disease), a detailed medication history (all current and recent medications, with particular attention to immunosuppressive agents, corticosteroids, cancer treatment, and cycles completed), recent or ongoing antibiotic use (whether therapeutic or prophylactic), use of invasive medical devices (e.g., central venous catheters, urinary catheters, feeding tubes), and a history of prior infections (including site, pathogen, and treatment response) can provide valuable insight (NCCN, 2025).

The assessment should also include epidemiologically relevant exposures that may predispose patients to infection. These include lifestyle factors such as marijuana use and tobacco smoking, both of which can compromise mucosal defenses, particularly in the respiratory tract. Exposure to infectious agents from household contacts or pets, recent travel (especially to regions with endemic or emerging infectious diseases), and recent administration of blood products should also be considered. Each of these factors may contribute to the overall risk profile for patients and influence diagnostic considerations and prophylactic or therapeutic strategies (NCCN, 2025).

Physical Examination

In addition to a thorough history, a complete physical examination is needed to identify the potential underlying cause of infection and to evaluate for symptoms consistent with sepsis. Focusing on high-risk sites of infection (e.g., skin, mouth, lungs, nasal sinus, GI and genitourinary tracts, perirectal and perivaginal sites) and areas of focal pain is necessary and should be performed at least every shift and with changes in condition (NCCN, 2025).

Early Intervention

Time-to-antibiotic administration can significantly impact outcomes for patients who have been identified as being at risk for developing sepsis. Rapid response processes in clinical practice settings should be implemented to reduce the time to antibiotic administration for patients with febrile neutropenia and sepsis.

Advanced Practice Considerations

Laboratory Studies

Laboratory findings are generally nonspecific and may reflect underlying hypoperfusion or organ dysfunction (see Table 15-3). Blood tests include a complete blood count with differential, with attention on a white blood cell count greater than 12,000 cells/mcl, less than 4,000 cells/mcl, or greater than 10% immature cells, which could be indicative of infection. However, in patients with cancer, alterations in white blood cell counts can be disease or treatment related. As ANC drops lower than 500 cells/mcl, the risks increase, and the frequency and severity of infection are inversely proportional to ANC (Neviere, 2025).

A complete chemistry panel and lactic acid measurement should be obtained. Lactate measurement is recommended to look for occult hypoperfusion because lactic acid is produced as a result of anaerobic metabolism (Meyer & Prescott, 2024). Lactate thresholds used to define elevated levels varied between 1.6–2.5 mmol/L; however, diagnostic performance remained consistent across this range. Reported sensitivities range from 66%–83%. In contrast, specificities are between 80%–85%. Although the presence of an elevated lactate level may significantly increase the likelihood of a sepsis diagnosis, lactate measurement alone lacks sufficient sensitivity and specificity to definitively confirm or exclude the diagnosis of sepsis (Evans et al., 2021).

TABLE 15-3
Diagnostic Evaluation of Patients With Sepsis

Diagnostic Study	Rationale
Abdominal ultrasound	This ultrasound is performed based on complaints of abdominal symptoms.
Arterial blood gases	These can assess oxygenation of patients; they are helpful in evaluating respiratory alkalosis and metabolic acidosis.
Biomarkers (proteins and cytokines that are released in response to infection and sepsis)	C-reactive protein is recommended for children but optional for adults. Elevated procalcitonin implicates poorer outcomes when combined with other predictive symptoms. Elevated high mobility group box 1 is correlated with the presence of sepsis.
Blood culture	To determine the pathogenic organisms responsible for sepsis, two sets of blood cultures (one set consists of two bottles, one aerobic and one anaerobic) are drawn, with one being from the central venous catheter and the other peripheral (but always at least two sets of cultures). Cultures should be drawn no more than every 24 hours thereafter and should be obtained from all potential sources prior to antibiotic administration, if possible.
Bronchoscopy or endoscopy	This procedure may be considered in patients who continue to show signs of infection despite treatment.
Chest computed tomography scan	This scan is performed based on a suspicious x-ray or unresolved symptoms of infection.
Chest radiographs	Radiographs are performed to rule out lung infection.
Coagulation tests	Prolonged prothrombin time and partial thromboplastin time, elevated D-dimer assay, and decreased fibrinogen and platelet count may reflect fibrinolysis or disseminated intravascular coagulation. Decreased prothrombin time may indicate hepatic failure.
Complete blood count with differential	Infection is indicated by a white blood cell count > 12,000 cells/mcl, < 4,000 cells/mcl, or > 10% bands. A high risk for infection exists with an absolute neutrophil count < 500 cells/mcl, with the highest risk at < 100 cells/mcl. Risk for opportunistic infections exists with an absolute lymphocyte count < 500 cells/mcl. A platelet count < 150,000 cells/mcl is included in Sequential (Sepsis-Related) Organ Failure Assessment criteria.

(Continued on next page)

TABLE 15-3
Diagnostic Evaluation of Patients With Sepsis *(Continued)*

Diagnostic Study	Rationale
Complete metabolic panel	Increased • Blood urea nitrogen, creatinine • Bilirubin Decreased • Low protein/albumin level–risk predictive of sepsis • Low phosphorus–risk predictive of sepsis • Low serum bicarbonate level–metabolic acidosis and risk predictive of sepsis • Serum glucose–implicated to predict the trajectory of sepsis
Cultures of body fluids, including urine, stool, and fluids from the throat, wound, sputum, and spine	Cultures are obtained before initiating antimicrobial therapy. Specific specimens are collected based on clinical findings.
Doppler ultrasound	This ultrasound is diagnostic for venous thrombosis based on fever.
Electrocardiogram or echocardiogram	This test is performed based on suspicion of a cardiac source of infection to evaluate the rate and rhythm.
Lumbar puncture	This procedure is initiated if a central nervous system infection is suspected.
$ScvO_2$ (central venous oxygen saturation)	This is a noninvasive way to obtain the essential readings needed for tissue perfusion without getting a blood gas; readings > 70% show perfusion; arterial blood gas is still required to obtain the blood pH level. It is recommended to evaluate the response to fluid resuscitation measures.
Serum lactate	If serum lactate is elevated, it indicates tissue hypoperfusion. It is helpful in evaluating metabolic acidosis (levels > 4 mmol/L are most predictive, as elevations can be false for multiple reasons, but a level > 2 mmol/L is guideline driven).
SvO_2 (mixed venous blood gas)	This is a noninvasive way to obtain essential readings needed for tissue perfusion without getting a blood gas; readings > 65% show perfusion; arterial blood gas is still required to obtain the blood pH level. It is recommended to evaluate the response to fluid resuscitation measures.
Thoracentesis	Thoracentesis assists in isolating a source of bacterial infection.
Venogram or spiral computed tomography scan	This scan is diagnostic for pulmonary embolus based on fever and symptoms.

Note. Based on information from National Comprehensive Cancer Network, 2025; Neviere, 2025.

N-terminal pro B-type natriuretic peptide has been shown to be a better predictor of ICU and 90-day mortality than cardiac troponin. However, because its levels are frequently elevated, even in the absence of overt cardiac dysfunction, its prognostic value may be limited when adjusted for illness severity (L'Heureux et al., 2020). Identification of the infectious pathogen is critical. Patients with cancer who have signs and symptoms consistent with infection, sepsis, or septic shock should have blood cultures drawn, as well as cultures from all other suspected infectious sites (e.g., urine, sputum), to help locate the source of infection. Obtaining antigen testing (e.g., tests for *Legionella* and *Streptococcal*), as well as polymerase chain reaction pathogen detection panels, is also helpful (Meyer & Prescott, 2024). NCCN (2025) guidelines recommend initially drawing two sets of blood cultures (one set consists of two bottles), preferably one from a peripheral site and the other from a central line catheter. If that is not possible, both cultures can be drawn from peripheral sites or both from central line catheters (NCCN, 2025).

Additional samples from other suspected sources may need to be obtained, including cerebrospinal fluid, pleural fluid, and bronchoalveolar lavage or bronchial brushings (NCCN, 2025).

Other Diagnostic Studies

No radiologic findings pathognomonic for sepsis exist; however, imaging may reveal evidence of infection at specific sites (e.g., infiltrates consistent with pneumonia on chest radiography, localized fluid collections on abdominal computed tomography suggestive of an abscess) (Neviere, 2025).

Treatment Modalities

Treatment Goals

The management of sepsis in patients with cancer includes preventive strategies, early identification, and prompt implementation of guidelines and evidence-based, goal-directed interventions. Although SSC interventions are not specific to oncology, they have been extrapolated and should be employed to quickly reverse the symptoms of sepsis. A one-hour bundle is highly encouraged to minimize the time to initiate treatment and emphasize the urgency of sepsis and septic shock. Goals are to be accomplished within three hours after the diagnosis of severe sepsis. The bundle includes the following elements (Evans et al., 2021):

- Recognize sepsis as early as possible.
- Look for signs of infection and organ dysfunction.
- Measure blood lactate level.
  - Lactate > 2 mmol/L suggests hypoperfusion.
  - Repeat measurement if the initial value is elevated.
- Obtain blood cultures before starting antibiotics. Collect at least two sets of blood cultures and other cultures as appropriate.

- Do not delay antibiotics.
  - Administer broad-spectrum antibiotics.
  - Start as soon as possible, ideally within the first hour after sepsis or septic shock recognition.
- Initiate fluid resuscitation of 30 ml/kg of IV crystalloids for hypotension or lactate ≥ 4 mmol/L.
- Start vasopressors if hypotension persists after fluids.
  - The goal is to maintain mean arterial pressure ≥ 65 mm Hg.
  - The first-line agent is norepinephrine (noradrenaline).

Gram-positive and Gram-negative organisms are the most common causes of sepsis, followed by viral or fungal infections (Meyer & Prescott, 2024). Viral infections, such as Middle East respiratory syndrome coronavirus, influenza, and severe acute respiratory syndrome coronavirus 2, have highlighted the role of viruses in sepsis, especially in patients who are critically ill. However, viral sepsis is often underdiagnosed due to the lack of routine viral testing in standard evaluations (Xu et al., 2024). Among bloodstream pathogens, the *Candida* species are the third most cultured (Meyer & Prescott, 2024; Timsit et al., 2020).

Preventive Strategies

Unique to patients being treated for cancer, the most frequently used evidence-based approach to prevent sepsis is the prophylactic use of antibiotics for those with the highest risk of infection. Extensive research has been conducted on the risk versus benefit of prophylactic antibiotics in patients with cancer who receive treatment that induces febrile neutropenia. Antibacterial prophylaxis is not recommended for patients at low risk of infection. In patients with neutropenia who have a lower risk of infectious complications, such as most individuals with solid tumor malignancies, the primary benefit of antibacterial prophylaxis is a reduction in fever rather than a decrease in documented infections (NCCN, 2025).

For patients with neutropenia expected to last fewer than seven days and not receiving immunosuppressive therapies (e.g., systemic corticosteroids), NCCN (2025) does not recommend antibiotic prophylaxis. However, in patients classified as intermediate or high risk, it advises considering fluoroquinolone prophylaxis, preferably with levofloxacin, for those with an expected duration of neutropenia (ANC ≤ 500 cells/mcl, or ≤ 1,000 cells/mcl with a predicted decline to ≤ 500 cells/mcl within 48 hours) lasting more than seven days. This recommendation aligns with the Infectious Diseases Society of America guidelines on antimicrobial use in patients with cancer and neutropenia. For patients intolerant to fluoroquinolones, trimethoprim–sulfamethoxazole or an oral third-generation cephalosporin may be considered as alternative options (NCCN, 2025).

Appropriate Antibiotic Selection

Identification of the underlying pathogen is essential to eradicate the infection and consequently the symptoms that cause sepsis. Antibiotic selection should be tailored to each individual and must consider a patient's history, comorbidities, potential immunodeficiencies, clinical context, existing invasive devices, and sites suspicious of infection (Schmidt et al., 2025).

Infections in patients with cancer vary by anatomical site, source, and treatment duration. Patients with solid tumors often develop infections from organisms reflecting the local microflora. Some infections follow seasonal patterns similar to the general population, whereas others are opportunistic, affecting individuals who are immunocompromised due to cytotoxic therapy. Treatment guidelines exist, and careful attention must be paid to interactions between antibiotics and cancer therapies (Delgado & Guddati, 2021).

About 80% of catheter-related infections are caused by Gram-positive organisms. Among patients with solid tumors, Gram-negative bloodstream infections are more prevalent. In hematologic malignancies, a lower incidence is likely due to postchemotherapy antibiotic prophylaxis; however, antibiotic-resistant strains are on the rise (Delgado & Guddati, 2021).

Gram-positive bacteria, fungi, and other opportunistic infections can cause sepsis, but they are not as common as Gram-negative bacteria. Antibiotic coverage for Gram-positive bacteria is usually added, either empirically or preemptively, for a prior history of Gram-positive infection, identification of Gram-positive bacteria, obvious skin infection, use of a central venous catheter, the presence of persistent fevers, or pneumonia. The addition of antibiotic coverage for Gram-positive fungal or other organisms is based on confirmation of organism identification or when a patient's condition is not improving on current therapy (Schmidt et al., 2025).

Transfer to the ICU is often initiated depending on a patient's condition and the level of monitoring and support that the nursing staff can provide. As oncology nurses infrequently care for these patients in this setting, staff who work in this unit will have extensive training on critical treatment modalities. Patients may require intubation or mechanical ventilator support, which should be considered early if progressing to septic shock, as well as intensive invasive monitoring, such as arterial lines or pulmonary arterial lines (Schmidt et al., 2025). Furthermore, SSC guidelines suggest that patients with sepsis or septic shock who require ICU admission should be transferred within six hours (Evans et al., 2021).

Adjuvant Therapeutic Treatments

Steroids

Corticosteroids attenuate the immune response to infection and have been shown to improve outcomes in various severe pulmonary infections (Pirracchio et al., 2024). Low-dose corticosteroids, defined as less than or equal to 400 mg of hydrocortisone or equivalent per day, are associated with reduced mortality in patients who have a severe case of COVID-19, community-acquired pneumonia, and *Pneumocystis pneumonia* (Pirracchio et al., 2024). Although steroids have also been found to decrease mortality from sepsis and reverse shock, they may increase the risk of muscle weakness, hypernatremia, and hyperglycemia (Pitre et al., 2024). Additionally, SSC guidelines regarding the use of corticosteroids provide a conditional recommendation for corticosteroid administration in septic shock with acute respiratory distress syndrome, a strong recommendation for severe community-acquired pneumonia, and a recommendation against the administration of high-dose and duration of corticosteroids in septic shock (Chaudhuri et al., 2024).

Coagulation Inhibitors

The use of coagulation inhibitors in sepsis, particularly recombinant thrombomodulin and antithrombin, aims to mitigate sepsis-induced coagulopathy. A meta-analysis suggested that recombinant thrombomodulin may reduce mortality and improve disseminated intravascular coagulation resolution without increasing bleeding risk (Kato et al., 2023). However, large trials, such as SCARLET, have reported mixed outcomes (Vincent et al., 2019). Randomized controlled trials showed no survival benefit from antithrombin. In contrast, observational studies in septic-associated disseminated intravascular coagulation reported improved outcomes; however, the risk for increased bleeding complications should necessitate careful benefit–risk evaluation (Tsuchida et al., 2024). Further research is needed to identify patient subgroups that may benefit the most.

Cytokines and Immune Modulators

Increasing evidence supports the role of immunosuppression in the pathogenesis of sepsis, and clinical trials are being established to determine if augmenting the immune system will provide benefit in treating sepsis. Research has identified promising and potential adjunctive immunotherapy agents for sepsis, including granulocyte–macrophage colony-stimulating factor, recombinant human IL-7, interferon gamma, programmed cell death protein 1 or programmed cell death-ligand 1 inhibitors, anti–tumor necrosis factor-alpha, and recombinant human IL-3 and IL-15 (Tavaci & Akgun, 2022).

Intravenous Immunoglobulin

Guidelines recommend against the routine use of IV immunoglobulin; however, some researchers support its consideration under certain circumstances, including in patients who are most immunosuppressed and have repeated sinopulmonary infections (Cui et al., 2019; Welte et al., 2018).

Glycemic Control

Evidence is conflicting regarding the benefits of normalization of blood glucose levels in sepsis. It has been found that strict glucose control can have a negative effect on outcomes in patients with sepsis, leading SSC to recommend maintaining a more liberal blood glucose level of less than 180 mg/dl, initiating insulin if it is greater than this value (Evans et al., 2021).

Transfusion Therapy

Blood product transfusion is often essential for multiple reasons in patients with sepsis. It is also a prevalent treatment for patients with cancer, particularly those with hematologic malignancies.

Packed red blood cells can be used as supportive therapy to increase low hemoglobin concentrations once tissue perfusion is adequate in patients with severe sepsis who do not have extenuating circumstances, such as myocardial ischemia, severe hypoxemia, or ischemic coronary artery disease. According to guidelines from the American College of Chest Physicians, a restrictive transfusion strategy should be used, with a threshold hemoglobin level of 7–8 g/dl (Yataco et al., 2025). SCC also recommends using a restrictive transfusion strategy in patients with sepsis or septic shock (Evans et al., 2021). Although the transfusion of packed red blood cells increases the hematocrit and oxygen delivery to the cells, it does not necessarily lead to increased oxygen consumption and uptake by cells because of oxygen transport abnormalities in patients with severe sepsis (Nicolescu et al., 2021).

Thrombocytopenia often accompanies postchemotherapy neutropenia or occurs as a result of hematologic disease. The frequent occurrence of thrombocytopenia in sepsis usually indicates a poor prognosis (Shannon, 2020). Per SCC guidelines, a platelet transfusion threshold of less than 10,000 cells/mcl is recommended in the absence of obvious bleeding, with a higher threshold of less than 20,000–50,000 cells/mcl for active bleeding or significant risk of bleeding (Rhodes et al., 2017). SSC guidelines do not recommend transfusion of fresh frozen plasma to reverse existing coagulopathies unless patients are actively bleeding or invasive procedures are planned (Evans et al., 2021).

Nursing Management

Early recognition of the risk for and detection of signs and symptoms of infection are important in preventing the progression to sepsis and septic shock. A stepwise approach to the nursing care of patients with sepsis is key, including preventive strategies, early recognition of symptoms, initiation of evidence-based interventions, implementation of general supportive care measures, and provision of emotional support and education to patients and caregivers at this critical time.

Prevention

When identifying preventive strategies for sepsis, nurses must consider the portals of entry for infections, such as the skin and the GI, genitourinary, and respiratory tracts. They should also implement evidence-based practices to minimize microbial exposure, including practicing strict hand hygiene, providing careful central venous catheter hub and site care in accordance with facility protocols (e.g., use of chlorhexidine), using appropriate patient placement in isolation rooms based on the type of infection (e.g., protective, airborne, contact, droplet), and, when possible, limiting the use of invasive devices (e.g., indwelling urinary catheters, arterial lines, pulmonary artery catheters). Because infections in patients with cancer often arise from their own normal flora, nurses should educate patients on personal hygiene, skin care, and good oral and rectal care. Oral hygiene is crucial in the management of oral complications during antineoplastic therapy for cancer (Suzuki et al., 2023).

General Supportive Nursing Care

Venous thromboembolism prophylaxis is recommended in SSC guidelines because it is essential for patients in the hospital who are acute or critically ill (Evans et al., 2021). Patients with sepsis, especially those being treated in an ICU, have a high risk for thrombus formation secondary to venous stasis resulting from immobility, vessel injury caused by invasive therapies, and sepsis-induced hypercoagulopathy.

Patients with sepsis who are critically ill and receiving antineoplastic therapy are at increased risk for ulceration of the GI tract because of hypoperfusion and tissue ischemia in the gut, leading to injury to the mucosal lining and loss of protective intestinal barrier functions (Haussner et al., 2019). SSC guidelines recommend using stress ulcer prophylaxis in patients at risk for GI bleeding (Evans et al., 2021).

The early initiation (commenced within 72 hours of ICU admission) of enteral nutrition in patients with sepsis and septic shock offers potential physiologic benefits, including the preservation of gut integrity, reduction of intestinal permeability, attenuation of the systemic inflammatory response, and modulation of metabolic processes, which may contribute to decreased insulin resistance (Evans et al., 2021; NCCN, 2025). Nursing assessment of nutritional intake and suggestions for nutritional sources that are well tolerated or palatable for patients are highly beneficial in maintaining adequate dietary requirements.

Emotional Support

Caring for the emotional health of patients and caregivers is integral to nursing practice. During acute and urgent clinical situations, nurses should make it a priority to support patients and families, as fear and anxiety are certain and can affect patient outcomes. The supportive environment provided by nurses is critical to patients' and caregivers' well-being and ability to cope. Nurses can serve as knowledgeable advocates and provide emotional support and listening skills as patients and caregivers face potential end-of-life issues. Referrals to interprofessional sources of support, such as spiritual care through a chaplaincy program, counseling from a psychologist or social worker, case management assistance, and patient or family support groups, may be beneficial.

Comprehensive nursing care can validate emotions, which can improve outcomes, enhance patient quality of life, and reduce length of stay and treatment costs (Shen et al., 2021).

Patient and Caregiver Education

Nurses should provide the bulk of education for patients and their caregivers and play a significant role in the overall education of patients. They should educate patients on their disease, its treatment, and the associated side effects. A major side effect of antineoplastic therapies is neutropenia. Nurses should facilitate education on the risks, timing, and preventive strategies. Evidence-based guidelines on how to prevent infection and on the appropriate use of colony-stimulating factors and prophylactic antibiotics are part of postchemotherapy education. Instructions should be provided to patients and caregivers about how to recognize the signs and symptoms of infection; the importance of notifying clinicians at the first sign of infection; the telephone numbers to call, particularly after business hours; and the logistics of where patients will go when they have signs of infection to expedite access to care. As patients become critically ill, nurses must provide patients and their caregivers with information about the next steps.

Summary

Sepsis and septic shock are life-threatening oncologic emergencies that can occur very quickly after the onset of infection. Because of the rapidity and severity of these conditions, early detection and intervention are imperative for better patient outcomes. Oncology nurses must assist in promptly recognizing and reporting aberrant vital signs or other signs of infection to allow for immediate initiation of appropriate therapies.

Although much is understood about the development and treatment of sepsis and septic shock, more research is needed to provide new insights into this complex syndrome and develop more effective targeted therapies. Oncology nurses are well positioned to research optimal evidence-based preventive strategies and contribute to the development of better risk models and nursing interventions for patients with infections that may progress to sepsis.

The authors would like to acknowledge Christine F. Rimkus, MSN, AOCN®, for her contribution to this chapter that remains unchanged from the previous edition of this book.

References

Akhmedov, M. (2021). Infectious complications in allogeneic hematopoietic cell transplant recipients: Review of transplant-related risk factors and current state of prophylaxis. *Clinical Transplantation, 35*(2), e14172. https://doi.org/10.1111/ctr.14172

Al-Khafaji, A.H., & Sharma, S. (2024, October 8). Multiple organ dysfunction syndrome in sepsis. *Medscape.* http://emedicine.medscape.com/article/169640-overview

Brent, A.J. (2021). Sepsis. *Medicine, 49*(11), 714–718. https://doi.org/10.1016/j.mpmed.2021.08.010

Chaudhuri, D., Nei, A.M., Rochwerg, B., Balk, R.A., Asehnoune, K., Cadena, R., … Pastores, S.M. (2024). 2024 focused update: Guidelines on use of corticosteroids in sepsis, acute respiratory distress syndrome, and community-acquired pneumonia. *Critical Care Medicine, 52*(5), e219–e233. https://doi.org/10.1097/CCM.0000000000006172

Chou, E.H., Mann, S., Hsu, T.C., Hsu, W.T., Liu, C.C., Bhakta, T., … Lee, C.C. (2020). Incidence, trends, and outcomes of infection sites among hospitalizations of sepsis: A nationwide study. *PLOS ONE, 15*(1), e0227752. https://doi.org/10.1371/journal.pone.0227752

Cui, J., Wei, X., Lv, H., Li, Y., Li, P., Chen, Z., & Liu, G. (2019). The clinical efficacy of intravenous IgM-enriched immunoglobulin (pentaglobin) in sepsis or septic shock: A meta-analysis with trial sequential analysis. *Annals of Intensive Care, 9*(1), 27. https://doi.org/10.1186/s13613-019-0501-3

Dantes, R.B., Kaur, H., Bouwkamp, B.A., Haass, K.A., Patel, P., Dudeck, M.A., … Prescott, H.C. (2023). Sepsis program activities in acute care hospitals—National Healthcare Safety

Network, United States, 2022. *Morbidity and Mortality Weekly Report, 72*(34), 907–911. https://doi.org/10.15585/mmwr.mm7234a2

Delgado, A., & Guddati, A.K. (2021). Infections in hospitalized cancer patients. *World Journal of Oncology, 12*(6), 195–205. https://doi.org/10.14740/wjon1410

Dellinger, R.P., Levy, M.M., Rhodes, A., Annane, D., Gerlach, H., Opal, S.M., ... Moreno, R. (2013). Surviving Sepsis Campaign: International guidelines for management of severe sepsis and septic shock 2012. *Critical Care Medicine, 41*(2), 580–637. https://doi.org/10.1097/CCM.0b013e31827e83af

Evans, L., Rhodes, A., Alhazzani, W., Antonelli, M., Coopersmith, C.M., French, C., ... Levy, M. (2021). Surviving Sepsis Campaign: International guidelines for management of sepsis and septic shock 2021. *Intensive Care Medicine, 47*(11), 1181–1247. https://doi.org/10.1007/s00134-021-06506-y

Giacobbe, D.R., Signori, A., Del Puente, F., Mora, S., Carmisciano, L., Briano, F., ... Bassetti, M. (2021). Early detection of sepsis with machine learning techniques: A brief clinical perspective. *Frontiers in Medicine, 8,* 617486. https://doi.org/10.3389/fmed.2021.617486

Haussner, F., Chakraborty, S., Halbgegauer, R., & Huber-Lang, M. (2019). Challenge to intestinal mucosa during sepsis. *Frontiers in Immunology, 10,* 891. https://doi.org/10.3389/fimmu.2019.00891

Herwanto, V., Shetty, A., Nalos, M., Chakraborty, M., McLean, A., Eslick, G.D., & Tang, B. (2019). Accuracy of quick sequential organ failure assessment score to predict sepsis mortality in 121 studies including 1,716,017 individuals: A systematic review and meta-analysis. *Critical Care Explorations, 1*(9), e0043. https://doi.org/10.1097/CCE.0000000000000043

Jarczak, D., Kluge, S., & Nierhaus, A. (2021). Sepsis—Pathophysiology and therapeutic concepts. *Frontiers in Medicine, 8,* 628302. https://doi.org/10.3389/fmed.2021.628302

Kato, H., Hagihara, M., Asai, N., Umemura, T., Hiari, J., Mori, N., ... Mikamo, H. (2023). Efficacy and safety of recombinant human soluble thrombomodulin in patients with sepsis-induced disseminated intravascular coagulation - A meta-analysis. *Thrombosis Research, 226,* 165–172. https://doi.org/10.1016/j.thromres.2023.05.009

Kochanek, M., Schalk, E., von Bergwelt-Baildon, M., Beutel, G., Buchheidt, D., Hentrich, M., ... Böll, B. (2019). Management of sepsis in neutropenic cancer patients: 2018 guidelines from the Infectious Diseases Working Party (AGIHO) and Intensive Care Working Party (iCHOP) of the German Society of Hematology and Medical Oncology (DGHO). *Annals of Hematology, 98*(5), 1051–1069. https://doi.org/10.1007/s00277-019-03622-0

Lewis, M.A., Hendrickson, A.W., & Moynihan, T.J. (2011). Oncologic emergencies: Pathophysiology, presentation, diagnosis, and treatment. *CA: A Cancer Journal for Clinicians, 61*(5), 287–314. https://doi.org/10.3322/caac.20124

L'Heureux, M., Sternberg, M., Brath, L., Turlington, J., & Kashiouris, M.G. (2020). Sepsis-induced cardiomyopathy: A comprehensive review. *Current Cardiology Reports, 22*(5), 35. https://doi.org/10.1007/s11886-020-01277-2

Li, A., Ling, L., Qin, H., Arabi, Y.M., Myatra, S.N., Egi, M., ... Phua, J. (2022). Epidemiology, management, and outcomes of sepsis in ICUs among countries of differing national wealth across Asia. *American Journal of Respiratory and Critical Care Medicine, 206*(9), 1107–1116. https://doi.org/10.1164/rccm.202112-2743OC

Liu, Z., Shu, W., Li, T., & Chong, W. (2025). Interpretable machine learning for predicting sepsis risk in emergency triage patients. *Scientific Reports, 15*(1), 887. https://doi.org/10.1038/s41598-025-85121-z

Manfredini, L.L., Conte, E.R., Santos, G.P.D., Leão, E.R., & Hamerschlak, N. (2024). Construction and validation of the Emergency Oncology Scale (EMOnco), a risk rating protocol for the triage of cancer patients in acute care settings. *Einstein, 22,* eAO0693. https://doi.org/10.31744/einstein_journal/2024AO0693

Meyer, N.J., & Prescott, H.C. (2024). Sepsis and septic shock. *New England Journal of Medicine, 391*(22), 2133–2146. https://doi.org/10.1056/NEJMra2403213

Multinational Association of Supportive Care in Cancer. (2015). *Identifying patients at low risk for FN complications: Development and validation of the MASCC Risk Index score.* https://mascc.memberclicks.net/index.php?option=com_dailyplanetblog&view=entry&year=2015&month=01&day=22&id=25:identifying-patients-at-low-risk-for-fn-complications-development-and-validation-of-the-mascc-risk-index-score

National Comprehensive Cancer Network. (2025). *NCCN Clinical Practice Guidelines in Oncology (NCCN Guidelines®): Prevention and treatment of cancer-related infections* [v.1.2025]. https://www.nccn.org

Nazer, L., Lopez-Olivo, M.A., Cuenca, J.A., Awad, W., Brown, A.R., Abusara, A., ... Nates, J.L. (2022). All-cause mortality in cancer patients treated for sepsis in intensive care units: A systematic review and meta-analysis. *Supportive Care in Cancer, 30*(12), 10099–10109. https://doi.org/10.1007/s00520-022-07392-w

Neviere, R. (2024). Pathophysiology of sepsis. In G. Finlay (Ed.), *UpToDate*. Retrieved May 28, 2025, from https://www.uptodate.com/contents/pathophysiology-of-sepsis

Neviere, R. (2025). Sepsis syndromes in adults: Epidemiology, definitions, clinical presentation, diagnosis, and prognosis. In G. Finlay (Ed.), *UpToDate*. Retrieved May 28, 2025, from https://www.uptodate.com/contents/sepsis-syndromes-in-adults-epidemiology-definitions-clinical-presentation-diagnosis-and-prognosis

Nicolescu, L.C., Nicolescu, C.M., Mihu, A.G., & Balta, C. (2021). The effect of red blood cell transfusion on peripheral tissue oxygen delivery and consumption in septic patients. *Transfusion Clinique et Biologique, 28*(1), 5–10. https://doi.org/10.1016/j.tracli.2020.12.002

Orhin, A.E., Gyato, A., Ohene, A., Otoo, S.D., Assabill, F., Akoto, N.A.Y., & Khanapara, D. (2024). National trends and disparities in sepsis-related mortality in adults with hematological cancers, 1999–2020. *Blood, 144*(1, Suppl.), 5176. https://doi.org/10.1182/blood-2024-204124

Owens, P.L., Miller, M.A., Barrett, M.L., & Hensche, M. (2024). *Overview of outcomes for inpatient stays involving sepsis, 2016–2021: HCUP Statistical Brief #306.* Agency for Healthcare Research and Quality. https://hcup-us.ahrq.gov/reports/statbriefs/sb306-overview-sepsis-2016–2021.pdf

Penack, O., Becker, C., Buchheidt, D., Christopeit, M., Kiehl, M., von Lilienfeld-Toal, M., ... Ostermann, H. (2014). Management of sepsis in neutropenic patients: 2014 updated guidelines from the Infectious Diseases Working Party of the German Society of Hematology and Medical Oncology (AGIHO). *Annals in Hematology, 93*(7), 1083–1095. https://doi.org/10.1007/s00277-014-2086-0

Pirracchio, R., Venkatesh, B., & Legrand, M. (2024). Low-dose corticosteroids for critically ill adults with severe pulmonary infections: A review. *JAMA, 332*(4), 318–328. https://doi.org/10.1001/jama.2024.6096

Pitre, T., Drover, K., Chaudhuri, D., Zeraaktkar, D., Menon, K., Gershengorn, H.B., ... Rochwerg, B. (2024). Corticosteroids in sepsis and septic shock: A systematic review, pairwise, and dose-response meta-analysis. *Critical Care Explorations, 6*(1), e1000. https://doi.org/10.1097/CCE.0000000000001000

Qiu, X., Lei, Y.P., & Zhou, R.X. (2023). SIRS, SOFA, qSOFA, and NEWS in the diagnosis of sepsis and prediction of adverse outcomes: A systematic review and meta-analysis. *Expert Review of Anti-Infective Therapy, 21*(8), 891–900. https://doi.org/10.1080/14787210.2023.2237192

Rhee, C., Jones, T.M., Hamad, Y., Pande, A., Varon, J., O'Brien, C., ... Klompas, M. (2019). Prevalence, underlying causes, and preventability of sepsis-associated mortality in US acute care hospitals. *JAMA Network Open, 2*(2), e187571. https://doi.org/10.1001/jamanetworkopen.2018.7571

Rhodes, A., Evans, L.E., Alhazzani, W., Levy, M.M., Antonelli, M., Ferrer, R., ... Dellinger, R.P. (2017). Surviving Sepsis Campaign: International guidelines for management of sepsis and septic shock: 2016. *Intensive Care Medicine, 43*(3), 304–377. https://doi.org/10.1007/s00134-021-06506-y

Royal College of Physicians. (2017). *National Early Warning Score (NEWS) 2: Standardising the assessment of acute-illness severity in the NHS. Updated report of a working party.* Royal College of Physicians. https://www.rcp.ac.uk/media/a4ibkkbf/news2-final-report_0_0.pdf

Rudd, K.E., Johnson, S.C., Agesa, K.M., Shackelford, K.A., Tsoi, D., Kievlan, D.R., ... Naghavi, M. (2020). Global, regional, and national sepsis incidence and mortality, 1990-2017: Analysis for the Global Burden of Disease Study. *Lancet, 395*(10219), 200–211. https://doi.org/10.1016/S0140-6736(19)32989-7

Schlapbach, L.J., Watson, R.S., Sorce, L.R., Argent, A.C., Menon, K., Hall, M.W., ... Bennett, T.D. (2024). International consensus criteria for pediatric sepsis and septic shock. *JAMA, 331*(8), 665–674. https://doi.org/10.1001/jama.2024.0179

Schmidt, G.A., Mandel, J., & Bell, T.D. (2025). Evaluation and management of suspected sepsis and septic shock in adults. In G. Findlay (Ed.), *UpToDate*. Retrieved May 28, 2025, from https://www

.uptodate.com/contents/evaluation-and-management-of-suspected-sepsis-and-septic-shock-in-adults

Shannon, O. (2020). The role of platelets in sepsis. *Research and Practice in Thrombosis and Haemostasis, 5*(1), 27–37. https://doi.org/10.1002/rth2.12465

Shen, G., He, Y., Ni, J., Jiang, L., Liu, H., Pan, S., ... Li, X. (2021). Effects of comprehensive nursing on negative emotion and prognosis of patients with sepsis. *American Journal of Translational Research, 13*(7), 8221–8227. https://pmc.ncbi.nlm.nih.gov/articles/PMC8340246

Subbe, C.P., Kruger, M., Rutherford, P., & Gemmel, L. (2001). Validation of a modified Early Warning Score in medical admissions. *QJM, 94*(10), 521–526. https://doi.org/10.1093/qjmed/94.10.521

Suzuki, K., Sasada, S., Nishi, H., Kimura, Y., Shintani, T., Emi, A., ... Okada, M. (2023). Impact of oral hygiene on febrile neutropenia during breast cancer chemotherapy. *Breast Cancer, 30*(1), 151–155. https://doi.org/10.1007/s12282-022-01410-9

Tavaci, T., & Akgun, N. (2022). Sepsis: Immunopathology, immunotherapies, and future perspectives. *Eurasian Journal of Medicine, 54*(1, Suppl.), S127–S132. https://doi.org/10.5152/eurasianjmed.2022.22314

Timsit, J.-F., Ruppé, E., Barbier, F., Tabah, A., & Bassetti, M. (2020). Bloodstream infections in critically ill patients: An expert statement. *Intensive Care Medicine, 46*(2), 266–284. https://doi.org/10.1007/s00134-020-05950-6

Tsuchida, T., Makino, Y., Wada, T., Ushio, N., Totoki, T., Fujie, N., ... Iba, T. (2024). Efficacy of antithrombin administration for patients with sepsis: A systematic review, meta-analysis, and meta-regression. *Acute Medicine and Surgery, 11*(1), e950. https://doi.org/10.1002/ams2.950

Vincent, J.-L., Francois, B., Zabolotskikh, I., Daga, M.K., Lascarrou, J.-B., Kirov, M.Y., ... Fineberg, D. (2019). Effect of a recombinant human soluble thrombomodulin on mortality in patients with sepsis-associated coagulopathy: The SCARLET randomized clinical trial. *JAMA, 321*(20), 1993–2002. https://doi.org/10.1001/jama.2019.5358

Welte, T., Dellinger, R.P., Ebelt, H., Ferrer, M., Opal, S.M., Singer, M., ... Torres, A. (2018). Efficacy and safety of trimodulin, a novel polyclonal antibody preparation, in patients with severe community-acquired pneumonia: A randomized, placebo-controlled, double-blind, multicenter, phase II trial (CIGMA study). *Intensive Care Medicine, 44*(4), 438–448. https://doi.org/10.1007/s00134-018-5143-7

Xu, J.-Q., Zhang, W.-Y., Fu, J.-J., Fang, X.-Z., Gao, C.-G., Li, C., ... Shang, Y. (2024). Viral sepsis: Diagnosis, clinical features, pathogenesis, and clinical considerations. *Military Medical Research, 11*(1), 78. https://doi.org/10.1186/s40779-024-00581-0

Yataco, A.O.C., Soghier, I., Hebert, P.C., Belley-Cote, E., Disselkamp, M., Flynn, D., ... Ouellette, D.R. (2025). Red blood cell transfusion in critically ill adults: An American College of Chest Physicians Clinical Practice Guideline. *Chest, 167*(2), 477–489. https://doi.org/10.1016/j.chest.2024.09.016

SECTION IV
ADVANCED PRACTICE

Megan O'Neil, DNP, APRN, FNP-C, OCN®,
Christina Matousek, DNP, RN, OCN®,
and Kristin Marie Ferguson, DNP, MBA, RN, OCN®, CGNC

CHAPTER 16

Hypersensitivity Reactions

FAST FACTS

- **Description:** Infusion-related reactions are systemic reactions that occur in response to infusions of IV agents that stimulate a variety of immunologic and nonimmunologic responses.
- **Incidence:** Infusion-related reaction incidence varies depending on the type of infusion, whether through chemotherapy or biologic agents.
- **Clinical Manifestations:** Symptoms associated with infusion-related reactions include itching, urticaria, wheezing, bronchospasm, angioedema, hypotension, pain, and a feeling of impending doom.
- **Risk Factors and Etiology:** Patients with prior drug allergies, multiple comorbidities, and those who are receiving platinum and taxane therapy are at higher risk for infusion-related reactions.
- **Pathophysiology and Patient Evaluation:** Diagnosis is based on signs and symptoms. Experienced and well-trained oncology infusion nurses are essential in assessing these symptoms, educating patients, notifying providers, and performing further treatments.
- **Advanced Practice Considerations:** Prevention and management of infusion-related reactions require a thorough risk assessment and awareness of reaction timing. Clinical approaches, such as the use of premedications and drug desensitization protocols, are effective measures to improve patient safety.
- **Treatment Modalities:** Treatment depends on the severity and cause of reactions associated with the infusion. Some measures include acetaminophen, antihistamines, corticosteroids, and epinephrine.
- **Nursing Management:** If a reaction occurs, nurses should stop the infusion, perform an accurate assessment (e.g., vital signs), remain with the patient, and administer rescue medications or symptom management.
- **Outcomes:** Prevention of infusion-related reactions is the goal when possible. If a reaction does occur, nurses should provide symptom relief. Prompt recognition and treatment are essential to ensure cardiopulmonary support.

Introduction

IV infusions, widely used in cancer settings, can result in serious patient harm. Severe, life-threatening hypersensitivity reactions (HSRs) can occur with chemotherapy, biotherapy, supportive medications (e.g., IV iron), and blood product transfusions. Antineoplastic agents are among the top causes of fatal infusion-related HSRs (Horita et al., 2021). HSRs have been documented for nearly every antineoplastic agent, and oncology nurses must be aware of the signs and take action when they occur (Seghers et al., 2023). Although not all infusion-related reactions constitute an emergency, seemingly mild symptoms can quickly progress to serious, life-threatening reactions that require immediate intervention.

British immunologists Philip George Houthem Gell and Robin Coombs published the first model for HSRs in 1968. They divided the reactions into four categories based on the body's immune response and the timing of the event after drug exposure: immunoglobulin (Ig) E, IgE, IgM, and T-cell mediated (Kozubek et al., 2024). However, since the development of the Gell and Coombs model, significant research has been completed, and more is understood about HSRs related to antineoplastics and immunotherapy; thus, this model is rarely used to describe HSRs related to chemotherapy. The *Common Terminology Criteria for Adverse Events* (*CTCAE*), which uses a five-point grading system for toxicities, has become the standard scale for classifying and grading the severity of adverse events resulting from cancer treatment (National Cancer Institute Cancer Therapy Evaluation Program, 2017; Olsen et al., 2023). Nurses should use their organization's standard *CTCAE*. Although it does not explicitly refer to medication reactions, the *CTCAE* section on immune system disorders includes general allergic reactions, anaphylaxis, cytokine release syndrome (CRS), and serum sickness.

Another commonly referenced scale regarding cancer treatment–related HSRs is the Brown grading system (Olsen et al., 2023). Although allergists most often use this scale, it focuses on the symptoms most frequently observed in HSRs and is pertinent for oncology care (Tsao et al., 2022). Because of the frequent use of premedications in the oncology setting to help prevent HSRs, it can be challenging for nurses to assess the frequency or degree of HSRs. Despite this challenge, a wealth of data exists on the medications used in oncology, providing a solid foundation for examining general risks, symptoms, and treatment.

Incidence

The exact incidence of HSRs related to chemotherapy and biotherapy is unknown but is believed to be underreported by clinicians, particularly for reactions that are not life threatening (Seghers, 2023). The most common antineoplastic agents causing HSRs are taxanes, platinum agents, and monoclonal antibodies. Literature also suggests that HSR rates are increasing, which may be a result of the increased number of antineoplastic medications that have been developed for the treatment of cancer (Cuartero et al., 2024).

Rates of HSRs for specific oncologic medications vary, and even rates for the same medication can have an extreme range depending on several variables. Although this inconsistency is multifactorial, most of the disparities are the result of whether premedications were given, the rate of infusion, whether it was a first or subsequent dose, and the grading system used to measure the reaction (Olsen et al., 2023). Thus, caution is advised when attempting to evaluate the HSR risk of a specific drug, particularly newly approved agents that have not yet accumulated the depth of postmarketing adverse infusion-related reaction data. Fortunately for patients with cancer, the number of drugs that result in HSRs—particularly severe HSRs—is relatively small.

Clinical Manifestations

Five organ systems are typically the target of HSRs: the integumentary (cutaneous), respiratory, cardiovascular, gastrointestinal, and central nervous systems (Price, 2021). Numerous adverse effects can occur in each of these systems; the number of involved organ sites and severity of symptoms can influence whether a HSR is considered mild or severe and whether it meets the criteria for anaphylaxis (Campbell & Kelso, 2024). Although many of these organ systems are affected by the same physiologic mechanisms, individual and multiple organ systems can be affected. Some symptoms (e.g., oral tingling) are much less obvious than others (e.g., respiratory distress). However, of the five target systems, cutaneous reactions merit further discussion because of their ubiquitous nature and high visibility.

Cutaneous Reactions

HSRs can present as seemingly innocuous cutaneous reactions, which may exist as isolated localized symptoms or as part of an anaphylactic reaction. Urticaria, also known as hives or wheals, is the hallmark dermatologic manifestation of a cutaneous reaction. It can be defined as a smooth, raised papule that blanches with pressure and can be as small as 1 mm or several centimeters in diameter (Asero, 2025). Patients with urticaria may complain of itching or pain in the affected areas. Other signs and symptoms of a cutaneous reaction include generalized rash, pruritus, flushing, and erythema. Reactions may begin on the abdomen, trunk, or neck and subsequently spread to other locations, including the conjunctiva and oral cavity, as seen with angioedema (Asero, 2025). By themselves, most cutaneous reactions are not life threatening; however, the presence of angioedema should be considered an emergency.

Angioedema involves deep dermal swelling in nondependent areas, typically affecting the face, tongue, and respiratory tract. It is mediated by vasoactive substances that result in capillary leakage into the surrounding tissues. In contrast to urticaria, angioedema has minimal or no pruritus (Asero, 2025).

Other, less common but equally life-threatening reactions include toxic epidermal necrolysis or Stevens-Johnson syndrome. Histamine activation results in vasodilation; dilated blood vessels cause the characteristic red or pink color associated with hives. Itching is thought to be caused by activation of the receptors H1 and H4. It is also believed that leukotriene C4 and prostaglandin D2 may play a role in the development of hives (Asero, 2025).

Anaphylaxis

Medications have been reported to be one of the most common sources of anaphylaxis in adults; antibiotics and nonsteroidal drugs are often the primary offenders (Campbell & Kelso, 2024). Because anaphylaxis typically involves multiple organs, it is considered a systemic response. Dermatologic findings are seen in up to 90% of all anaphylactic reactions, and a respiratory component is present in up to 70% (Campbell & Kelso, 2024). However, dermatologic findings may be completely absent. As many as 45% of all patients will have cardiac and gastrointestinal symptoms (Campbell & Kelso, 2024). Anaphylaxis can occur at any time during an infusion or may be delayed until after the infusion is over (Olsen et al., 2023). A delayed reaction has additional implications, as more infusions are performed on an outpatient basis, shifting the location of the reaction to a patient's home and away from trained professionals.

One challenge for bedside nurses is that anaphylaxis can be progressive, beginning with mild dermatologic symptoms (e.g., urticaria, pruritus) or mild upper respiratory symptoms (e.g., rhinitis), and progressing to wheezing, coughing, shortness of breath, nausea, vomiting, and additional life-threatening signs and symptoms (e.g., hypotension, cardiovascular collapse) (Campbell & Kelso, 2024). In the early stages of anaphylaxis, patients may display sudden anxiety with a feeling of impending doom or indicate that "something does not feel right" without being able to articulate specific symptoms. Although not all patients will progress, a rapid diagnosis with prompt treatment is a priority.

Risk Factors and Etiology

Nurses should be aware of the risk factors associated with the development of an HSR and understand that multiple factors may contribute. A history of general allergies increases the risk for patients receiving platinum agents, and obesity and pulmonary dysfunction increase the risk for patients receiving paclitaxel (Price, 2021). Other known risk factors include age, comorbidities (e.g., chronic cardiopulmonary diseases), mast cell disorders, and severe atopic conditions (Demir et al., 2019). IV medications are more likely to cause a reaction when compared to the intramuscular, subcutaneous, or oral routes (Demir et al., 2019), an important consideration for patients receiving agents such as bleomycin and L-asparaginase, which can be administered by more than one route. In general, females tend to be at higher risk than males, and anaphylaxis is more common in Black individuals and older patients (Demir et al., 2019). Concurrent medications also present a potential HSR risk and underscore the importance of performing medication reconciliation or, at a minimum, a thorough review of a patient's home medications. For example, angiotensin-converting enzyme inhibitors can blunt the body's response to hemodynamic instability during anaphylaxis (Demir et al., 2019). Beta-blockers interfere with the breakdown of bradykinin, which is responsible for vasodilation, and lead to more profound hypotension. They also enhance the release of vasoactive substances from mast cells and inhibit the effects of epinephrine (Campbell & Kelso, 2025).

Pathophysiology and Patient Evaluation

Physiologic Mechanisms of Reactions

The complex diversity in causative pathways involved with HSRs provides the rationale for combining different classes of premedications for prophylaxis (e.g., an antihistamine and a corticosteroid). It also helps explain why some HSRs occur on the first dose, whereas others occur after several administrations. Understanding the physiologic mechanisms is important in risk assessment, prophylaxis, and treatment. HSRs can be placed into two distinct but related groups or pathways: nonimmunologic and immunologic.

Nonimmunologic

Nonimmunologic reactions are caused by direct activation of complement or mast cells or by direct cytokine release (Castells & Solensky, 2023). They typically occur on the first dose without the presence of drug-specific antibodies and often respond to titration of the medication—two hallmarks of this type of reaction (Olsen et al., 2023).

Although nonimmunologic and immunologic reactions produce similar signs and symptoms, immunologic HSRs tend to be more severe but less common in the oncology setting. Nonimmunologic reactions are typically less severe but occur more frequently (Seghers et al., 2023). Within the nonimmunologic category, CRS is a unique type of reaction.

Immunologic

Despite the differences in how the responses are initiated, the immunologic pathway recruits portions of the nonimmunogenic pathway. Immunologic reactions are classic examples of type I reactions in which patients are sensitized to the medication, resulting in the production of IgE antibodies with subsequent activation of the nonimmunologic pathway. These antibodies attach to mast cells and basophils, which can remain quiescent until patients are reexposed to the antigen during a subsequent dose of the offending agent. Adjacent IgE antibodies become cross-linked to the sensitized IgE antibodies and cause mast cell degranulation and the release of cytokines and mediators (Allergy and Asthma Network, 2025).

Immunologic reactions can be divided into three phases (Bernstein et al., 2024):

- The first phase involves sensitization to the foreign protein or drug.
- The second phase occurs with reexposure and involves mast cell degranulation, resulting in the release of histamine, leukotrienes, and other chemical mediators.
- The final phase involves the influence of mast cells on organ systems primarily responsible for immune defense.

Only a small amount of the drug is required to initiate a severe HSR in patients who are sensitized. Reactions can begin within seconds of administration and may first appear as urticaria and progress to a more serious cardiopulmonary event. However, nurses should remember that not all patients will follow this sequence of events. Because IgE antibodies are already present, immunologic reactions cannot be prevented by titration or the administration of premedication (AlMuhizi, Ton-Leclerc, et al., 2022). However, temporary tolerance can sometimes be induced by desensitization, allowing patients to continue receiving therapy. Desensitization exposes patients, in a controlled environment, to the agent that caused a previous reaction to produce temporary tolerance (Olsen et al., 2023). This subsequently allows patients to safely receive the remainder of their treatment course.

Cross-Reactivity

Although biologic therapies are designed to target specific antigens on tumor cells, healthy tissues may exhibit the same or similar antigens, causing unintended reactions. For example, dermatologic manifestations seen with cetuximab result from epidermal growth factor receptor unintentionally targeting healthy skin tissues (Popa et al., 2021). These cross-reactive antigens can produce HSRs, as observed in patients who have never received cetuximab but possess IgG antibodies, which precipitate anaphylaxis. Nurses need to understand that patients who are drug-naïve are responsible for the majority of acute HSRs (Seghers et al., 2023).

Typically, the complement system remains inactive until sufficient stimuli initiate a complex series of cascading reactions (see Table 16-1). Each biochemical step must meet a threshold before activation can occur, preventing inappropriate triggering of an immune response. This helps explain why patients may tolerate a drug (e.g., rituximab) when the infusion is given over a more extended period or slowly titrated upward instead of being initiated at the fastest possible rate (Olsen et al., 2023).

Once complement activation has occurred, vasoactive substances are produced that act as potent anaphylatoxins because of their ability to cause the release of histamine and produce severe cardiopulmonary changes (Ghebrehiwet et al., 2024). Although the complement system also plays a major role in B-cell differentiation, activation of the complement cascade can occur independently of the presence of antibodies, explaining why patients may react to a drug they have never received; antibody development typically requires prior exposure or cross-linking.

Mast Cells

Similar to other human immune cells, mast cells originate from pluripotent stem cells within the bone marrow. They arise from the granulocyte–monocyte progenitor, which is responsible for the development of basophils and monocytes, and their production is stimulated by stem cell factor (Castells & Dwyer, 2023). However, mast cells are unique in several respects.

For one, mature mast cells do not circulate and are stationed in strategic anatomic locations where they can intercept potential foreign invaders. Mast cells can also be found in epithelial tissues throughout the skin, lungs, gastrointestinal tract, and blood vessels. These organs and their proximity to other organs (e.g., lungs) help explain the symptoms associated with anaphylactic reactions (Castells & Dwyer, 2023). Additionally, mast cells can survive for years with the unique ability to release potent biologically active mediators (i.e., granules) contained within the cytoplasm of the cell, and they are also able to replenish these mediators when needed (Castells & Dwyer, 2023).

These immunoreactive mediators can be divided into three distinct categories: preformed mediators within the granules, synthesized mediators produced

TABLE 16-1
Overview of the Complement System

Feature	Description
Definition	A part of the innate immune system, complement proteins bind to antigens to make them more visible to other immune cells (e.g., phagocytes) and can lyse both foreign and host cells.
Main functions	• Opsonization: marks pathogens for phagocytosis • Cell lysis: forms the membrane attack complex to destroy cells • Inflammation: produces anaphylatoxins (C3a, C5a) that trigger histamine release and cardiopulmonary changes • Homeostasis: clears damaged or altered self-components to maintain tissue health
Pathways of activation	• Classical pathway: triggered by antibody–antigen complexes • Lectin pathway: activated by mannose-binding lectin binding to microbial surfaces • Alternative pathway: spontaneously activated on pathogen surfaces
Regulation	Complement activation remains inactive until sufficient stimuli trigger a cascading reaction. Each biochemical step must meet a threshold to prevent inappropriate immune responses.
Clinical relevance	• Overactivation: causes diseases such as rheumatoid arthritis, multiple sclerosis, and ischemic stroke • Underactivation: leads to infections and autoimmune diseases (e.g., systemic lupus erythematosus) • Drug infusions: slow rates (e.g., rituximab), preventing excessive immune response
Effects of activation	Activation of the complement system produces vasoactive substances that act as potent anaphylatoxins, leading to histamine release and severe cardiopulmonary changes.
Antibody independence	The complement cascade can be activated without antibodies, explaining why patients may react to a drug they have never received. Antibody development typically requires prior exposure.
Potential risks	Because complement proteins opsonize or lyse cells, excessive or improper activation can lead to the destruction of healthy tissue. Regulation failures contribute to inflammatory and autoimmune diseases.

Note. Based on information from Liszewski & Atkinson, 2024; Olsen et al., 2023.

on demand, and cytokines. Some mediators, such as the cytokine tumor necrosis factor-alpha, are both preformed and made on demand. Because of their stationary location and ability to express high-affinity Fc receptors binding to IgE, mast cells are considered "first responders" to a foreign invader or inflammatory response. Release of granules (degranulation) can occur within seconds of antigen detection.

Mast cells can be activated by complement C3a and C5a, cytokines, and IgE (Castells & Bankova, 2024).

Mast cell granules include the proteases tryptase-β2, chymase, mast cell carboxypeptidase, and cathepsin G. Of these, tryptase-β2 is the most abundant and generates complement C3a while enhancing the respiratory effects of histamine, promoting bronchoconstriction, and recruiting neutrophils and other inflammatory cells to the area (Castells & Bankova, 2024). Release of tryptase-β2 results in further mast cell degranulation in a positive feedback loop. Other cytokines, such as tumor necrosis factor-alpha, chemokines CXCL8 and CXCL11, and vascular endothelial growth factor, are produced and cause increased vascular permeability. Chymase converts angiotensin I to angiotensin II, enhances the effects of histamine, stimulates interleukin (IL)-1β production, and potentiates local inflammation (Castells & Bankova, 2024). In addition to proteases, mast cells contain heparin and histamine.

Histamine

Although four classes of histamine receptors exist, allergic reactions have been primarily associated with the H1 receptor (Olsen et al., 2023). Medications such as diphenhydramine (histamine receptor antagonists) block the H1 receptor but do not prevent the generation or release of histamine. H2 receptor secretion is associated with gastric acid production. The H3 and H4 receptors have been implicated in allergic and immune reactions in animal models and cause itching. They also contribute to the inflammatory response (Castells & Bankova, 2024).

Histamine is produced in mast cells and basophils and is associated with several significant biologic effects, including the following (Castells & Bankova, 2024):

- Production of prostacyclin and nitric oxide, resulting in vasodilation
- Constriction of bronchioles and smooth muscles, resulting in dyspnea, shortness of breath, and abdominal cramps
- Stimulation of peristalsis and gastric acid secretion, resulting in diarrhea and dyspepsia
- Stimulation of H1 and H2 dermal receptors, resulting in itching and hives

H1 receptor stimulation in particular is responsible for rash and urticaria, vagal nerve stimulation, increased mucus production, and bronchospasm (Asero, 2025).

Release of histamine can result in extremely high local tissue concentrations, which may help to explain why the administration of antihistamines during anaphylaxis is ineffective (Plaut, 1979). Although the circulating half-life of histamine is only approximately two minutes, its release is proportional to the number of mast cells involved; increased levels of histamine equate to more mast cell degranulation (Asero, 2025). Histamine levels peak approximately 10 minutes after the initiation of an HSR and drop rapidly within 30 minutes (Schwartz, 2024).

Basophils

Basophils are also implicated in HSRs, but in a less active role than mast cells. Although similar in some respects, the two cells differ in marked ways. Basophils have a relatively short life span of one to three days and are found in the circulation after maturing in the bone marrow. Migration of basophils to an inflammatory response is thought to be mediated by IL-3 and thymic stromal lymphopoietin (Kemp, 2024).

Basophils contain many of the same granules but also produce platelet-activating factor; cluster of differentiation 40 ligand, which allows T cells to initiate B-cell antibody production; and chemokine CCR3, which is involved with the migration of eosinophils during an allergic response (Kemp, 2024). Basophils are activated by several cytokines, including IL-3, IL-5, IL-18, and IL-33, as well as complements C3a and C5a and IgE (Kemp, 2024; Olsen et al., 2023) (see Table 16-2).

Cytokine Release Syndrome

First coined in 1991, CRS involves the release of proinflammatory cytokines into systemic circulation. Common cytokines involved include IL-1, IL-2, IL-6, IL-10, and interferon gamma (Porter & Maloney, 2024). In its most severe form, CRS can develop into a potentially fatal cytokine storm. This type of life-threatening reaction can be seen in patients receiving chimeric antigen receptor T-cell therapy; reactions may last from hours to seven days following the infusion (Cobb & Lee, 2021). Monoclonal antibodies, used for the treatment of hematologic malignancies, are implicated in most occurrences of CRS because of how they interact with host immune cells by liberating cytokines after cell death from both tumor and immune cells and by

TABLE 16-2
Other Types of Activation Mediators

Mediator	Function
Cytokines	Act as messengers in the immune system; involved in local and systemic immune responses
Proinflammatory cytokines	Potentiate inflammation; includes ILs and interferons
• IL-1β	The inflammatory gatekeeper; regulates other proinflammatory cytokines
• IL-2	Induces fever; used therapeutically in melanoma and other cancers
• IL-4	Stimulates T cells, promotes IgE production, and blunts steroid effectiveness in anaphylaxis
• IL-5	Interacts with B cells to produce IgA; promotes basophil differentiation along with IL-3
• IL-6	Implicated in hypersensitivity reactions
• IL-8 and IL-16	Promotes migration of T cells and dendritic cells to inflammatory sites
• IL-13	Works with IL-4 to promote IgE production, leading to antibody-mediated allergic responses
TNF-α	Regulates immune responses, upregulates T cells, and is involved in mast cell degranulation

Ig—immunoglobulin; IL—interleukin; TNF—tumor necrosis factor

Note. Based on information from Fajgenbaum & June, 2020.

cross-linkage of antibody–antigen complexes and T cells. Increased levels of interferon gamma and IL-6 have been reported during CRS (Porter & Maloney, 2024). As with the complement activation–related pseudoallergy, CRS typically occurs with the first dose and decreases or disappears entirely with subsequent infusions. Signs and symptoms include general flu-like symptoms, respiratory distress, hypotension, fever and chills, nausea, swelling of the tongue, itching, and rash. They can appear during or several hours after the infusion (Cobb & Lee, 2021).

The involvement of multiple systems in homeostasis underscores the complexity of human physiology. Symptoms associated with these immune system components can overlap based on several causes, and other mechanisms can potentiate existing symptoms or initiate unique symptoms.

Patient Assessment

The prevention of HSRs is pivotal to ensuring that patient safety is maintained during all aspects of oncology care (Zhu et al., 2021). Nurses must fully understand their patients' risk factors and the risks associated with specific medications, as clinical management and patient monitoring will be determined based on this assessment. Further, it is crucial to know at what point during treatment an agent may produce a reaction. For example, for platinum-based chemotherapy agents, the likelihood of reactions increases with subsequent doses, whereas with rituximab, reactions tend to occur with the first or second dose (Barroso et al., 2024). Patients who have reacted to a prior infusion should be thoroughly assessed to determine the nature of the reaction, differentiating between an anticipated side effect (e.g., nausea, vomiting) and an HSR. Baseline vital signs and assessments should note the presence of preexisting cutaneous symptoms (e.g., rash, pruritus), respiratory difficulties (e.g., wheezing, shortness of breath), and altered mental state (e.g., confusion, somnolence) (Cuartero et al., 2024).

Advanced Practice Considerations

In addition to performing an initial risk assessment, three clinical approaches are used to prevent or lessen the likelihood of an HSR: premedication, intradermal skin testing, and rapid drug desensitization (AlMuhizi, De Las Vecillas Sanchez, et al., 2022; Zwimpfer et al., 2023).

Premedication

Premedications can be beneficial in preventing many HSRs. Without premedications, HSRs occur in 25%–42% of patients (AlMuhizi, De Las Vecillas Sanchez, et al., 2022). Nurses must allow sufficient time for the medications to take effect, particularly for oral premedications.

Although no standard premedication regimen is available for the prevention of HSRs, antihistamines and corticosteroids are commonly prescribed. Because the release of histamine plays a significant role in most HSRs, antihistamines are often the mainstay in preventing reactions. For some antineoplastic agents, an H1 receptor antagonist, typically diphenhydramine, is sufficient (AlMuhizi, De Las Vecillas Sanchez, et al., 2022). Furthermore, for infusions that may cause a fever, acetaminophen may be added prophylactically (see Table 16-3).

Skin Testing

Intradermal skin testing and epicutaneous skin prick testing can be used to identify patients who may be at risk of experiencing an HSR. Intradermal skin testing involves injecting a small amount of the potential allergen into the dermis. In contrast, epicutaneous skin prick testing involves puncturing the upper layers of the skin through a drop of the allergen extract (Galateanu et al., 2023). This usage of intradermal skin testing and epicutaneous skin prick testing has proven to be valuable in the evaluation of IgE-mediated chemotherapy reactions, specifically for platinum and taxane

TABLE 16-3
Types of Premedications to Prevent Hypersensitivity Reactions

Medication Type	Example	Route	Purpose	Onset of Action
Antihistamines; H1 receptor antagonist	Diphenhydramine	Oral or IV	Prevent the occurrence of hypersensitivity reactions by blocking the immunoglobulin E–mediated release of histamines.	Oral: 15–30 minutes IV: immediate
H2 receptor antagonists	Famotidine	IV	Prevent the occurrence of hypersensitivity reactions by blocking the effects of histamine released; they are given concurrently with an H1 receptor antagonist to provide comprehensive protection against hypersensitivity reactions.	30 minutes
Corticosteroids	Dexamethasone	Oral or IV	Reduce the inflammatory effects of proinflammatory genes.	Varies, depending on dose
	Hydrocortisone	IV		
	Prednisone	Oral		
Antipyretics	Acetaminophen	Oral	Prevent fever.	30–60 minutes

Note. Based on information from Barrett et al., 2022; Goodman et al., 2023.

agents (Galateanu et al., 2023). Skin tests should be performed at least two weeks following an HSR to reduce false-negative results. A positive result is defined as a raised wheal with a diameter of at least 3 mm larger than the control injection (Villarreal-González et al., 2023).

Despite their usefulness, intradermal skin testing and epicutaneous skin prick testing for platinum agents have yielded inconsistent results, and their usage varies in practice between institutions. Although an intradermal skin test can have a negative predictive value of 81%–92%, the positive predictive value is difficult to ascertain, given the concerns challenging a patient with a positive skin test (Galateanu et al., 2023). However, opinions differ regarding oxaliplatin and the reliability of skin testing, with studies failing to find a relationship between positive skin tests and HSRs (Silver et al., 2020). Further, intradermal skin testing can be used to rule out cross-reactivity between platinum agents, which is particularly useful if therapy needs to be changed because of a severe HSR to one platinum agent (Galateanu et al., 2023).

Rapid Desensitization

Drug desensitization comprises administering multiple diluted incremental infusions of the offending medication. Although the exact mechanism for building temporary tolerance in this manner is not fully understood, it has been suggested that the binding of IgE along with the inhibition of specific tyrosine kinase signaling pathways is responsible (Ali et al., 2024). The mechanism of desensitization for reactions not mediated by IgE is unclear. Desensitization induces a temporary tolerance, lasting for hours or days; therefore, patients generally need to be desensitized prior to their next cycle of chemotherapy. Rapid drug desensitization has become an increasingly common practice, but it also carries a high risk of a repeated reaction (Villarreal-González et al., 2023). Although traditional drug desensitization can require several months to achieve tolerance, rapid desensitization procedures typically take 4–12 hours and may span 1–2 days. Patients with severe HSRs may require a longer procedure. The advantage of rapid desensitization is that it allows patients to continue with oncologic therapies without prolonged delays in treatment that could adversely affect disease progression and survival (Villarreal-González et al., 2023).

Several successful desensitization protocols have been developed, particularly for carboplatin. Each desensitization protocol may use different dilutions of the drug depending on the severity of the initial HSR; patients who have experienced a severe HSR tend to tolerate a more gradual increase in drug concentration or rate of infusion (Villarreal-González et al., 2023). Due to the increased likelihood of subsequent HSRs, the facility must be able to support one-to-one nursing care and have emergency equipment available (Portz & Froggatt, 2022).

Treatment Modalities

Each facility should have its own HSR and anaphylaxis protocols, and nurses must be familiar with the medications, route of administration, and dosages (see Table 16-4).

TABLE 16-4
Types of Hypersensitivity Reactions and Their Treatment Modalities

Type of Reaction	Treatment Modalities
Cutaneous	H1 and H2 receptor antagonist (diphenhydramine); famotidine, IV Short-acting corticosteroids (hydrocortisone)
Anaphylaxis and anaphylactoid	Epinephrine intramuscularly, vastus lateralis; can give a second dose after 5 minutes if symptoms do not subside Glucagon intramuscularly; patients on beta-blockers not responding to epinephrine IV fluid bolus if hypotension occurs Supplemental oxygen therapy, if hypoxia occurs Nebulizer treatments based on symptoms
Biphasic	Same treatment as uniphasic reactions, depending on symptoms and presentation

Note. Based on information from Corbett et al., 2022; Jao et al., 2024.

Nursing Management

Although nurses are not called on to diagnose the physiologic etiology of a reaction, a basic understanding of the potential mechanisms is essential for providing patient education and successfully managing HSRs. Similarly, the ability to accurately assess the signs and symptoms of HSRs can aid in treating the reaction and determining what changes may need to be made for subsequent infusions. As cancer treatments continue to shift from inpatient to outpatient settings, nurses will play an increasingly important role in ensuring the safety of patients receiving these therapies.

Medication Administration

Techniques for the administration and safe handling of hazardous medications are beyond the scope of this chapter; however, the methods used for infusing drugs can affect how closely patients are monitored for a reaction and when the reaction is likely to be observed. IV tubing setups vary depending on pump manufacturer and institutional policies. Chemotherapy guidelines often recommend administering drugs using a secondary IV line in addition to a primary line. This provides a safer method of priming the tubing with a neutral solution and allows for flushing of the tubing once the chemotherapy is completed, thereby preventing potential hazardous drug exposure (Olsen & Walton, 2024). The use of low-volume primary and secondary tubing can also significantly decrease the time delay. Approvals for newer monoclonal antibodies have allowed subcutaneous injection (Davis et al., 2024). Although studies comparing subcutaneous and IV administration show time savings for administration and cost savings, the need to monitor for infusion-related reactions remains; often patients must stay at the site of care (infusion center) for monitoring for acute reactions after the first dose (McCloskey et al., 2023). Whichever system is used, nurses must be cognizant of when medication reaches their patients.

Regardless of the clinical setting, emergency equipment and experienced personnel must be available during the administration of medications known to produce HSRs (Olsen & Walton, 2024). Standing orders are recommended for the management of reactions by decreasing delays in initiating immediate treatment measures (Hall et al., 2023). In lieu of standing orders, some institutions have implemented HSR protocols within the electronic health record (Chichelo & Colopoulos, 2025). All emergency supplies should be conveniently located, and nursing staff should be familiar with their use. Simulations have been highly beneficial for nursing education, specifically in crises such as codes and oncologic emergencies (LeBoeuf & Pritchett, 2020).

Infusion-Related Reaction Management

Even mild reactions can progress quickly. According to the Allergy and Asthma Network (2025), anaphylaxis can cause death in less than 15 minutes if untreated. Nurses must be able to assess the subtleties of an impending reaction. This is particularly salient when, in the absence of other signs and symptoms, patients say, "Something does not feel right." Although the symptoms are vague and potentially easily dismissed, nurses must further evaluate any patients who display these early warning signs. Institutions should have a written policy and procedure in place for nurses to use when handling these emergencies. This type of policy is significant for office and clinic practices, which may have limited resources.

At the first sign of a reaction, nurses should stop the infusion and maintain IV patency (Barroso et al., 2024; Olsen et al., 2023). If the offending medication has been administered via the secondary set into another fluid (e.g., normal saline), nurses should stop infusion of that fluid to avoid infusing the rest of the offending medication remaining in the tubing. For this reason, it is preferable to connect normal saline to a Y-site closest to the patient or to another lumen of a multilumen catheter. Staff should ensure that emergency equipment is available, functional, and not expired, and they should be aware of its location (Olsen et al., 2023).

At this point, decisions need to be made regarding how to proceed. For patients clearly displaying overt signs of anaphylaxis, the standard procedure is to administer epinephrine first. However, nurses must carefully assess the situation to provide critical information to the responding physician or licensed independent practitioner. Assessment must include the medication that patients are or were receiving, what premedications (if any) were administered, and the onset of symptoms, noting both subjective and objective assessments. Assessment is crucial; epinephrine is not warranted for patients who are ambulatory with a small hive and no other symptoms, but it would be appropriate if the assessment demonstrates that multiple organ systems have been affected (e.g., respiratory distress, hypotension).

Depending on the assessment, nurses should then follow basic life support guidelines. Determining the oxygen saturation level is beneficial in assessing pulmonary status. Patients should be seated in the supine position during administration (Olsen et al., 2023). If they are having respiratory difficulty, they should be kept sitting up. If patients have hypotension, then they should be placed in the supine position and legs elevated if possible (Barroso et al., 2024; Olsen et al., 2023).

Additional assessment should include auscultation of lung sounds for the presence of wheezing or crackles and evaluation of level of consciousness. Patients should remain under continuous nursing observation until the determination of whether the reaction is life threatening (Olsen et al., 2023). Although no standardized practice for the frequency of vital signs exists for all agents, patients should be monitored as clinically indicated and according to institutional guidelines during an emergency event (Barroso et al., 2024; Olsen et al., 2023).

Depending on the degree and type of HSR, antihistamines, both H1 and H2 receptor antagonists, may be given along with a corticosteroid such as hydrocortisone. Most nurses are familiar and comfortable with the administration of H1 and H2 receptor antagonists, as the use of IV diphenhydramine has become ubiquitous. However, it is important to remember that histamine receptor antagonists cannot stop the physiologic process responsible for an HSR and that other interventions may be warranted. Hospitals may develop their own protocols or adopt those established by professional organizations (Barroso et al., 2024). IV hydration may be ordered, particularly in cases of hypotension. If respiratory distress is present, bronchodilators may be given, and supportive measures should be available for immediate use, including supplemental oxygen, suction equipment, and an oximeter.

For HSRs occurring in the outpatient setting, admission to the hospital for 24-hour observation may be required until patients have completely stabilized (Barosso et al., 2024). Careful monitoring during the postreaction period is crucial, as anaphylaxis may suddenly recur if the epinephrine wears off before the offending agent has been eliminated from circulation. Depending on the drug and severity of the reaction, it may be possible to restart the infusion at a slower rate after administering corticosteroids and H1 and H2 receptor antagonists.

Regardless of the type or severity of a reaction, nurses should meticulously document the event per institution guidelines. Best practices include documenting when the reaction began; signs and symptoms; initial interventions, such as stopping the infusion and notifying the physician; measures to support airway, breathing, and circulation; vital signs, including oxygen saturation; additional interventions, such as oxygen and medication administration; patient monitoring; resolution of symptoms; and admission to the hospital or transfer to another inpatient unit. Some electronic health record systems allow for the creation of a specialized infusion-related reaction note, which is stored in a separate electronic folder within the record. This feature enables nurses caring for new patients to quickly see if they have had an HSR to a drug and what interventions were taken without having to read through every note to find a previous reaction.

Patient and Caregiver Education

Prior to the infusion, nurses must educate patients and caregivers regarding potential adverse reactions. This preemptive education may be key in helping patients identify early signs and symptoms of an evolving reaction. They should understand that reactions can occur during and after the infusion. Accordingly, specific nursing processes should be in place for providing written postinfusion educational materials to outpatients, including symptoms to watch for and telephone numbers to call if symptoms return. All patient education should be appropriately documented in the medical record. In addition to assisting other clinicians regarding what information patients are given, failure to include thorough documentation may have legal ramifications if a serious event occurs (Olsen et al., 2023).

Nurses should be aware that patients and caregivers may experience anxiety related to infusion-related reactions or nonhemolytic transfusion reactions (e.g., fever, chills, hives) (Barasso et al., 2024). The same drug may be continued at a lower dose, or existing premedication may be given at an increased dose, and new medications may be added. In these situations, patients may be reluctant to receive a second dose when the traumatic memory of the first dose still lingers. When premedication fails to prevent an HSR, rapid drug desensitization may be initiated to allow patients to proceed with the desired therapy (Price, 2024). Desensitization has been shown to be incredibly effective at limiting further HSRs (Villarreal-González, 2023). Nurses should explain to patients undergoing desensitization the basic concept of drug tolerance and the rationale for the procedure and reassure them that they will be closely monitored throughout the process. Providing information and emotional support can help decrease the fear and anxiety surrounding the desensitization procedure. Nurses need to be aware of the emotional effects that an HSR has on patients.

In the event of an HSR, nurses should facilitate an open dialogue between patients, caregivers, and medical providers regarding the plan for continued therapy. The type and severity of the HSR will dictate whether the treatment plan can be continued or will need to be modified.

Several drugs used in oncology can produce a wide range of reactions. Specific drug information, types of adverse effects (including HSRs), and percentage of HSR in patients can be found on the prescribing package insert or on the specific drug website.

Summary

Many of the therapies used for cancer treatment and supportive care can produce life-threatening infusion-related reactions or pose a serious risk of morbidity. Nurses caring for patients with cancer must be familiar with risk factors, prevention strategies, etiology, and treatment options to facilitate safe infusions of chemotherapy, biotherapy, and blood products. They also must be alert to the signs and symptoms of infusion-related reactions and ensure that patients and caregivers receive the requisite information about potential reactions and understand the importance of alerting the healthcare team to the presence of symptoms.

The authors would like to acknowledge Seth Eisenberg, RN, ADN, OCN®, BMTCN®, for his contribution to this chapter that remains unchanged from the previous edition of this book.

References

Ali, S., Nedelcu, D.-M., Serescu, R., & Bumbacea, R.S. (2024). Successful desensitization to irinotecan in a patient with metastatic esophageal squamous cell carcinoma and a history of anaphylaxis in response to irinotecan: Case report and literature review. *Journal of Clinical Medicine, 13*(24), 7824. https://doi.org/10.3390/jcm13247824

Allergy and Asthma Network. (2025). *Anaphylaxis.* https://allergyasthmanetwork.org/anaphylaxis

AlMuhizi, F., De Las Vecillas Sanchez, L., Gilbert, L., Copaescu, A.M., & Isabwe, G.A.C. (2022). Premedication protocols to prevent hypersensitivity reactions to chemotherapy: A literature review. *Clinical Reviews in Allergy and Immunology, 62*(3), 534–547. https://doi.org/10.1007/s12016-022-08932-2

AlMuhizi, F., Ton-Leclerc, S., Fein, M., Tsoukas, C., Garvey, L.H., Lee, D., ... Copaescu, A.M. (2022). Successful desensitization to mRNA COVID-19 vaccine in a case series of patients with a history of anaphylaxis to the first vaccine dose. *Frontiers in Allergy, 3.* https://doi.org/10.3389/falgy.2022.825164

Asero, R. (2025). New-onset urticaria (hives). In Z. Hussain & A.M. Feldweg (Eds.), *UpToDate.* Retrieved April 23, 2025, from https://www.uptodate.com/new-onset-urticara-hives

Barrett, C., Park, S.J., Edmondson, L., & Monga, D. (2022). Incidence of hypersensitivity reactions in patients with H1-receptor antagonists receiving oxaliplatin-based chemotherapy. *Journal of Oncology Pharmacy Practice, 28*(3), 577–581. https://doi.org/10.1177/10781552211003958

Barroso, A., Estevinho, F., Hespanhol, V., Teixeira, E., Ramalho-Carvalho, J., & Araújo, A. (2024). Management of infusion-related reactions in cancer therapy: Strategies and challenges. *ESMO Open, 9*(3), 102922. https://doi.org/10.1016/j.esmoop.2024.102922

Bernstein, J.A., Bernstein, J.S., Makol, R., & Ward, S. (2024). Allergic rhinitis: A review. *JAMA, 331*(10), 866–877. https://doi.org/10.1001/jama.2024.0530

Campbell, R.L., & Kelso, J.M. (2024). Anaphylaxis: Acute diagnosis. In A.M. Feldweg (Ed.), *UpToDate.* Retrieved April 23, 2025, from https://www.uptodate.com/contents/anaphylaxis-acute-diagnosis

Campbell, R.L., & Kelso, J.M. (2025). Anaphylaxis: Emergency treatment. In A.M. Feldweg & M. Ganetsky (Eds.), *UpToDate.* Retrieved September 29, 2025, from https://www.uptodate.com/contents/anaphylaxis-emergency-treatment

Castells, M.C., & Bankova, L. (2024). Mast cell-derived mediators. In A.M. Feldweg (Ed.), *UpToDate.* Retrieved April 23, 2025, from https://uptodate.com/contents/mast-cell-derived-mediators

Castells, M.C., & Dwyer, D.F. (2023). Mast cells: Development, identification and physiologic roles. In A.M. Feldweg (Ed.), *UpToDate.* Retrieved April 23, 2025, from https://www.uptodate.com/contents/mast-cells-development-identification-and-physiologic-roles

Castells, M.C., & Solensky, R. (2023). Rapid drug desensitization for immediate hypersensitivity reactions. In A.M. Feldweg (Ed.), *UpToDate.* Retrieved April 22, 2025, from https://www.uptodate.com/contents/rapid-drug-desensitization-for-immediate-hypersensitivity-reactions

Chichelo, L., & Colopoulos, K. (2025). Hypersensitivity infusion reaction management: A time sensitive solution to a common problem. *American Nurse Journal, 20*(1). https://doi.org/10.51256/ANJ012522

Cobb, D.A., & Lee, D.W. (2021). Cytokine release syndrome biology and management. *Cancer Journal, 27*(2), 119–125. https://doi.org/10.1097/PPO.0000000000000515

Corbett, M., Scullion, B., & Nesbitt, M. (2022). Implementation of an evidence-based hypersensitivity algorithm revision in an adult ambulatory oncology clinic. *Oncology Nursing Forum, 49*(2), E17. https://doi.org/10.1188/22.onf.e2

Cuartero, J.B., Gorriz, M.C.T., Coronado, C.I.S., Sanchez, A.G., Mendez, C.G.P., Ibanez, M.D.L., & Enrique, E. (2024). The increasing role of the allergist in the management of infusion reactions at the oncology infusion center. *Frontiers in Allergy, 5,* 1–10. https://doi.org/10.3389/falgy.2024.1479469

Davis, J.D., Padros, M.B., Conrado, D.J., Ganguly, S., Guan, X., Hassan, H.E., ... Zhu, M. (2024). Subcutaneous administration of monoclonal antibodies: Pharmacology, delivery, immunogenicity, and learnings from applications to clinical development. *Clinical Pharmacology and Therapeutics, 115*(3), 422–439. https://ascpt.onlinelibrary.wiley.com/doi/pdf/10.1002/cpt.3150

Demir, S., Erdenen, F., Gelincik, A., Unal, D., Olgac, M., Coskun, R., ... Buyukozturk, S. (2019). Evaluation of the potential risk factors for drug-induced anaphylaxis in adult patients. *International Archives of Allergy and Immunology, 178*(2), 167–176. https://doi.org/10.1159/000494130

Fajgenbaum, D.C., & June, C.H. (2020). Cytokine storm. *New England Journal of Medicine, 383*(23), 2255–2273. https://doi.org/10.1056/NEJMra2026131

Galateanu, B., Puscasu, A.I., Tircol, S.A., Tanase, B.C., Hudita, A., Negrei, C., ... Ginghina, O. (2023). Allergy in cancer care: Antineoplastic therapy-induced hypersensitivity reactions. *International Journal of Molecular Sciences, 24*(4), 3886. https://doi.org/10.3390/ijms24043886

Ghebrehiwet, B., Joseph, K., & Kaplan, A.P. (2024). The bradykinin-forming cascade in anaphylaxis and ACE-inhibitor induced angioedema/airway obstruction. *Frontiers in Allergy, 5,* 1302605. https://doi.org/10.3389/falgy.2024.1302605

Goodman, R.S., Johnson, D.B., & Balko, J.M. (2023). Corticosteroids and cancer immunotherapy. *Clinical Cancer Research, 29*(14), 2580–2587. https://doi.org/10.1158/1078-0432.CCR-22-3181

Hall, T.R., MacDonald, J.E., Bylinowski, K.M., Alvarez, E.A., Hardesty, M.M., & Smith, J.A. (2023). Management of chemotherapy hypersensitivity reactions and desensitization: An SGO clinical practice statement. *Gynecologic Oncology, 177,* 180–185. https://doi.org/10.1016/j.ygyno.2023.08.017

Horita, N., Miyagi, E., Mizushima, T., Hagihara, M., Hata, C., Hattori, Y., ... Kaneko, T. (2021). Severe anaphylaxis caused by intravenous anti-cancer drugs. *Cancer Medicine, 10*(20), 7174–7183. https://doi.org/10.1002/cam4.4252

Jao, M.E., Indorf, A.L., Segal, E.-M., Miske, A., Eaton, K.D., Marsolini, T., & Ghuman, S. (2024). Impact of institutional interventions on the rate of paclitaxel hypersensitivity reactions. *Journal of Oncology Pharmacy Practice, 30*(1), 105–111. https://doi.org/10.1177/10781552231168594

Kemp, S.F. (2024). Pathophysiology of anaphylaxis. In A.M. Feldweg (Ed.), *UpToDate.* Retrieved April 23, 2025, from https://www.uptodate.com/contents/pathophysiology-of-anaphylaxis

Kozubek, P., Kopeć, S., Drewko, K., Kuźniar, J., Orłowski, M., & Gomułka, K. (2024). Variety of allergic symptoms in the therapy of selected respiratory and autoimmune diseases. *Environmental Medicine/Medycyna Środowiskowa, 27*(3), 131–136. https://doi.org/10.26444/ms/190784

LeBoeuf, J., & Pritchett, W. (2020). Mock drills: Implementation for emergency scenarios in the outpatient setting. *Clinical Journal of Oncology Nursing, 24*(1), E7–E12. https://doi.org/10.1188/20.CJON.E7-E12

Liszewski, M.K, & Atkinson, J.P. (2024). Overview and clinical assessment of the complement system. In A.M. Feldweg (Ed.), *UpToDate.* Retrieved April 23, 2025, from https://www.uptodate.com/contents/overview-and-clinical-assessment-of-the-complement-system

McCloskey, C., Ortega, M.T., Nair, S., Garcia, M.J., & Manevy, F. (2023). A systematic review of time and resource use costs of subcutaneous versus intravenous administration of oncology biologics in a hospital setting. *PharmacoEconomics Open, 7*(1), 3–36. https://doi.org/10.1007/s41669-022-00361-3

National Cancer Institute Cancer Therapy Evaluation Program. (2017). *Common Terminology Criteria for Adverse Events* [v.5.0]. https://dctd.cancer.gov/research/ctep-trials/for-sites/adverse-events/ctcae-v5-5x7.pdf

Olsen, M.M., LeFebvre, K.B., Walker, S.L., & Dunphy, E.P. (Eds.). (2023). *Chemotherapy and immunotherapy guidelines and recommendations for practice* (2nd ed.). Oncology Nursing Society.

Olsen, M.M., & Walton, A.M.L. (2024). *Safe handling of hazardous drugs* (4th ed.). Oncology Nursing Society.

Plaut, M. (1979). Histamine, H1 and H2 antihistamines, and immediate hypersensitivity reactions. *Journal of Allergy Clinical Immunology, 63*(6), 371–375. https://doi.org/10.1016/0091-6749(79)90208-2

Popa, C.-M., Ianoşi, S.L., & Săftoiu, A. (2021). Cutaneous toxicity in oncologic patients receiving epidermal growth factor receptor inhibitors. *Current Health Sciences Journal, 47*(4), 516–522. https://doi.org/10.12865/CHSJ.47.04.06

Porter, D.L., & Maloney, D.G. (2024). Cytokine release syndrome (CRS). In A.G. Rosmarin (Ed.), *UpToDate.* Retrieved April 23, 2025, from https://www.uptodate.com/contents/cytokine-release-syndrome-crs

Portz, D., & Froggatt, N. (2022). Moving out: Oncology nurses transition chemotherapy desensitization out of the intensive care unit. *Oncology Nursing Forum, 49*(2), E39–E40. https://doi.org/10.1188/22.onf.e2

Price, M. (2021). Acute infusion-related reactions: How to recognize and intervene when these reactions occur in practice. *Clinical Journal of Oncology Nursing, 25*(5), 591–594. https://doi.org/10.1188/21.cjon.591-594

Price, M. (2024). Drug reactions and desensitization to chemotherapeutic agents: An overview and case study. *Clinical Journal of Oncology Nursing, 28*(4), 360–365. https://doi.org/10.1188/24.cjon.360–365

Schwartz, L.B. (2024). Laboratory tests to support the clinical diagnosis of anaphylaxis. In A.M. Feldweg (Ed.), *UpToDate.* Retrieved April 23, 2025, from https://www.uptodate.com/contents/laboratory-tests-to-support-the-clinical-diagnosis-of-anaphylaxis

Seghers, S., Teuwen, L.-A., Beyens, M., De Blick, D., Sabato, V., Ebo, D.G., & Prenen, H. (2023). Immediate hypersensitivity reactions to antineoplastic agents – A practical guide for the oncologist. *Cancer Treatment Reviews, 116,* 102559. https://doi.org/10.1016/j.ctrv.2023.102559

Silver, J., Garcia-Neuer, M., Lynch, D.-M., Pasaoglu, G., Sloane, D.E., & Castells, M. (2020). Endophenotyping oxaliplatin hypersensitivity: Personalizing desensitization to the atypical platin. *Journal of Allergy and Clinical Immunology in Practice, 8*(5), 1668–1680. https://doi.org/10.1016/j.jaip.2020.02.013

Tsao, L.R., Young, F.D., Otani, I.M., & Castells, M.C. (2022). Hypersensitivity reactions to platinum agents and taxanes. *Clinical Reviews in Allergy and Immunology, 62*(3), 432–448. https:/doi.org/10.1007/s12016-021-08877-y

Villarreal-González, R.V., González-Diaz, S., Vidal-Gutiérrez, O., de la Cruz-de la Cruz, C., Pérez-Ibave, D.C., & Garza-Rodríguez, M.L. (2023). Hypersensitivity reactions to anticancer chemotherapy and monoclonal antibodies: Safety and efficacy of desensitization. *Journal of Oncology Pharmacy Practice, 30*(5), 811–822. https://doi.org/10.1177/10781552231189461

Zhu, L., Li, H., Du, Q., Ye, X., Yu, S., Luo, X., & Zhai, Q. (2021). Meta-analysis of risk factors associated with oxaliplatin hypersensitivity reactions in cancer patients. *International Journal of Clinical Oncology, 26*(12), 2194–2204. https://doi.org/10.1007/s10147-021-02034-3

Zwimpfer, T.A., Scherer, K., Schötzau, A., Heinzelmann-Schwarz, V., Hartmann, K., Vetter, M., & Montavon, C. (2023). Desensitization in patients with hypersensitivity to platinum and taxane in gynecological cancers. *Cancer Medicine, 13*(1), e6840. https://doi.org/10.1002/cam4.6840

Vivian Huang, MS, RN, CNS, AGCNS-BC, OCN®, TCTCN™,
and Whitney Houser, MSN, RN, OCN®

CHAPTER 17

Immune-Related Adverse Events

FAST FACTS

- **Description:** Immune checkpoint inhibitors have revolutionized cancer treatment. However, they come with a unique adverse effect profile compared to traditional chemotherapy, necessitating different management strategies. Immune checkpoint inhibitors enhance the immune system's ability to attack cancer cells, which can lead to an overactive immune response and damage to healthy tissues.
- **Incidence:** Up to 90% of patients undergoing immune checkpoint inhibitor therapy experience immune-related adverse events, with severe toxicities leading to hospitalization or death in approximately 30% of cases.
- **Clinical Manifestations:** Compared to adverse events from traditional cytotoxic chemotherapy, immune-related adverse events typically have a later onset and an inflammatory or autoimmune picture. Driven by the inflammatory response, immune-related adverse events can present with a wide range of symptoms affecting different organ systems, requiring a thorough patient history and awareness for early recognition.
- **Risk Factors and Etiology:** Immune-related adverse event risk and severity are affected by the type and dose of immune checkpoint inhibitor therapy, underlying medical conditions, genetic predisposition, and other factors.
- **Pathophysiology and Patient Evaluation:** Immune-related adverse events are driven by immune system overactivation caused by immune checkpoint inhibitors disrupting immune system regulation. They should be considered in the differential during or after immune checkpoint inhibitor therapy. Diagnosis can be complex because of the unpredictable nature and similarity of immune-related adverse events to other disease processes, necessitating a comprehensive diagnostic approach. Testing includes bloodwork and imaging of symptomatic areas.
- **Advanced Practice Considerations:** Frontline providers may implement diagnostic and treatment protocols for immune-related adverse events based on severity. Collaboration with oncologists, nurses, and specialists on the care team ensures prompt and effective patient management.
- **Treatment Modalities:** Treatment of immune-related adverse events involves close monitoring, corticosteroids, and other localized therapies. Institutional or society guidelines should be followed for grading and managing symptoms. Dose reduction, interruption, or discontinuation of immune checkpoint inhibitor therapy may be indicated.
- **Nursing Management:** Nurses play a critical role in early recognition of immune-related adverse events, patient education, supportive care, and symptom management.

- **Outcomes:** Mitigation of immune-related adverse events and continuation of immune checkpoint inhibitor therapy for oncologic treatment are the goals. As immune-related adverse events are common, prevention may not be possible. Still, early recognition and intervention are key to moderating the severity of immune-related adverse events and preventing lasting toxicity.

Introduction

The use of immune checkpoint inhibitors (ICIs) has become a rapidly expanding cornerstone in the treatment of numerous cancers, including both solid tumors and blood cancers. In 2019, 40% of patients with cancer in the United States were eligible for ICI therapy (Haslam et al., 2020). ICIs, as with other immunotherapies, have a significantly different adverse effect profile compared to traditional cytotoxic chemotherapy.

Immune-related adverse events (irAEs) are a complex set of side effects that can occur in patients receiving immunotherapy, primarily with ICI therapy. These events arise from an overactive immune response, which can lead to damage to healthy tissues, particularly in the internal organs. The presence of irAEs has been linked to improved overall response and survival in some patients.

Adoptive T cells and bispecific T-cell engager antibodies have different mechanisms of action and thus different side effect profiles than more traditional irAEs, such as cytokine release syndrome and immune effector cell–associated neurotoxicity syndrome. More information on these immunotherapies and their unique adverse effects, as well as nonemergent irAEs, can be found in the Oncology Nursing Society publication *Guide to Cancer Immunotherapy* (second edition) and its joint efforts with Elsevier, *Core Curriculum for Oncology Nursing* (seventh edition).

Although immunotherapy has revolutionized cancer treatment, understanding and managing irAEs is essential for optimizing patient outcomes and minimizing morbidity. Most irAEs can be managed effectively with high-dose corticosteroids. Prompt recognition and treatment are crucial to mitigate the severity of these adverse events.

Incidence

The incidence of irAEs varies depending on the specific immunotherapy agent and the underlying cancer type, as well as the patient's individual immune response. The overall incidence is high, with up to 90% of patients undergoing ICI therapy experiencing some degree of irAEs. Severe toxicities requiring hospitalization or leading to death occur in approximately 30% of cases (Gould Rothberg et al., 2022).

Most often, irAEs affect the dermatologic, gastrointestinal, hepatic, endocrine, or respiratory systems; however, they can impact any organ. Common emergent irAEs are colitis, hypophysitis, pneumonitis, nephritis, diabetes, uveitis, myocarditis, and encephalitis (Cooksley et al., 2020; Dougan et al., 2020; Shannon et al., 2020) (see Table 17-1). The incidence of these irAEs often peaks within the first three to

TABLE 17-1
Incidence of the Most Common Emergent Immune-Related Adverse Events

Immune-Related Adverse Event	Incidence			
	Overall	Anti–Programmed Cell Death Ligand 1 ICI	Anti–Cytotoxic T-Lymphocyte Antigen 4 ICI	Combination ICIs
Colitis	8%–27%	1% (1% grade ≥ 3)	8% (5% grade ≥ 3)	16% (11% grade ≥ 3)
Hypophysitis	1%–10%	1% (0% grade ≥ 3)	4% (2% grade ≥ 3)	10%
Nephritis	2%–5%	2%	2%	4.5%
Pneumonitis	3%–5%	4% (1% grade ≥ 3)	1% (1% grade ≥ 3)	7% (2% grade ≥ 3)

ICI—immune checkpoint inhibitor

Note. Based on information from Cooksley et al., 2020; Dougan et al., 2020; Shannon et al., 2020.

four months of treatment, but they can manifest earlier or later, even after therapy has concluded.

Clinical Manifestations

Clinicians in the emergency department and acute care clinic settings receive patients presenting with a myriad of potential irAE symptoms. An awareness and knowledge of this class of events based on patient history is critical for early recognition. The pharmacodynamics and pharmacokinetics of ICIs are distinct from those of traditional cytotoxic chemotherapy, and thus have different toxicity profiles, a later onset, and generally an inflammatory or autoimmune picture. Although patients may have atypical presentation or absence of classic symptoms, nurses should know the common signs and symptoms of emergent irAEs (see Table 17-2).

Onset may be delayed by months or years, and duration may be prolonged. An irAE may also occur or recur months after discontinuation of immunotherapy. All irAEs should be considered in the differential, even if ICI therapy ended over 12 months prior.

Multiple professional organizations, such as the National Comprehensive Cancer Network (NCCN), American Society of Clinical Oncology, Society for Immunotherapy of Cancer, Multinational Association of Supportive Care in Cancer, and European Society for Medical Oncology, have published clinical guidelines for ICI-related irAEs. Adverse events, including irAEs, are graded according to a standard scale of severity, such as the National Cancer Institute (NCI) Cancer Therapy Evaluation Program publication *Common Terminology Criteria for Adverse Events.* Institutional standards or protocols should be followed in regard to which version of this documentation should be used. Figure 17-1 details the Society for Immunotherapy of Cancer terminology and definitions used to categorize irAEs for management.

TABLE 17-2
Emergent Immune-Related Adverse Event Manifestations and Assessments

Adverse Event	Common Manifestations	Assessment
Colitis	Watery diarrhea, abdominal pain, abdominal cramping, mucus or blood in stool, fever	Abdominal tenderness, abdominal distension, guarding, rigidity, rebound tenderness, watery stool
Hypophysitis	Fatigue, headache, nausea, vomiting, weakness, photophobia, gonadotrophic deficiency (loss of libido, erectile dysfunction), secondary adrenal insufficiency (nausea, loss of appetite, weight loss, light-headedness, hypoglycemia, hypotension)	Hormone levels, imaging studies (e.g., thyroid ultrasound)
Diabetes	New or worsening diabetes mellitus, hyperglycemia, diabetic ketoacidosis, polyuria, polydipsia, general weakness, vomiting, confusion, abdominal pain, dry skin, dry mouth, tachycardia, fruity odor on the breath, fatigue, blurred vision	Blood glucose, ketones
Encephalitis	Confusion, altered behavior, agitation, fatigue, headache, tremors, seizures, short-term memory loss, depressed level of consciousness, focal weakness, speech abnormality, difficulty swallowing, respiratory compromise	Neurologic examination
Nephritis	Oliguria, edema, anuria, electrolyte disorders	Urinalysis, renal function, electrolytes
Pneumonitis	Dyspnea, new or worsening cough, hypoxia, chest pain, tachypnea, cyanosis, fatigue, general weakness, fever	Lung sounds (e.g., crackles, loss of adventitious sounds, egophony, dullness to percussion) Decrease in oxygen saturation
Uveitis	Eye pain, floaters, photophobia, blurry vision, conjunctival redness, eyelid swelling	Ocular assessment
Myocarditis	Chest pain, dyspnea, arrhythmia, fatigue, syncope, generalized weakness	Electrocardiogram

Note. Based on information from Schneider et al., 2021; Suarez-Almazor et al., 2020.

FIGURE 17-1. Consensus Definitions for Immune-Related Adverse Event Terminology

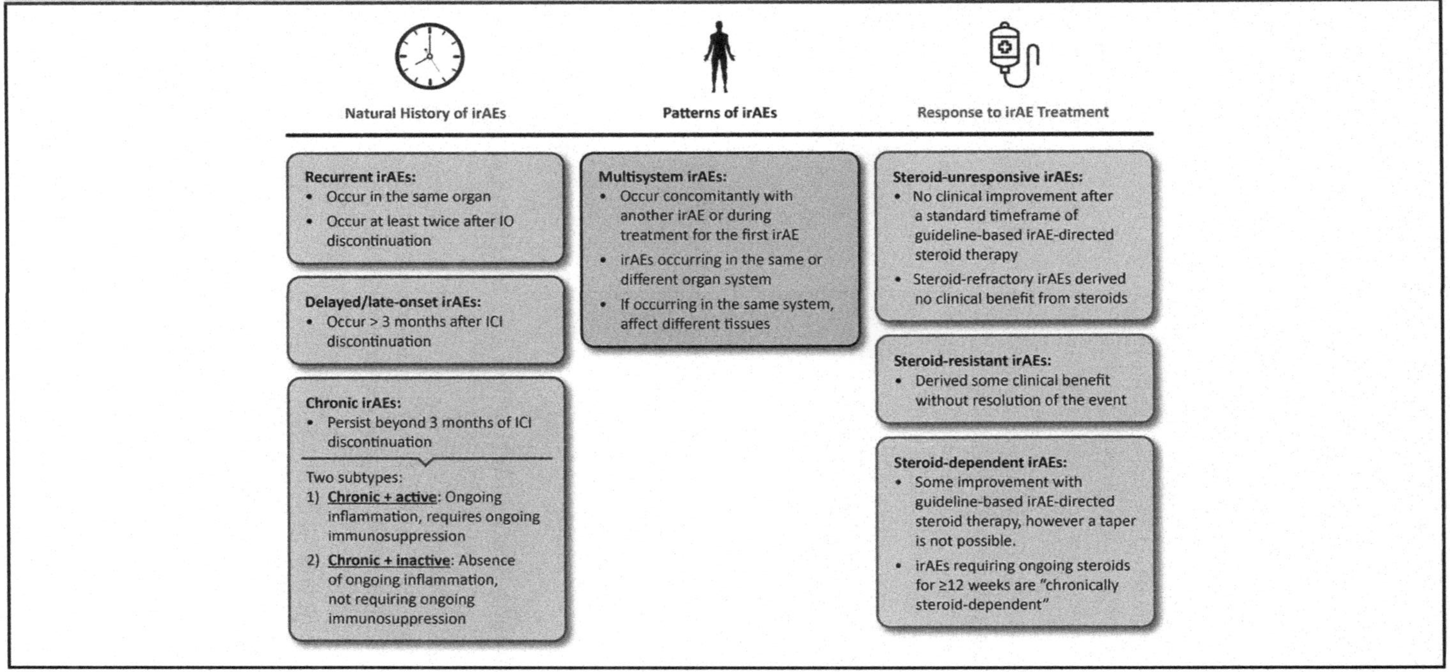

ICI—immune checkpoint inhibitor; IO—immuno-oncology; irAE—immune-related adverse event

Note. From "Society for Immunotherapy of Cancer (SITC) Consensus Definitions for Immune Checkpoint Inhibitor-Associated Immune-Related Adverse Events (irAEs) Terminology," by J. Naidoo, C. Murphy, M.B. Atkins, J.R. Brahmer, S. Champiat, D. Feltquate, ... L.C. Cappelli, 2023, *Journal for Immunotherapy of Cancer, 11*(3), p 2. (https://doi.org/10.1136/jitc-2022-006398). Licensed under CC BY-NC-ND 4.0 (https://creativecommons.org/licenses/by-nc-nd/4.0).

Risk Factors and Etiology

The following factors can affect the risk of developing irAEs by amplifying immune activation, lowering the threshold for autoimmunity, disrupting immune tolerance, or creating tissue environments more susceptible to immune-mediated damage (Arnaud-Coffin et al., 2019; Haslam et al., 2020; Naidoo et al., 2023; Raschi et al., 2020):

- Immunotherapy regimen (class and dose)
  - Higher incidence and severity with anti–cytotoxic T-lymphocyte antigen 4 compared to anti–programmed cell death-ligand 1
    * Anti–programmed cell death-ligand 1 ICI = 74% (14% grade ≥ 3)
    * Anti–cytotoxic T-lymphocyte antigen 4 ICI = 89% (34% grade ≥ 3)
  - Higher incidence, severity, and onset with combinations: combination ICIs = 90% (55% grade ≥ 3)
- Underlying medical conditions (e.g., autoimmune disorders, inflammatory conditions)
- Organ-specific immune checkpoint expression (e.g., cytotoxic T-lymphocyte antigen 4 on pituitary tissues, programmed cell death-ligand 1 in renal epithelium)
- Concomitant medications (e.g., nonsteroidal anti-inflammatory drug use associated with an increase in enterocolitis, corticosteroids)
- Tumor mutational burden
- Genetic predisposition
- Gut microbiota composition
- Presence of thymic tumors
- Elevated body mass index
- Specific human leukocyte antigen genotypes
- Cytokine level abnormalities (e.g., interleukin-6, interleukin-17)

Pathophysiology and Patient Evaluation

Immune System Activation and Mechanism of Action

An irAE is a common toxicity caused by ICIs and driven by the inflammatory response in one or more organ systems. ICIs are a subclass of monoclonal antibodies, which are a further subclass of antineoplastic agents that interfere with oncogenesis pathways. As one of the hallmarks of cancer is evasion of the immune system, ICIs treat cancer by enhancing the immune system's ability to recognize and preferentially attack cancer cells. This activation of the immune system causes these irAEs (Gould Rothberg et al., 2022) (see Figure 17-2).

Immune checkpoints are natural regulatory mechanisms that help to maintain a balanced immune response. They regulate the immune system and prevent overactivity from causing damage to healthy tissues. Cancer cells can exploit these checkpoints to evade detection and destruction by the immune system (Choi & Lee, 2020; NCI, 2022; Schneider et al., 2021).

By targeting specific immune checkpoints, ICIs can stimulate a stronger antitumor response. Some tumor cells present checkpoint proteins that engage immune

FIGURE 17-2. Mechanisms of Targeted Therapeutic Toxicities

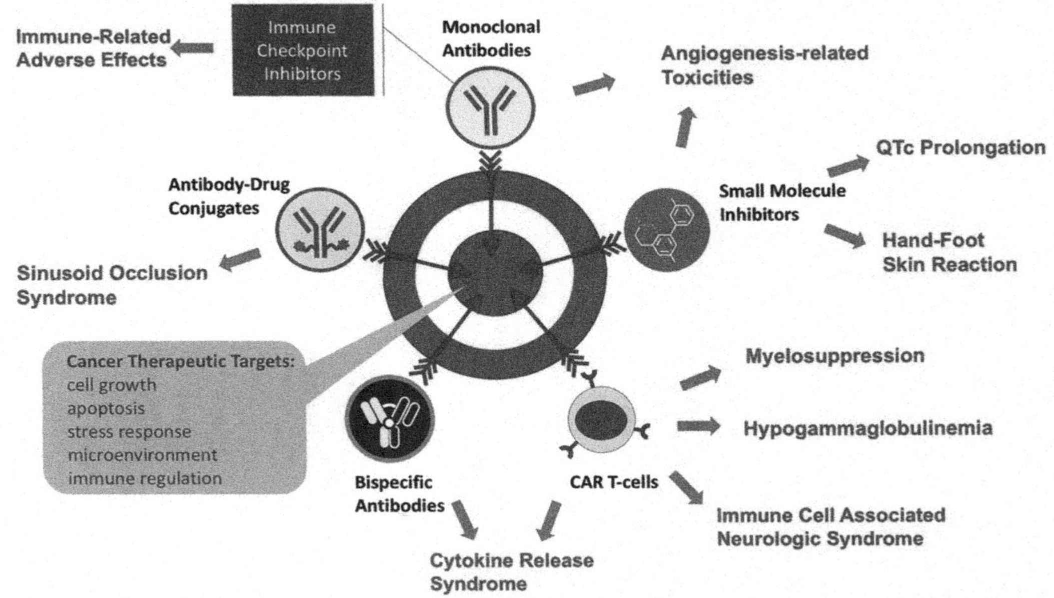

Targeted therapies can be subdivided into small molecules, cell-based therapies (e.g., chimeric antigen receptor [CAR] T-cells), and antibody-based therapies, with the latter including the specific subclasses of antibody-drug conjugates and immune checkpoint inhibitors. Although some toxicities, such as immune-related adverse events, QTc prolongation, and sinusoidal occlusion syndrome, are class-specific, angiogenesis-related toxicities and cytokine release syndrome are demonstrated with multiple classes.

Note. From "Oncologic Emergencies and Urgencies: A Comprehensive Review," by B.E. Gould Rothberg, T.E. Quest, S.J. Yeung, L.C. Pelosof, D.E. Gerber, J.A. Seltzer, ... D.N. Kyriacou, 2022, *CA: A Cancer Journal for Clinicians, 72*(6), p. 582. (https://doi.org/10.3322/caac.21727). Licensed under CC BY-NC-ND 4.0 (https://creativecommons.org/licenses/by-nc-nd/4.0).

checkpoints on T cells, thereby turning off the immune response. ICIs block these tumor proteins from binding at T-cell checkpoints, reactivating the T cell to mount an appropriate immune response and kill the cancer cell (NCI, 2022).

Examples of immune checkpoint targets and their associated inhibitors include the following (Cooksley et al., 2020; Dougan et al., 2020; Shannon et al., 2020):

- Cytotoxic T-lymphocyte antigen 4: ipilimumab, tremelimumab
- Programmed cell death-ligand 1: atezolizumab, avelumab, durvalumab
- Programmed cell death protein 1: cemiplimab, nivolumab, pembrolizumab, toripalimab
- Lymphocyte-activation gene 3: relatimab

Additional agents may be approved or under investigation.

This heightened immune activity often leads to irAEs in different organs, ranging from mild to severe. Although irAEs are potentially dangerous side effects, they also serve as a biomarker of treatment response. The presence of irAEs has been linked to improved treatment response and overall survival (Fan et al., 2021).

The exact mechanisms driving irAEs are not fully understood. However, it is believed that ICIs disrupt the regulation of the immune system, and irAEs are primarily caused by the activation of the immune system against self-antigens. This can lead to a variety of immune-mediated inflammatory responses, such as the following (Naidoo et al., 2023):

- Cytotoxic T lymphocyte–associated cytotoxicity
  - Self-reactive T cell escapes from central tolerance.
  - T-cell overactivation attacks healthy organs.
- Humoral immunity
  - Autoantibody production puts targets on specific organs.
  - Cross-reactivity mistakenly targets healthy tissues that share similarities with tumor antigens.
  - Epitope spreading broadens the immune response to target additional self-antigens.
- Inflammation: T-cell activation increases cytokines in healthy tissue.

Patient Evaluation

An irAE can be challenging to diagnose because of its ability to affect any tissue or organ system. Inflammation caused by immunotherapy can be unpredictable, making symptom prediction, monitoring, and precise diagnosis complex. Additionally, many inflammatory symptoms mimic other disease processes, leading to diagnostic uncertainty, particularly for nurses who may be less experienced with oncology or ICI therapies (Gerber et al., 2024).

The diagnostic approach for irAEs varies depending on the organ or tissue involved. A general infection workup should always be considered as part of the evaluation.

Advanced Practice Considerations

Advanced practice providers are key contributors to the diagnosis, management, and long-term monitoring of patients experiencing irAEs. Their expertise in recognizing subtle or atypical symptoms is vital for early identification of irAEs, particularly in settings where oncologists may not be immediately available.

The diagnostic approach should include a tailored system-specific evaluation to confirm irAE diagnosis and rule out infections or other underlying conditions (Choi & Lee, 2020):

- Laboratory assessments: complete blood count, electrolyte panels, and other organ-specific biomarkers
- Imaging: targeted imaging studies based on suspected organ involvement (e.g., abdominal computed tomography scan for gastrointestinal symptoms)
- Specialized tests: stool analysis for colitis and diarrhea, or other tests relevant to the affected system

More information regarding diagnostics appears in the Treatment Modalities section of this chapter.

The combination of symptoms, diagnostic findings, and severity (graded based on established guidelines) will steer the development of the care plan. This plan may include additional diagnostic evaluations, specialty consultations, treatment interventions, and considerations for the future use of ICI therapy.

Acute or chronic implications of irAEs must also be factored into the long-term management strategy. Advanced practice providers are uniquely positioned to assist patients with ongoing care after irAE resolution, including regular follow-up to monitor for recurrence or residual organ dysfunction, continued shared decision-making regarding treatment options, and reinforcement of patient education.

Treatment Modalities

General Systemic Toxicity Treatment Guidelines

For general systemic toxicity related to ICIs, all new symptoms should be assumed to be treatment related. Management includes close monitoring for grade 1 toxicities and escalating interventions, such as holding ICIs, initiating corticosteroids, and possibly using biologic agents for grade 2–4 toxicities. Grade 5 indicates death. Permanent discontinuation is recommended for most grade 4 toxicities except endocrinopathies managed with hormone replacement (see Table 17-3).

Some irAEs are considered oncologic emergencies because they can develop rapidly and lead to life-threatening organ damage or failure if not promptly recognized and treated. These events, such as colitis, hypophysitis, diabetes mellitus, encephalitis, nephritis, pneumonitis, uveitis, and myocarditis, can escalate quickly, leading to critical organ dysfunction or failure if not identified and managed without delay.

Specific Systemic Toxicity Diagnosis and Treatment Guidelines

Table 17-4 details the diagnostic and treatment guidelines for the adverse events described in this section.

TABLE 17-3
General Systemic Toxicity Treatment Guidelines

	Grade 1	Grade 2	Grade 3	Grade 4
Diagnostics	Monitor closely, except for cardiac, hematologic, and neurologic toxicities.	Consider holding the immune checkpoint inhibitor. Resume when symptoms or diagnostics return < grade 1. Consider low-dose corticosteroids (0.5–1 mg/kg).	Hold the immune checkpoint inhibitor. Initiate high-dose corticosteroids (1–2 mg/kg). Taper within 4–6 weeks. If no improvement is seen with high-dose steroids, consider biologic agents. Consider rechallenging with caution when symptoms or diagnostics return to < grade 1. Consider inpatient admission.	Discontinue permanently (except endocrinopathies monitored with hormone replacement). Inpatient admission is likely.

The *Common Terminology Criteria for Adverse Events* 1–4 grading scale is shown. Grade 5 is often used in diagnostic and treatment guidelines and represents death. Grade 5 was omitted intentionally.

Note. Based on information from National Cancer Institute Cancer Therapy Evaluation Program, 2017; National Comprehensive Cancer Network, 2025; Schneider et al., 2021.

TABLE 17-4
Immune-Related Adverse Event Diagnostic and Treatment Guidelines

	Grade 1	Grade 2	Grade 3	Grade 4
Colitis				
Description	< 4 bowel movements above baseline, no colitis symptoms	4–6 bowel movements above baseline Colitis symptoms present but ADLs unaffected	> 6 bowel movements above baseline, colitis symptoms, interference with ADLs, hemodynamic instability, hospitalization, serious conditions (e.g., megacolon, ischemic bowel, perforation)	
Diagnostics	Evaluate stool for *Clostridium difficile* (c-diff), nucleic acid amplification tests, bacteria, viruses, para/ovasites, and lactoferrin/calprotectin. If fecal lactoferrin/calprotectin test is positive, perform grade 2 diagnostics.	Complete all diagnostic recommendations for irAE-related colitis grade 1 and obtain a computed tomography scan of the abdomen and pelvis with contrast. Initiate referral to gastroenterology for advanced management and colonoscopy or endoscopy with biopsies. This should be performed within 2 weeks with a positive fecal lactoferrin /calprotectin.	Complete all diagnostic recommendations for irAE-related grade 1–2 colitis.	

(Continued on next page)

TABLE 17-4

Immune-Related Adverse Event Diagnostic and Treatment Guidelines *(Continued)*

	Grade 1	Grade 2	Grade 3	Grade 4
Colitis *(Cont.)*				
Treatment	Consider holding ICI. Closely monitor, with check-ins every 3 days. For hydration, consider symptom management medications after infection has been ruled out, with caution to avoid masking of symptoms; discontinue if diarrhea persists. Dietary modifications include lactose-free, low-fiber, and BRAT (bananas, rice, apple sauce, toast) diets. If the lactoferrin/calprotectin test is positive, treat as grade 2. If this test is negative, add mesalamine or cholestyramine as needed.	Hold ICI. For pathologically confirmed colitis, consider budesonide 9 mg/day prior to systemic steroids. Initiate oral corticosteroids 1–2 mg/kg/day until symptoms ≤ grade 1. If no response to oral corticosteroids, consider IV corticosteroids. If no symptom improvement is seen after 72 hours of corticosteroids, consider biologic agents (e.g., infliximab, vedolizumab). If endoscopy shows significant ulceration or extensive nonsignificant inflammation, consider adding infliximab or vedolizumab. Consider tofacitinib or ustekinumab for infliximab/vedolizumab-refractory colitis.	Discontinue ICI therapy and admit to inpatient setting for management of dehydration and/or electrolyte imbalances. Initiate IV methylprednisolone 1–2 mg/kg/day. If no response after 1–2 days or unable to transition to oral steroids, add additional immunosuppression. If no symptom improvement after 72 hours of corticosteroids, consider biologic agents (e.g., infliximab, vedolizumab). If endoscopy shows significant ulceration or extensive nonsignificant inflammation, consider adding infliximab or vedolizumab. Consider tofacitinib or ustekinumab for infliximab/vedolizumab-refractory colitis.	

(Continued on next page)

TABLE 17-4
Immune-Related Adverse Event Diagnostic and Treatment Guidelines *(Continued)*

	Grade 1	Grade 2	Grade 3	Grade 4
Colitis *(Cont.)*				
Treatment *(Cont.)*		For persistent diarrhea that does not resolve, consider other etiologies (e.g., pancreatic disorder, exocrine insufficiency, celiac disease).		
Rechallenge considerations	Permanently discontinue for serious, life-threatening colitis symptoms. If the patient cannot taper off steroids, ICI may be resumed if the patient is ≤ 10 mg prednisone/day (or equivalent). Consider concurrent vedolizumab.	Consider resuming ICI after symptoms are < grade 1. Permanently discontinue for serious, life-threatening colitis symptoms. If the patient cannot taper off steroids, ICI may be resumed if the patient is ≤ 10 mg prednisone/day (or equivalent). Consider concurrent vedolizumab.	If combination ICI was used, consider monotherapy with anti–programmed cell death-ligand 1 ICI or anti–programmed cell death protein 1 ICI. Permanently discontinue for serious, life-threatening colitis symptoms. If the patient cannot taper off steroids, ICI may be resumed if the patient is ≤ 10 mg prednisone/day (or equivalent). Consider concurrent vedolizumab.	Permanently discontinue for serious, life-threatening colitis symptoms. If the patient cannot taper off steroids, ICI may be resumed if the patient is ≤ 10 mg prednisone/day (or equivalent). Consider concurrent vedolizumab.

(Continued on next page)

TABLE 17-4
Immune-Related Adverse Event Diagnostic and Treatment Guidelines *(Continued)*

	Grade 1	Grade 2	Grade 3	Grade 4
Hypophysitis				
Description	Asymptomatic, mild symptoms	Moderate symptoms, able to perform ADLs	Severe symptoms, life-threatening consequences, unable to perform ADLs	
Diagnostics	Refer to endocrinology for further evaluation and management. Evaluate morning ACTH, morning cortisol, thyroid-stimulating hormone, Free T4, complete metabolic panel, and sex hormones. Morning ACTH and cortisol levels should be evaluated in accordance with institutional policies or procedures. Consider ACTH stimulation testing. Consider MRI of the brain with or without contrast.			
Treatment	Consider holding ICI. Consider initiating corticosteroid replacement therapy (hydrocortisone preferred) if adrenal insufficiency is present. Follow endocrinology guidance for hormone replacement. Educate on stress dosing, emergency injectables, and medical alert bracelets.	Hold ICI until stable on replacement hormones. Follow endocrinology guidance for hormone replacement.	Hold ICI until stable on replacement hormones. Assess fluid and steroid needs; admit as necessary. Follow endocrinology guidance for hormone replacement. For MRI findings of swelling or threatened optic chiasm compression, initiate oral steroid pulse dosing (1 mg/kg/day). Taper over 2 weeks and switch to an oral maintenance dose.	Hold ICI until stable on replacement hormones. Admit to the emergency department or inpatient setting for hydration or IV stress dose steroids.
Rechallenge considerations	ICI may be resumed with resolution of symptoms and/or stable on controlled steroid or hormone replacement.			

(Continued on next page)

TABLE 17-4
Immune-Related Adverse Event Diagnostic and Treatment Guidelines *(Continued)*

	Grade 1	Grade 2	Grade 3	Grade 4
Diabetes Mellitus				
Description	Asymptomatic, mild symptoms Fasting glucose > upper limit of normal to 160 mg/dl	Moderate symptoms, able to perform ADLs Fasting glucose > 160–250 mg/dl	Severe symptoms, significant or life-threatening consequences Unable to perform ADLs Fasting glucose 250–500 mg/dL Ketoacidosis	Severe symptoms, significant or life-threatening consequences Unable to perform ADLs Fasting glucose > 500 mg/dl Ketoacidosis
Diagnostics	Assess for new-onset type 1 diabetes mellitus, diabetic ketoacidosis, and/or ICI-associated diabetes mellitus. Initiate referral to endocrinology for further evaluation and management. Evaluate C-peptide with repeat serum glucose, blood pH, basic metabolic panel, and urine/serum ketones. Consider autoantibodies, such as antiglutamic acid decarboxylase (e.g., islet cell antibody, islet antigen-2, anti-insulin, zinc transporter 8).			
Treatment	Monitor closely. Continue ICI. Monitor glucose and hemoglobin A1c frequently. Refer to a primary care provider for a new diagnosis of type 2 diabetes mellitus or worsening type 2 diabetes mellitus. Diet and lifestyle interventions may be necessary.	Continue ICI. Start insulin. If unable to start insulin, send to the emergency department for hospital admission.	Hold ICI. Admit for diabetic ketoacidosis, hypovolemia, impaired electrolytes, and insulin initiation.	
Rechallenge considerations	Consider resuming once diabetic ketoacidosis and/or glucose have stabilized.			

(Continued on next page)

TABLE 17-4
Immune-Related Adverse Event Diagnostic and Treatment Guidelines *(Continued)*

	Grade 1	Grade 2	Grade 3	Grade 4
Encephalitis				
Description	Mild symptoms, no effect on ADLs and symptoms not concerning to the patient	Moderate symptoms, interference in ADLs Any cranial nerve symptoms or involvement	Severe symptoms, unable to perform ADLs	
Diagnostics	Initiate referral to neurology for further evaluation and management. Complete workup to rule out leptomeningeal disease. Evaluate complete blood count, complete metabolic panel, erythrocyte sedimentation rate, C-reactive protein, antineutrophil cytoplasmic antibody, thyroid panel with thyroid peroxidase antibody and thyroglobulin, morning ACTH, morning cortisol, GQ1B antibody, celiac antibodies, and paraneoplastic and autoimmune encephalitis panels. Morning ACTH and cortisol levels should be evaluated in accordance with institutional policies or procedures. Complete brain and spine MRI with or without contrast and electroencephalogram testing. Perform lumbar puncture with cerebrospinal fluid analysis, opening pressure, cell count, differential, cell cytology protein, glucose, Gram stain, infection cultures, oligoclonal bands, autoimmune encephalopathy, and paraneoplastic panels.			
Treatment	Hold ICI. Start acyclovir until aseptic meningitis is ruled out through lumbar puncture and/or imaging. Initiate IV methylprednisolone 1–2 mg/kg/day. If severe or progressive symptoms or oligoclonal bands are present in lumbar puncture tests, initiate methylprednisolone 1g IV daily for 3–5 days and 2 g/kg IVIG for 5 days or plasmapheresis.		Complete all treatment recommendations for irAE-related encephalitis grade 1–2. Arrange for hospital admission. Initiate methylprednisolone IV 1 g/day and 2 g/kg IVIG or plasmapheresis for 3–5 days. If positive for autoimmune encephalopathy antibody or there is no improvement after 7–14 days, consider rituximab.	
Rechallenge considerations	Consider ICI resumption with neurology involvement	Consider ICI resumption with neurology involvement.	Permanently discontinue ICI.	Permanently discontinue ICI.

(Continued on next page)

TABLE 17-4

Immune-Related Adverse Event Diagnostic and Treatment Guidelines *(Continued)*

	Grade 1	Grade 2	Grade 3	Grade 4
Myocarditis				
Description	Abnormal cardiac biomarkers without symptoms and no ECG abnormalities	Abnormal cardiac biomarkers with mild symptoms and/or new ECG abnormalities without conduction delay	Abnormal cardiac biomarkers with moderate symptoms and/or new ECG abnormalities with conduction delay	Moderate to severe decompensation, life-threatening care required
Diagnostics	Conduct concurrent myasthenia gravis and myositis irAE workup. Complete ECG, echocardiogram, chest x-ray, and cardiac MRI. Arrange for continuous telemetry monitoring. Evaluate troponin, B-type natriuretic peptide, and creatine phosphokinase cardiac biomarkers. Initiate urgent referral to cardiology for further evaluation and management.			
Treatment	Discontinue ICI. Treatment will be guided by clinical severity at presentation. Admission to the intensive care unit and/or temporary or permanent cardiac pacing may be necessary. Initiate methylprednisolone IV 1g/day for 3–5 days. If responsive, switch to oral prednisone 1 mg/kg/day, then taper slowly over 6–12 weeks based on response and cardiac biomarker improvement. If there is no improvement within 24–48 hours on steroids, initiate additional immunosuppression agents, such as abatacept, alemtuzumab, antithymocyte globulin, infliximab, IVIG, methotrexate, mycophenolate mofetil, or plasmapheresis. Infliximab should be used with extreme caution in patients with reduced left ventricular ejection fraction. Manage acute or prolonged symptoms with American Heart Association recommendations.			
Rechallenge considerations	Risk versus benefit should be highly evaluated with the patient and cardiology before reinitiation of ICI.	Permanently discontinue ICI.	Permanently discontinue ICI.	Permanently discontinue ICI.

(Continued on next page)

TABLE 17-4
Immune-Related Adverse Event Diagnostic and Treatment Guidelines *(Continued)*

	Grade 1	Grade 2	Grade 3	Grade 4
Nephritis				
Description	Creatinine level > 0.3 mg/dl or 1.5–2 × above baseline	Creatinine 2–3 × above baseline	Creatinine > 3 × above baseline or > 4 mg/dl	Life-threatening consequences, creatine 6 × above baseline
Diagnostics	Monitor closely. Rule out other causes (e.g., recent computed tomograph contrast, medications, fluid status, urinary tract infection, acute obstructive etiology). Evaluate complete metabolic panel, urine protein/creatinine ratio, microalbumin/creatinine ratio, urine electrolytes, and urinalysis.		Complete all diagnostic recommendations for irAE-related grade 1 nephritis. Initiate referral for nephrology for further evaluation and management.	
Treatment	Monitor closely. Hold ICI and other nephrotoxic medications.	Complete all treatment recommendations for irAE-related grade 1 nephritis. Initiate oral corticosteroids 0.5–1 mg/kg/day. If worsening or no improvement after 1 week, start IV methylprednisolone 1–2 mg/kg/day.	Permanently discontinue ICI and consider inpatient admission. Initiate IV methylprednisolone (or equivalent) 1–2 mg/kg/day. If elevation persists for greater than 3–5 days, consider additional immunosuppression.	Complete all treatment recommendations for irAE-related grade 1–3 nephritis. Arrange hospital admission for renal replacement therapy or hemodialysis.

(Continued on next page)

TABLE 17-4
Immune-Related Adverse Event Diagnostic and Treatment Guidelines *(Continued)*

	Grade 1	Grade 2	Grade 3	Grade 4
Nephritis *(Cont.)*				
Rechallenge considerations	–	Once diagnostics return to ≤ grade 1, evaluate risks versus benefits of ICI therapy. Only restart ICI therapy if steroids are reduced to < 10 mg/day with routine creatinine monitoring, and ICI has been held for at least 2 months.	Once diagnostics return to ≤ grade 1, evaluate risks versus benefits of ICI therapy. Only restart ICI therapy if steroids are reduced to < 10 mg/day with routine creatinine monitoring, and ICI has been held for at least 2 months. Consider permanent discontinuation in the setting of grade 3–4 proteinuria.	Consider permanent discontinuation in the setting of grade 3–4 proteinuria.
Pneumonitis				
Description	Asymptomatic, confined to 1 lobe and/or < 25% lung parenchyma affected	New or worsening symptoms	Severe symptoms with involvement of all lung lobes or > 50% of lung parenchyma, resulting in limitation of ADLs and requiring supplemental oxygen	Life-threatening respiratory compromise

(Continued on next page)

TABLE 17-4
Immune-Related Adverse Event Diagnostic and Treatment Guidelines *(Continued)*

	Grade 1	Grade 2	Grade 3	Grade 4
Pneumonitis *(Cont.)*				
Diagnostics	Monitor closely with weekly assessments and pulse oximetry. Assess pulse oximetry at rest and ambulation. Complete computed tomography scan of chest with contrast, and reassess every 1–2 weeks; if no improvement, treat as grade 2. Conduct a history and physical examination, with a focused lung assessment.	Complete all diagnostic recommendations for irAE-related grade 1 pneumonitis. Consider initiating referral to pulmonology and infectious disease for further evaluation and management. Obtain sputum, blood, urine, and respiratory cultures to assess for infection; evaluate need for prophylactic antibiotics.	Complete all diagnostic recommendations for irAE-related grade 1–2 pneumonitis. Initiate referral to pulmonology for further evaluation and management. Arrange urgent hospital admission.	
Treatment	Consider holding ICI.	Hold ICI. Initiate oral prednisone 1–2 mg/kg/day. If no improvement after 48–72 hours, treat as grade 3.	Discontinue ICI. Arrange for hospital admission. Initiate IV methylprednisolone 1–2 mg/kg/day. Assess response in 48 hours. If improvement, transition to oral steroids and taper steroids over 6 weeks. If no improvement after 48 hours, consider an immunosuppressant (e.g., IVIG, mycophenolate, tocilizumab, infliximab).	

(Continued on next page)

TABLE 17-4
Immune-Related Adverse Event Diagnostic and Treatment Guidelines *(Continued)*

	Grade 1	Grade 2	Grade 3	Grade 4
Pneumonitis *(Cont.)*				
Rechallenge considerations	Consider resuming on radiographic evidence of improvement.	Resume once pneumonitis has resolved to ≤ grade 1 and the patient is on a steroid dose of ≤ 10 mg/day of prednisone.	–	Permanent discontinuation is warranted.
Uveitis				
Description	Anterior or intermediate uveitis		Posterior or panuveitis	Uveitis causing worse than 20/200 vision
Diagnostics	Initiate referral to ophthalmology for further evaluation, including fundoscopic and slit lamp examinations. Assess vision, color, red reflex, pupil size, shape, and reactivity in each eye separately.			
Treatment	Continue ICI. Recommend artificial tears for comfort.		Hold ICI until opthalmology guidance is complete. Complete all treatment recommendations for irAE-related grade 1 uveitis. Follow ophthalmology guidance for possible initiation of topical and/or systemic steroids.	Hold ICI. Follow ophthalmology guidance for initiation of topical and/or systemic steroids. If little or no improvement with steroids, consider adding infliximab or methotrexate.

(Continued on next page)

TABLE 17-4
Immune-Related Adverse Event Diagnostic and Treatment Guidelines *(Continued)*

	Grade 1	Grade 2	Grade 3	Grade 4
Uveitis *(Cont.)*				
Rechallenge considerations	Consider ICI resumption with ophthalmology involvement, symptoms ≤ grade 1 with only one ocular irAE, and if the patient is on a steroid dose of ≤ 10 mg/day of prednisone.			

ACTH—adrenocorticotropic hormone; ADL—activity of daily living; ECG—electrocardiogram; ICI—immune checkpoint inhibitor; irAE—immune-related adverse event; IVIG—intravenous immunoglobulin; MRI—magnetic resonance imaging

The Common Terminology Criteria for Adverse Events 1–4 grading scale is shown. Grade 5 is often used in diagnostic and treatment guidelines and represents death. Grade 5 was omitted intentionally.

Note. Based on information from National Cancer Institute Cancer Therapy Evaluation Program, 2017; National Comprehensive Cancer Network, 2025; Schneider et al., 2021.

Colitis

Colitis is a severe inflammation of the colon, as evidenced by watery diarrhea, abdominal pain or cramping, mucus or blood in stool, fever, and potentially severe complications, such as megacolon or perforation (NCCN, 2025). Diagnosis and management involve performing targeted gastrointestinal assessment, laboratory testing, imaging, holding ICIs, ruling out infections, and escalating from symptom monitoring and dietary changes to corticosteroids and biologic agents (e.g., infliximab, vedolizumab). Rechallenge may be considered for lower-grade cases if symptoms resolve, but ICIs should be permanently discontinued for life-threatening events (NCCN, 2025; Schneider et al., 2021).

Hypophysitis

Hypophysitis is an inflammatory condition affecting the pituitary gland and presents with nonspecific symptoms, such as fatigue, headache, nausea, and more severe endocrine deficiencies (e.g., secondary adrenal insufficiency). Diagnosis involves hormone evaluation and imaging, with treatment focused on hormone replacement, corticosteroids, and endocrinology guidance. ICIs should be held until patients are stable, and rechallenge may be considered once symptoms are controlled and replacement therapy is initiated (NCCN, 2025; Schneider et al., 2021).

Diabetes Mellitus

Diabetes mellitus can occur from the destruction of pancreatic beta cells, which are responsible for insulin production and can lead to autoimmune diabetes (Barroso-Sousa et al., 2018). When related to ICIs, diabetes mellitus presents as new-onset or worsening hyperglycemia or diabetic ketoacidosis, with symptoms such as polyuria, polydipsia, fatigue, abdominal pain, and confusion. Diagnosis includes blood glucose levels, ketone testing, electrolytes, and an endocrinology consultation. Treatment involves insulin therapy, IV fluids for diabetic ketoacidosis, and close glucose monitoring; ICIs may be resumed once blood sugars are well-controlled, with or without insulin, based on endocrinology guidance (NCCN, 2025; Schneider et al., 2021).

Encephalitis

Encephalitis is a life-threatening inflammation of the brain, as evidenced by impaired neurologic function. ICI-related encephalitis can cause a range of neurologic symptoms, including confusion, seizures, memory loss, and speech or swallowing difficulties (NCCN, 2025). Diagnosis requires an extensive neurologic workup, including laboratory testing, imaging, lumbar puncture, and electroencephalogram. Treatment involves holding ICIs, initiating steroids and antivirals, and escalating to IV immunoglobulin or plasmapheresis if severe. Rechallenge may be considered for grade 1 cases with neurology guidance, but it is not recommended for grade 3–4 cases (NCCN, 2025; Schneider et al., 2021).

Nephritis

Nephritis is an inflammation of the kidneys, indicated by impaired renal function. ICI-related nephritis can present with oliguria, edema, or electrolyte disturbances and is graded based on creatinine elevation (NCCN, 2025). Diagnosis includes ruling out other causes, urine studies, imaging, and nephrology consultation. Treatment ranges from close observation to high-dose corticosteroids and potential inpatient care. Rechallenge may be cautiously considered for grade 2–3 cases if laboratory values normalize and steroids are successfully tapered, but permanent discontinuation is recommended for severe or proteinuria-associated cases (NCCN, 2025; Schneider et al., 2021).

Pneumonitis

Pneumonitis is an inflammation of the lungs, manifested by impaired lung or respiratory function. ICI-related pneumonitis presents as dyspnea, cough, and hypoxia, and ranges from asymptomatic localized inflammation to life-threatening respiratory compromise (NCCN, 2025). Diagnosis includes imaging, pulse oximetry, and infectious workup, with treatment escalating from corticosteroids and monitoring to hospitalization and immunosuppressants for severe cases. Rechallenge may be considered once symptoms and imaging improve for grade 1–2 cases, but grade 4 pneumonitis warrants permanent ICI discontinuation (NCCN, 2025; Schneider et al., 2021).

Uveitis

Uveitis is an inflammatory condition affecting the uvea (i.e., iris, ciliary body, and choroid) or middle layer of the eye, as evidenced by impaired eye function. ICI-related uveitis presents with eye pain, photophobia, and vision changes, ranging from mild anterior involvement to severe vision loss (NCCN, 2025). Diagnosis requires ophthalmology consultation and a detailed eye examination. Treatment includes artificial tears, topical and systemic steroids, and possible methotrexate or biologics for refractory cases. Resumption of ICI therapy should be considered in collaboration with ophthalmology if the irAE has improved to grade 1 or lower, involves only one ocular site, and the patient is receiving a steroid dose less than or equal to 10 mg/day of prednisone (or equivalent) (NCCN, 2025; Schneider et al., 2021).

Myocarditis

Myocarditis is an inflammation of the heart muscle (myocardium) that can impair its ability to pump blood and may lead to arrhythmias, heart failure, or sudden death. ICI-related myocarditis presents with symptoms such as chest pain, dyspnea, arrhythmia, and fatigue. It may occur alongside myositis (inflammation of the skeletal muscles) or myasthenia gravis (weakness and fatigue of voluntary muscles), which must be ruled out (NCCN, 2025). Diagnosis requires a complete cardiac workup and specialist consultation. Treatment involves discontinuing ICIs, initiating high-dose steroids, and possibly adding immunosuppressive agents if no improvement is seen within 48 hours. Rechallenge with ICIs is not recommended for grade 2 or higher events, and grade 1 cases require a careful risk–benefit discussion (NCCN, 2025; Schneider et al., 2021).

Nursing Management

An irAE is a significant concern in patients receiving ICI therapy, requiring vigilant nursing management to ensure early identification and appropriate intervention

(Wood et al., 2019). Nurses are pivotal in quickly assessing and monitoring patients for side effects of ICI therapy and intervening with supportive care. Key nursing management for all irAEs includes the following (Kottschade, 2021; Wood et al., 2019):

- Importance of early irAE identification
- Understanding of ICI treatment and side effect continuum: acute versus chronic and early and delayed onset of potential irAEs
- Clinical assessments for irAE signs and symptoms: both face-to-face and via telecommunication
- Initial and ongoing patient and caregiver education
- Supportive care medications and interventions
- Corticosteroid education: dosing, administration, side effects (e.g., sleeplessness, agitation, hyperglycemia), and precise directions regarding when and how to taper
- Gastrointestinal prophylaxis
- Infection prevention
- Comprehensive baseline evaluation: full-body physical and mental nursing assessments, laboratory tests, psychosocial status, preferred learning and education styles, current medications, and history of autoimmune diseases

In addition to the core management principles, nurses should include the following focused assessment and education points when monitoring for specific irAEs.

- Colitis (Nicolaides & Boussioutas, 2023)
  - A focused gastrointestinal assessment should include baseline bowel habits, bowel sounds, abdominal pain or tenderness, nausea, vomiting, and rectal bleeding. Assess diarrhea frequency and volume, noting if blood or mucus is present in the stool.
  - Monitor and assess for signs and symptoms of dehydration and malnutrition, including skin turgor, dry mucous membranes, electrolyte imbalances, strict input and output documentation, orthostatic hypotension, dizziness, and weight loss.
  - Safety precautions include fall and skin breakdown prevention.
- Hypophysitis (Cooksley et al., 2023)
  - A focused endocrine assessment includes fatigue, vision changes, headaches, mental status changes, and hypotension.
  - Monitor fluids and electrolytes for signs and symptoms of hyponatremia and dehydration, including thirst, dizziness, fatigue, dry mucous membranes, decreased skin turgor, sunken eyes, hypotension, and tachycardia.
- Diabetes (Zhou et al., 2024)
  - Closely monitor serum glucose.
  - Adhere to strict and accurate input and output documentation and tracking.
  - Monitor electrolytes, specifically potassium, sodium, phosphorus, and magnesium.
  - Monitor and assess for signs and symptoms of hypervolemia or hypovolemia, including dizziness, weight changes, dry mucous membranes, skin turgor, fluid retention, lung sounds, and vital signs.
  - Monitor for signs and symptoms of diabetic ketoacidosis, including fruity breath or urine, abdominal pain, nausea, vomiting, shortness of breath, and mental status changes.
  - Provide education on signs and symptoms of hypoglycemia, insulin administration, emergency hypoglycemia interventions, diet, and exercise.

  - Recommend a dietary consultation for enhanced education on diabetic carbohydrate counting, increased protein intake, and suggested meal times.
- Encephalitis (Reynolds & Guidon, 2018)
  - A focused neurologic assessment includes changes in mental status or behaviors from baseline, lethargy, headache, muscle weakness, tremor, numbness or tingling, and vision or speech changes.
  - Take seizure precautions.
  - Provide caregiver psychosocial support for patient behavioral changes.
- Nephritis (Pirovano et al., 2025)
  - A focused renal assessment includes strict input and output tracking and documentation, changes in urine output (increase or decrease), blood in urine, fluid retention, and flank or back pain.
  - Monitor for signs and symptoms of decreased kidney function, including decreased urine output, swelling in the lower extremities, electrolyte imbalances, lethargy, and confusion.
  - Avoid nephrotoxic medications.
- Pneumonitis: A focused lung assessment includes baseline respiratory assessment, breathing pattern, respiratory rate, new or worsening cough, chest pain, activity intolerance, and oxygen saturation (Li et al., 2025; Naidoo et al., 2020).
- Uveitis: A focused eye assessment includes eye pain, redness, sensitivity to light, blurred vision, and vision changes (Duplechain et al., 2023).
- Myocarditis (Ganatra & Neilan, 2018)
  - A focused cardiac assessment includes new or worsening chest pain, shortness of breath, heart palpitations, fatigue, activity intolerance, fever, jugular venous distention, peripheral edema, vital signs, and/or new anxiety or restlessness.
  - Monitor telemetry for conduction abnormalities, including arrhythmias, ST wave changes, QTc prolongation, or QRS widening.
  - Monitor electrolytes and cardiac biomarkers.
  - Accurate input and output documentation and tracking are essential.

Patient and Caregiver Education

Patient and caregiver education is vital for early diagnosis, effective symptom management, and the continuation of ICI therapy (Dougan et al., 2020; Naidoo et al., 2023; Schneider et al., 2021; Shannon et al., 2020). Both patients and their caregivers must be thoroughly informed about potential irAEs (Olsen et al., 2023). They should also understand when and how to contact their healthcare providers. Patients and caregivers should be provided access to 24/7 contact information for their oncology team.

Nurses should begin patient and caregiver education before initiating ICI therapy, with verbal discussions to outline what symptoms to monitor for and acute versus chronic symptoms. These should be complemented by written handouts for ongoing reference (Olsen et al., 2023). In addition to any institution-specific patient education, resources are available through NCCN, NCI, the Oncology Nursing Society, the American Cancer Society, and Blood Cancer United. This information can be shared with non-oncology healthcare providers and institutions to facilitate appropriate diagnostic workups and treatments (Gould Rothberg et al., 2022; Naidoo et al., 2023).

It is common for patients to underreport symptoms due to the fear of treatment delays or discontinuation, putting them at risk for severe irAE complications (Arnaud-Coffin et al., 2019; Naidoo et al., 2023; Schneider et al., 2021). Therefore, education should emphasize the importance of reporting all symptoms, no matter how minor they may seem. Nurses should continue patient education after initiation of ICI therapy, especially with modifications in the treatment plan (Olsen et al., 2023). They must reassure patients that holding ICI therapy temporarily does not mean it is ineffective; these therapies can continue working for weeks to months and may be restarted once symptoms are resolved (Haslam et al., 2020; Schneider et al., 2021).

As another consideration, adolescents and young adults with cancer may have unique concerns for irAE management. They may experience specific psychosocial challenges related to body image, fertility, and future life plans, which should be discussed in shared decision-making conversations (Olsen, 2023; Schneider et al., 2021). Age-appropriate education and support may be required.

Summary

An irAE is a significant consideration in the management of patients receiving immunotherapy, particularly ICIs. Nurses play a vital role in the prevention and management of irAEs, including patient and caregiver education on potential side effects, close monitoring for signs and symptoms of irAEs, accurate and timely reporting of adverse events, and the implementation of treatment plans.

Early recognition and prompt management of irAEs are crucial for optimizing patient outcomes and minimizing morbidity. This requires an interprofessional approach involving oncologists, nurses, and other healthcare professionals. Nurses must always consult institutional clinical guidelines as well as those published by professional societies, such as NCCN, the American Society of Clinical Oncology, and the Society for Immunotherapy of Cancer.

References

Arnaud-Coffin, P., Maillet, D., Gan, H.K., Stelmes, J.J., You, B., Dalle, S., & Péron, J. (2019). A systematic review of adverse events in randomized trials assessing immune checkpoint inhibitors. *International Journal of Cancer, 145*(3), 639–648. https://doi.org/10.1002/ijc.32132

Barroso-Sousa, R., Barry, W.T., Garrido-Castro, A.C., Hodi, F.S., Min, L., Krop, I.E., & Tolaney, S.M. (2018). Incidence of endocrine dysfunction following the use of different immune checkpoint inhibitor regimens: A systematic review and meta-analysis. *JAMA Oncology, 4*(2), 173–182. https://doi.org/10.1001/jamaoncol.2017.3064

Choi, J., & Lee, S.Y. (2020). Clinical characteristics and treatment of immune-related adverse events of immune checkpoint inhibitors. *Immune Network, 20*(1), e9. https://doi.org/10.4110/in.2020.20.e9

Cooksley, T., Girotra, M., Ginex, P., Gordon, R.A., Anderson, R., Blidner, A., … Rapoport, B.L. (2020). Multinational Association of Supportive Care in Cancer (MASCC) 2020 clinical practice recommendations for the management of immune checkpoint inhibitor endocrinopathies and the role of advanced practice providers in the management of immune-mediated toxicities. *Supportive Care in Cancer, 28*(12), 6175–6181. https://doi.org/10.1007/s00520-020-05709-1

Cooksley, T., Knight, T., Lindsay, D., Gupta, A., Ho, J.H., Higham, C., ... Adam, S. (2023). *Immune checkpoint inhibitor-mediated hypophysitis: No place like home. Clinical Medicine, 23*(1), 81–84. https://doi.org/10.7861/clinmed.2022-0429

Dougan, M., Blidner, A.G., Choi, J., Cooksley, T., Glezerman, I., Ginex, P., ... Rapoport, B.L. (2020). Multinational Association of Supportive Care in Cancer (MASCC) 2020 clinical practice recommendations for the management of severe gastrointestinal and hepatic toxicities from checkpoint inhibitors. *Supportive Care in Cancer, 28*(12), 6129–6143. https://doi.org/10.1007/s00520-020-05707-3

Duplechain, A., Conrady, C.D., Patel, B.C., & Baker, S. (2023). Uveitis. In *StatPearls*. StatPearls Publishing. https://www.ncbi.nlm.nih.gov/books/NBK540993

Fan, Y., Xie, W., Huang, H., Wang, Y., Li, G., Geng, Y., ... Zhang, Z. (2021). Association of immune-related adverse events with efficacy and survival among patients with cancer treated with immune checkpoint inhibitors: A systematic review and meta-analysis. *Frontiers in Oncology, 11*, 633032. https://doi.org/10.3389/fonc.2021.633032

Ganatra, S., & Neilan, T.G. (2018). Immune checkpoint inhibitor–associated myocarditis. *Oncologist, 23*(8), 879–886. https://doi.org/10.1634/theoncologist.2018-0130

Gerber, D.E., Bermas, B.L., & Meara, A. (2024). Acknowledging and addressing real-world challenges to treating immune-related adverse events. *Journal for Immunotherapy of Cancer, 12*(7), e009540. https://doi.org/10.1136/jitc-2024-009540

Gould Rothberg, B.E., Quest, T.E., Yeung, S.J., Pelosof, L.C., Gerber, D.E., Seltzer, J.A., ... Kyriacou, D.N. (2022). Oncologic emergencies and urgencies: A comprehensive review. *CA: A Cancer Journal for Clinicians, 72*(6), 570–593. https://doi.org/10.3322/caac.21727

Haslam, A., Gill, J., & Prasad, V. (2020). Estimation of the percentage of US patients with cancer who are eligible for immune checkpoint inhibitor drugs. *JAMA Network Open, 3*(3), e200423. https://doi.org/10.1001/jamanetworkopen.2020.0423

Kottschade, L.A. (2021, September 14). Don't delay when managing irAEs from immune checkpoint inhibitors. *ONS Voice*. https://www.ons.org/publications-research/voice/conferences/09-2021/dont-delay-when-managing-iraes-immune-checkpoint

Li, C., Faiz, S.A., Boysen-Osborn, M., Sheshadri, A., & Wattana, M.K. (2025). Immune checkpoint inhibitor–associated pneumonitis: A narrative review. *Western Journal of Emergency Medicine, 26*(2), 210–218. https://doi.org/10.5811/westjem.20305

Naidoo, J., Cottrell, T.R., Lipson, E.J., Forde, P.M., Illei, P.B., Yarmus, L.B., ... Suresh, K. (2020). Chronic immune checkpoint inhibitor pneumonitis. *Journal for Immunotherapy of Cancer, 8*(1), e000840. https://doi.org/10.1136/jitc-2020-000840

Naidoo, J., Murphy, C., Atkins, M.B., Brahmer, J.R., Champiat, S., Feltquate, D., ... Cappelli, L.C. (2023). Society for Immunotherapy of Cancer (SITC) consensus definitions for immune checkpoint inhibitor–associated immune-related adverse events (irAEs) terminology. *Journal for Immunotherapy of Cancer, 11*(3), e006398. https://doi.org/10.1136/jitc-2022-006398

National Cancer Institute. (2022). *Immune checkpoint inhibitors*. https://www.cancer.gov/about-cancer/treatment/types/immunotherapy/checkpoint-inhibitors

National Cancer Institute Cancer Therapy Evaluation Program. (2017). *Common Terminology Criteria for Adverse Events* [v.5.0]. https://dctd.cancer.gov/research/ctep-trials/for-sites/adverse-events/ctcae-v5-5x7.pdf

National Comprehensive Cancer Network. (2025). *NCCN Clinical Practice Guidelines in Oncology (NCCN Guidelines®): Management of immune checkpoint inhibitor–related toxicities* [v.1.2026]. https://www.nccn.org

Nicolaides, S., & Boussioutas, A. (2023). Immune-related adverse events of the gastrointestinal system. *Cancers, 15*(3), 691. https://doi.org/10.3390/cancers15030691

Olsen, M.M., LeFebvre, K.B., Walker, S.L., & Dunphy, E.P. (Eds.). (2023). *Chemotherapy and immunotherapy guidelines and recommendations for practice (2nd ed)*. Oncology Nursing Society.

Pirovano, M., Hanna, P., Hassanein, M., & Gupta, S. (2025). Immune checkpoint inhibitor–associated acute kidney injury. In *StatPearls*. StatPearls Publishing. https://www.ncbi.nlm.nih.gov/books/NBK611983

Raschi, E., Gatti, M., Gelsomino, F., Ardizzoni, A., Poluzzi, E., & De Ponti, F. (2020). Lessons to be learnt from real-world studies on immune-related adverse events with checkpoint inhibitors: A clinical perspective from pharmacovigilance. *Targeted Oncology, 15*(4), 449–466. https://doi.org/10.1007/s11523-020-00738-6

Reynolds, K.L., & Guidon, A.C. (2018). Diagnosis and management of immune checkpoint inhibitor–associated neurologic toxicity: Illustrative case and review of the literature. *Oncologist, 24*(4), 435–443. https://doi.org/10.1634/theoncologist.2018-0359

Schneider, B.J., Naidoo, J., Santomasso, B.D., Lacchetti, C., Adkins, S., Anadkat, M., ... Bollin, K. (2021). Management of immune-related adverse events in patients treated with immune checkpoint inhibitor therapy: ASCO Guideline update. *Journal of Clinical Oncology*, 39(36), 4073–4126. https://doi.org/10.1200/JCO.21.01440

Shannon, V.R., Anderson, R., Blidner, A., Choi, J., Cooksley, T., Dougan, M., ... Rapoport, B.L. (2020). Multinational Association of Supportive Care in Cancer (MASCC) 2020 clinical practice recommendations for the management of immune-related adverse events: Pulmonary toxicity. *Supportive Care in Cancer, 28*(12), 6145–6157. https://doi.org/10.1007/s00520-020-05708-2

Suarez-Almazor, M.E., Pundole, X., Abdel-Wahab, N., Johnson, D.B., Gupta, D., Glezerman, I., ... Rapoport, B.L. (2020). Multinational Association of Supportive Care in Cancer (MASCC) 2020 clinical practice recommendations for the management of immune-mediated cardiovascular, rheumatic, and renal toxicities from checkpoint inhibitors. *Supportive Care in Cancer, 28*(12), 6159–6173. https://doi.org/10.1007/s00520-020-05710-8

Wood, L.S., Moldawer, N.P., & Lewis, C. (2019). *Immune checkpoint inhibitor therapy: Key principles when educating patients. Clinical Journal of Oncology Nursing*, 23(3), 271–280. https://doi.org/10.1188/19.CJON.271-280

Zhou, L., Yang, S., Li, Y., Xue, C., & Wan, R. (2024). A comprehensive review of immune checkpoint inhibitor–related diabetes mellitus: Incidence, clinical features, management, and prognosis. *Frontiers in Immunology, 15,* 1448728. https://doi.org/10.3389/fimmu.2024.1448728

Index

The letter *f* after a page number indicates that relevant content appears in a figure; the letter *t*, in a table

C

D

E

F

G

H

I

J

K

L

Q

R

S

V

W

Z

T

U